Family-Focused Care

Family-Focused Care

Jean R. Miller, Ph.D., R.N.

Professor and Chairperson
Department of Nursing
State University of New York
College at Brockport
Brockport, New York

Ellen H. Janosik, M.S., R.N.

Assistant Professor
Psychiatric-Mental Health Nursing
College of Nursing and Health Care
Alfred University
Alfred, New York

Adjunct Professor of Nursing
School of Nursing
Roberts Wesleyan College
Rochester, New York

McGraw-Hill Book Company

New York   St. Louis   San Francisco   Auckland   Bogota´ Hamburg
Johannesburg   London   Madrid   Mexico   Montreal   New Delhi
Panama   Paris   São Paulo   Singapore   Sydney   Tokyo   Toronto

FAMILY-FOCUSED CARE

Copyright © 1980 by McGraw-Hill, Inc. All rights reserved. Printed in the United States of America. No part of this publication may be reproduced, stored in a retrieval system, or transmitted, in any form or by any means, electronic, mechanical, photocopying, recording, or otherwise, without the prior written permission of the publisher.

2 3 4 5 6 7 8 9 0   DODO   8 3 2 1 0

See Acknowledgments on pages xx and xxi. Copyrights included on this page by reference.

Library of Congress Cataloging in Publication Data
Main entry under title:

Family-focused care.

    Bibliography: p.
    Includes index.
    1. Nursing—Social aspects.   2. Family—Health and hygiene.   3. Community health nursing.
I. Miller, Jean R.   II. Janosik, Ellen.
RT86.5.F36   362.8 '2   79-14168
ISBN 0-07-042060-2

This book was set in English Times by Allen Wayne Technical Corp.
The editor was David P. Carroll;
the cover was designed by Joseph Gillians;
the production supervisor was Jeanne Selzam.
R. R. Donnelley & Sons Company was printer and binder.

To our parents

Contents

1
FAMILY PERSPECTIVES

2

FAMILY DEVELOPMENTS

3
FAMILY CHALLENGES

4
FAMILY INTERVENTIONS

5
FAMILY DIRECTIONS

List of Contributors

JOAN E. BOWERS, R.N., Ed.D.
Assistant Professor
Department of Psychosocial Nursing
School of Nursing
University of Washington
Seattle, Washington

ANN CAIN, R.N., Ph.D.
Professor
Graduate Program in Psychiatric
  Nursing
University of Maryland
Baltimore, Maryland

BIANCA M. CHAMBERS, R.N., M.S.
Candidate for M.S.
Community Health Nursing
School of Nursing
Boston University
Boston, Massachusetts

SANDRA A. CHENELLY, R.N., M.S.
Gerontological Nurse Clinician
Rochester, New York

MARILYN L. DeGIVE, R.N. , M.S.
Senior Associate in Community Health
School of Nursing
University of Rochester
Rochester, New York

CARLOS FRIAS, M.D.
Clinical Assistant Professor
Department of Psychiatry
School of Medicine and Dentistry
University of Rochester
Rochester, New York

ELTA GREEN, M.S.W., A.C.S.W.,
   C.S.W.
Associate Director
Family and Marriage Clinic
Assistant Professor of Psychiatry
   (Social Work)
School of Medicine and Dentistry
University of Rochester
Rochester, New York

JOHN Q. GRIFFIN, B.A.
Formerly Managing Editor
Exceptional Parent Magazine
Boston, Massachusetts

ELLEN H. JANOSIK, M.S., R.N.
Assistant Professor
Psychiatric-Mental Health Nursing
College of Nursing and Health Care
Alfred University
Alfred, New York

Adjunct Professor of Nursing
Department of Nursing
Roberts Wesleyan College
Rochester, New York

BETTY JANE KINSINGER, R.N.,
   Ph.D.
Associate Professor
College of Nursing
University of Texas
El Paso, Texas

KATHLEEN KUHN, R.N., M.S.
Family Health Nurse Clinician
Private Practice
Bath, New York

MARY-'VESTA MARSTON, Ph.D.,
   F.A.A.N.
Professor, Graduate Program
Community Health Nursing
School of Nursing
Boston University
Boston, Massachusetts

SUSANNE J. McNALLY, Ph.D.
Assistant Professor of History
Hobart and William Smith Colleges
Geneva, New York

IDA M. MARTINSON, R.N., Ph.D.
Professor and Director of Research
School of Nursing
University of Minnesota
Minneapolis, Minnesota

JEAN R. MILLER, R.N., Ph.D.
Family counselor, researcher, and
   consultant
Rochester, New York

Professor and Chairperson
Department of Nursing
State University of New York
College at Brockport
Brockport, New York

JUDITH ANN MOORE, R.N., M.S.
Assistant Clinical Professor
Department of Mental Health and
   Community Nursing
School of Nursing
University of California
San Francisco, California

ELIZABETH G. MORRISON, R.N.,
   M.S.
Associate Professor, School of Nursing
Instructor, Department of Psychiatry
School of Medicine
University of Alabama
Birmingham, Alabama

SALLY M. O'NEILL, R.N., Ph.D.
Professor and Chairperson
Maternal and Child Nursing
School of Nursing
University of Washington
Seattle, Washington

LENORE BOLLING PHIPPS,
  R.N., M.S.
Assistant Professor
Psychiatric-Mental Health Nursing
College of Nursing and Health Care
Alfred University
Alfred, New York

DOROTHY R. POPKIN,
  Ph.D., C.G.P., C.F.T.
Associate Professor
Mental Health Practitioner Program
School of Nursing
State University of New York
Long Island, New York

PHYLLIS NOERAGER STERN,
  D.N.S.
Assistant Professor
Department of Nursing in Biological
  Dysfunction
School of Nursing
University of California
San Francisco, California

MARILYN PEDDICORD WHITLEY,
  R.N., M.A.
Lecturer
Department of Psychosocial Nursing
School of Nursing
University of Washington
Seattle, Washington

Preface

The fundamental premise of this book is that all individuals belong to family systems. The family is the transmitter of biological and genetic endowment, and a contributor to the psychological strength or vulnerability of its members. Furthermore, the family shapes social and moral values, whether these values are a function of ethnicity, socioeconomic class, or personal preference. Each of us is intimately affected by experiences in our family of origin, experiences that influence the nature of events in the family systems we later establish. The importance of family influences is a forceful argument for a book which places the physiological, psychological, and social aspects of health and illness within the framework of family theory.

The relationships between physical illness and psychological stress are complex. Somatic illness may be aggravated by psychosocial factors, but illness may also be the means of relieving psychological or social tension. For many individuals, a diagnosis of physical disability is more acceptable than the recognition of psychological distress. In many instances, the physical disability of persons seeking treatment may constitute a response to psychosocial strain, and thus cannot be regarded as only physiological. It follows that health professionals involved in family care must be prepared to deal with a wide range of physical, psychological, and social factors. Often, in dealing with physical or mental illness, health professionals adhere to an artificial distinction between the physical and the psychological. It is our hope that this book on the family will help bridge the artificial gulf between physical and mental health care.

The book has been written for upper-level undergraduate students and for students enrolled in masters' programs in nursing, social work, counseling, or community service. Because it combines family theory with concepts related to physical and mental health, the book will be useful in a variety of courses. Areas for which the book is recommended include: community health; psychiatric-mental health; maternal and child health; medical-surgical nursing; and nurse-practitioner programs.

The trend toward collaboration between health care providers in a variety of disciplines points to the need for a book such as this one. Consultation and cooperation between the major health disciplines are increasing with the objective of providing total care in one clinical facility, and viewing health care in terms of its meaning to the family as well as the individual. A distinctive feature of this book is the integration of conceptual theories common to more than one discipline or clinical speciality.

The book is divided into 24 chapters, most of which include clinical examples which apply the theoretical concepts discussed within the chapter. These clinical examples are based on actual situations encountered in our practice. Names, dates, and other details have been altered to protect confidentiality. Finally, each chapter contains a short summary in which salient points are emphasized.

Part 1: Family Perspectives. In the first part, the family is examined from several vantage points, beginning with an explication of general systems theory relevant to the study of families. The structural-functional aspects of systems theory, which are used throughout the book, are described. A historical overview of changes in family structure and function is presented in the context of the environment in which families exist. Contributing theories related to family assessment, planning, intervention, and evaluation are introduced as ways in which to examine and understand family systems. Ethnicity and socioeconomic class are discussed as variables that affect the durability or fragility of family systems.

Part 2: Family Developments. In Part 2 the progressive nature of family life is stressed. The Eriksonian explanation of a critical time of ascendance for individual developmental tasks is combined with Duvall's sequence of family developmental tasks. Physical maturation, psychological needs, and cultural expectations are perceived as a triumvirate that impels the individual toward success or failure in mastering each developmental task in turn. Superimposed on family developmental issues are the needs and aspirations of individual members. Sometimes there is conflict between individual needs and family needs, and compromise must be negotiated. This part of the book begins with a discussion of the establishment of the marital dyad, and moves chronologically through the entry, rearing, launching, and eventual departure of children from the family. The stresses of postparental couples arising from the "empty nest" are included, as well as the inevitable losses sustained by aging family systems. The cyclic nature of family life is presented as a universal process experienced by all of us.

Part 3: Family Challenges. Part 3 deals with events which test the family system to its limits, and sometimes beyond. Attention is shifted from the normal developmental crises that occur in any family to cataclysmic events that threaten the system. The ramifications of physical and mental illness in a family member are presented, and differences in the consequences of acute, chronic, and terminal illness are contrasted so that the student or practitioner may identify family problems ensuing from each type of physical illness. The family may sometimes be the matrix for mental illness, with pathology residing as much in the family system as in the identified patient; however, this in no way negates the pain of a family with a mentally ill member. Physical and mental illnesses are perceived as stressors which challenge and disrupt the operation of the family system, yet at times maintain the system. Crisis is depicted as both a danger and an opportunity, in the sense that crisis resolution sometimes impairs and sometimes improves the coping skills of a beleaguered family. Crisis intervention is accorded the attention its importance deserves in family work.

Part 4: Family Interventions. The earlier chapters of the book deal largely with assessing the family system. However, at its later stages, family therapy consists of planning and implementing appropriate interventions and these are dealt with in Part 4. The wisdom of seeking family participation in planning the therapeutic process cannot be overstated. Interventions based on the manipulation of structural family variables are noted, as well as interventions that attempt to modify extreme or problematic family functioning. Behavioral intervention as a family treatment modality is also described. The behavioral method is viewed as humanistic rather than a mechanistic approach.

Part 5: Family Directions. This part is less concerned with individual families than with surveying the larger dimensions of family needs. The evaluation of community needs is suggested in order to identify families at risk and justify programs which reduce or eliminate risk factors. Problem solving is presented as a technique which practitioners can teach to families as a form of anticipatory guidance. Attention is given to subjective and objective evaluation of treatment outcomes, and the need for more rigorous work in this area is acknowledged.

Further refinement of family theory, family practice, and family research is essential. Until adequate instruments and techniques are developed for assessing and working with families, and measuring treatment outcomes, efforts toward theory building must continue. However, the need for additional family theory does not detract from the value of this comprehensive text, which provides a theoretical foundation for the clinical use of family-focused care.

ACKNOWLEDGMENTS

We should like to acknowledge the interest and assistance of contributors and colleagues during the preparation of the book. The efforts of Patricia Hopkins, our typist, allowed us to meet deadlines which sometimes appeared impossible. Her unfailing good humor and dependability were as important as her technical skills. We should like to mention the patience and forbearance of our own families and friends, to whom we are most grateful. We also should like to thank Elta Green for allowing us to photograph her sycamore tree painted by Bobbie Dunnington and used on the cover of our book to symbolize the family tree. Dr. Salvador Minuchin graciously allowed us to adapt the key used in the figures in his book, *Families and Family Therapy,* published by Harvard Press, for use in *Family-Focused Care.* Finally, we gratefully acknowledge the authors and publishers listed below for permission to reprint selected materials from their copyrighted works.

Behmer, M. Children with disabilities. *The Exceptional Parent,* 1976, **6**(1), 35.

Biddle, E. H. The American Irish-Catholic family. In C. H. Mendel & R. W. Habenstein (Eds.), *Ethnic families in America.* New York: Elsevier, 1976, p. 98.

Bowen, M. Family and family group psychotherapy. In H. I. Kaplan & B. J. Sadock (Eds.), *Comprehensive group psychotherapy.* Baltimore: Williams & Wilkins, 1971, pp. 395–396.

Cain, A. The role of the therapist in family systems therapy. *The Family,* 1976, **3**(2), 66.

Duvall, Evelyn Millis. *Marriage and family development* (5th ed.). Philadelphia: J. B. Lippincott Company, copyright © 1957, 1962, 1967, 1971, 1977, Table 7-3, p. 144 and text pp. 176–177. Reprinted by permission of Harper & Row, Publishers, Inc.

Engel, G. L. Psychological responses to major environmental stress. Grief and mourning; danger, disaster and deprivation. In G. L. Engel (Ed.), *Psychological development in health and disease.* Philadelphia: Saunders, 1962, pp. 278–279.

Giacquinta, B. Helping families face the crisis of cancer. *American Journal of Nursing,* 1977, **77**(10), 1587.

Group for the Advancement of Psychiatry. *The joys and sorrows of parenthood.* New York: Scribner's, 1973, p. 117.

Hamburg, D., & Adams, J. A perspective on coping behavior. *Archives of General Psychiatry,* 1967, **17**, 277.

Hill, Wm. Fawcett. Group cognitive map. In *Learning thru discussion: Guide for leaders and members of discussion groups.* Beverly Hills/ London: Sage Publications, Inc., © copyrighted 1977, 1969, 1962 by the author, p. 23. By permission of the publisher.

Janosik, E. H., & Miller, J. R. Theories of family development. In D. P. Hymovich & M. U. Barnard (Eds.), *Family health care* (2nd ed., Vol. 1). New York: McGraw-Hill, 1979, Fig. 1-2, p. 10. Originally adapted from E. M. Duvall, *Marriage and family development* (5th ed.). Philadelphia: Lippincott, 1977, Table 7-3, p. 144.

Light, N. The family with a psychotic child. In J. Haer, A. Leach, S. M. Schurdy, & B. F. Sideleau (Eds.), *Comprehensive psychiatric nursing.* New York: McGraw-Hill, 1978, p. 567.

Neugarten, B. L. The awareness of middle age. In B. L. Neugarten (Ed.), *Middle age and aging.* Chicago: University of Chicago Press, 1968, p. 98.

Novak, M. *Rise of the unmeltable ethnics.* New York: Macmillan, 1972, p. 44.

Speigel, J. *Transactions: The interplay between individual, family and society.* New York: Science House, 1971, p. 38.

Jean R. Miller
Ellen H. Janosik

Part One

Family
Perspectives

Chapter 1

The Family as a System

Jean R. Miller

Health professionals concerned with family functioning are faced with an increasingly difficult challenge in light of the complexity and variations in present family systems. Problems within a family are seldom the result of a single cause. Similarly, a family problem seldom has a single effect. Although the health professional may intuitively understand the relationships among causes and effects in a particular family, the use of a theoretical framework ensures that complexities within families will be subjected to rational analysis.

APPLYING A THEORETICAL FRAMEWORK

Clearly a theoretical framework is needed to guide the health professional in assisting families to obtain optimal health. Because of the complexity of family functioning, it is helpful initially to combine a large number of variables into a single explanatory model that shows the relationship among the major categories of variables. The importance of the theoretical model or framework to each step of the therapeutic process is discussed in the following paragraphs.

First, a theoretical framework guides the health professional in determining what information or data should be obtained. Usually it is helpful to select general categories of variables, moving gradually toward gathering more specific information within each category as dictated by the particular theory being used and the needs of the family in question. For instance, one broad category might be the organizational structure of the family. Within this category, information would be obtained concerning what members comprise the family and the position of each member within the family hierarchy. Organizational structure can be viewed as a category which refers to membership and positions in the family. It tells us who fills what positions, but not how these positions are filled. A theoretical framework, then, specifies what information should be obtained and what should be excluded.

Secondly, a theoretical framework assists the health professional in assessing information after it has been collected. The same general categories that were used for data gathering can be used for assessment. Here the main task is to examine, compare, and interpret the collected information. For example, if a mother tells a health professional that her husband is a devoted father, but is seldom at home due to occupational demands, the health professional might compare the ambiguous structure of this family with the structure of other families which do not experience excessive father absences. An interpretation of the information may reveal that in reality no one enacts the father role despite the presumed influence of the father.

The third step for which a theoretical framework is helpful is the diagnosis of the problem(s) within the broad categories. The problems are defined and explained on the basis of several assumptions and propositions derived from the theoretical framework. Within each of the categories the main problems need to be classified. Using our previous example, the diagnosis might be structural stress due to cyclic adjustments and readjustments of the family arising from the father's absences from and reentries into the family system. The resultant lack of clarity regarding family roles and how they are enacted provides data within the broad category of organizational structure for the diagnosis of the problem(s). Although health professionals tend to deal mostly with family deficiencies, diagnosis by major categories may also disclose unsuspected family strengths. For example, in this case, the willingness of the mother to sustain the father in his role of provider and to acknowledge his ongoing importance to the family despite his absences would constitute a strength available for problem solving.

Fourth, the health professional, in conjunction with the family, plans appropriate actions which strengthen the family system and alleviate its problems. This step can also be taken on the basis of the theoretical framework selected, since the framework indicates which variables or conditions within the system can be manipulated, and to what extent. For instance, if the father's absence hindered his children's accomplishment of expected developmental tasks, a prescription might be to utilize a caring father substitute, such as an uncle or grandfather, who could fill in while the father was absent. If the family tended to exclude the father from a position of influence despite his wish to participate more fully, efforts could be directed toward interpreting the father's absence as indicative of his involvement with the family, and as a form of giving rather than withholding.

Implementing the plan which has been developed collaboratively by family members and health professionals is the next step in the therapeutic process. A theoretical framework will guide the health professional and the family in knowing how, when, and under what circumstances the intervention should be applied. For example, suggesting a father substitute might be appropriate in one ethnic group but not in another. For some absentee fathers and their families, a surrogate male parent would provide tension relief, whereas other fathers would resent the suggestion that their place might be filled even temporarily by another.

The final step in the therapeutic process is the evaluation of family outcomes resulting from the therapeutic actions. Obviously, the theoretical framework tells what to evaluate and under what conditions. Outcomes should reflect subjective satisfaction by the family as well as objective progress. Use of a theoretical framework guides the evaluation by offering criteria against which to measure progress.

To summarize, the theoretical framework is applicable throughout the therapeutic process. It assists the health professional in data gathering, assessment, diagnosis, planning and implementation, and evaluation. It also provides a guide for assessing family strengths and weaknesses, a manual for planning interventions, and a standard by which to evaluate therapeutic outcomes. Further information on this process can be obtained from Glennin (1974) and Yura (1973).

The theoretical framework used in this text is largely based on general systems theory. This framework was chosen because it enables the health professional to deal with the complexities of family social systems, because it is general enough for wide use, and because it can easily be integrated into other theoretical frameworks. The major concepts of systems theory will be discussed in this chapter, with further explanations in later chapters.

THE FAMILY AS A SOCIAL SYSTEM

The family can be viewed as a social system, since it is a structural complex of elements among which there are patterned relationships. As a social system the family has characteristic properties—wholeness, nonsummativity and equifinality. Wholeness or unity in the family is reflected in the interdependence of its members. It is not possible to assess the needs and strengths of one family member without also assessing how these needs and strengths relate to the total family unit.

Family social systems are characterized by *nonsummativity,* or the interrelatedness among the system parts. *Interrelatedness* means that the health professional cannot assess family members individually and then add the obtained scores in order to obtain the degree of interrelatedness among the members. To assess nonsummativity, assessments must be made of every possible interaction pattern. Thus, in a family in which there are two members there is one prevailing interaction pattern, while in a four-member family there are six possible interaction patterns. Family interdependence is crucial to family survival, since interdependence allows self-interest and family interest to be mutually dependent in many respects.

Interactions between family members are circular in the sense that there are few simple cause-effect relationships. The behavior of one member affects the behavior of another, who in turn affects the behavior of the first member, and so forth. This progressive complexity of interaction patterns in the family is known as *equifinality.* One value to the clinician of this characteristic is that an assessment of family interaction patterns may be initiated at any of a number of starting points and approached in different ways. The patterns of interaction remain similar regardless of the vantage point from which they are approached (von Bertalanffy, 1968).

FAMILY GOALS

All families have implicit and explicit goals, although families may lack conscious awareness of these goals. Family goals can be classified as biological, psychological, economic, and social, and each of these categories can be broken down into more specific goals. A biological goal could be as broad as producing children and ensuring their survival. There are many specific goals, however, toward which a family may socialize its young and which consequently ensure family survival. In many families, the exchange of love and affective support is a main goal, whereas in other families economic survival is the most important objective. Society needs families with one or more functioning members who exchange resources with other members of the larger society. The emphasis which each family places upon general and specific goals within each broad category is a function of the family's values. Family values often are a reflection of the family's cultural background in combination with contemporary societal demands. The normative influence of society will vary, however, according to the openness of the family system to societal values.

Family goals may vary according to the stage in the family life cycle. Socialization of children may be an important goal in the early stages of the life cycle, but this goal may cease to exist in the later stages. Socioeconomic status affects family goals. Economic survival is more likely to be a goal for families at lower socioeconomic levels than for middle and upper socioeconomic families. The physical health of family members also may affect the selection of goals as will such changes in the system as the loss or addition of family members (Ford and Herrick, 1974).

Considerations should be made in goal setting for the individual family members, the marital dyad, and the family as a whole. Each family member needs to develop and thrive, but not to the detriment of other members. Similarly, the husband and wife may seek stability, satisfaction, and love from each other but this should ideally not be at the expense of the children's goals. Family goals, therefore, include the goals of the individual and those of subgroups, as well as the goals of the total family unit. Examples of general family goals are those related to the physical and emotional environment within the home or to the overall economic resources available for individual, subgroup, and family needs. Goal setting may be conscious or unconscious, but the goals of a family are closely associated with the family structure and the activities of everyday living.

FAMILY STRUCTURE

Structure refers to family organization and the pattern of relationships among family members. An organizational structure such as the one shown in Figure 1-1 is likely to reveal relationship patterns between the mother and the children and between the father and the children. In the structure illustrated in Figure 1-2, there is likely to be more interaction between the mother and the children than between the father and the children, because the father is separated from the children by the mother.

Family structure usually consists of subsystems which are linked by members who hold overlapping memberships in two or more groups. This multiple overlapping of subsystem structure facilitates communication among the family members. For instance, the mother in a parent-child subsystem is also a wife in the husband-wife subsystem and a daughter in the mother-daughter subsystem of her family of origin. Therefore she has

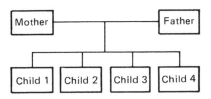

Figure 1-1 Structure in which the leadership is shared.

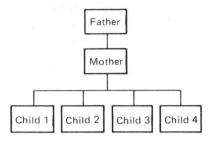

Figure 1-2 Structure in which the father is dominant.

knowledge of characteristics and events pertaining to several subsystems. A family member is likely to function differently in each subsystem, and to exert varying levels of influence and power.

Subsystems contribute to effective family functioning in several ways. Their members usually engage in activities which help the family system achieve its goals. For example, loving communication between husband and wife enhances the marital subsystem and most likely will contribute to the attainment of a warm and emotionally gratifying home environment. Subsystems tend to work cooperatively, and do not usually seek to defeat the efforts of other subsystems. Cooperation and clear communication between subsystems are obviously important for maintaining a feeling of cohesion among the parts.

Any change in one member of a subsystem affects other members of that subsystem, as well as other subsystems and the family as a whole. Change may stem from an illness or death in the family or from the addition of a new member such as a newborn child or a grandparent who comes to live in the home. Alterations in memberships change the family structure, since they affect the patterns regarding who talks to whom, and when and how members interact with one another. The necessary adjustments might be made with greater ease if families were aided professionally to respond constructively to changes in family membership.

Boundaries

Individual family members, subsystems, and the total family unit are protected by boundaries (see Figure 1-3). *Boundaries* resemble rules which specify who can participate in the system or subsystem and the extent to which one can interact with members in the system or subsystem. Boundaries also refer to the degree to which members allow input or information into the system from other systems.

According to Chin (1969) boundaries are like a ''line forming a closed circle around selected variables, where there is less interchange of energy (or communication, etc.) across the line of the circle than within the delimiting circle.'' Boundaries, therefore, separate the family system, subsystem, or individual from the surrounding environment.

   Boundaries may serve unhealthy as well as healthy functions. For example, a mother and son may form a subsystem around which a boundary exists. The rest of the family members find it difficult to overcome the boundary in order to interact with mother or son. In most "normal" families, a boundary exists around the mother and father as subsystem rather than around one of the parents and a child.

   An important characteristic of boundaries is their degree of permeability. Boundaries may vary from rigid (disengaged) to diffuse (enmeshed), with an excess on either side being undesirable. When family subsystems have rigid boundaries there is little communication among subsystems and minimal involvement among members in terms of stress. On the other hand, families with diffuse boundaries contain overinvolved members and do not encourage individual growth. Diffuse boundaries allow little opportunity for individuation and separation of family members.

   Boundaries, then, maintain the family system in a state of equilibrium and permit the family to adapt to changes and growth. They regulate the input of energy or information according to the ability of the system to cope with inputs from outside the system. When a family system is in a state of instability or change (for example, because of the illness or loss of a family member) there is need to communicate and coordinate information within the system and to monitor interaction so as to protect family equilibrium (balance) from being upset by disturbing inputs from the environment. Family boundaries which are overly rigid, however, hinder the family from receiving the help and information required to deal with crisis in an efficient manner.

   The concept of boundaries can be utilized by health professionals for diagnosing, predicting, and treating family problems. Families can in turn assist the professional in exploring the causes of disequilibrium within the

Figure 1-3   Family feedback mechanism with other systems.

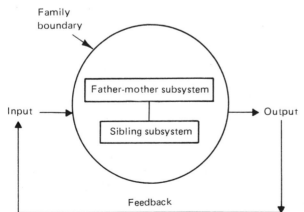

system. Assessment of certain variables can be temporarily delayed, but introduced for diagnosis later, in order to determine the effects, if any, of each variable on the interrelationships within the system. Knowledge of boundary functioning also helps a professional to predict a family's response to the environment and to stress. The more permeable or open a system is, the greater the amount of input it will receive from the environment and the more difficult it will be to specify the exact source of the system's response to the environment. On the other hand, the more rigid or closed a system is, the less likely it is that input will be received from the environment and the more predictable the families' response to the limited input from the environment. Finally, the health professional can facilitate growth in families by assisting them with boundary maintenance. Families can be guided so that they obtain information appropriate to their needs while shielding themselves from information which may cause disequilibrium within the system.

FUNCTION

Family function is the process by which a family operates. The effectiveness with which a family meets its goals depends upon all the processes that take place within the family and its subsystems. Analysis of the processes would normally include a description of communication, environment, and resources.

Communication is a complex process whereby family members relate to one another. Families have both affective and instrumental patterns of communication. Members transmit feelings through *affective* communication, and information through *instrumental* communication. Messages are transmitted with varying degrees of clarity and directness. Disturbed families usually have difficulty with clarity and directness of communication in both the affective and instrumental areas.

It is difficult for families to function efficiently without resources, and some families lack sufficient strengths or resources with which to meet their goals. Examples of available resources include health, education, problem-solving skills, money, emotional and physical support from relatives and friends, religious faith, and information regarding how to obtain and use resources within the community. The number and nature of resources change over different periods of the family life cycle and are affected by circumstances such as illness or recovery. In adverse circumstances, the role of the health professional would be to help the family utilize existing resources in order to reestablish equilibrium.

Feedback

Feedback is the process whereby the family gathers information about its usual level of system functioning. Through this process, the system provides output to the environment in the form of information, behavior, or energy; the environment in turn responds by sending input back into the system. The family system must evaluate from the input the disparity between its actual functioning and expected or ideal functioning. For example, a family in an apartment building may transmit output in the form of arguments and quarrels which are audible to its neighbors. Input from the neighbors in relation to the output could come back in the form of bangs on the wall to indicate that the family is too noisy. A sensitive family would receive and interpret the banging message, realizing that there was great disparity between their family activity and the type of activity required of them from their neighbors.

The overt response of the disharmonious family might be (1) to move away, (2) to attempt to solve problems in a different way, or (3) to unite against the common enemy, the neighbors. Adjustment in the level of activity is termed *negative feedback* because the process is intended to decrease the difference between ideal and actual behavior.

In diagnosing family feedback systems, the health professional must assess (1) the adequacy of the family's feedback procedures, (2) impediments to effective use of the procedures, and (3) family skills in gathering data, and coding and using the returned information. Professional intervention in the feedback process should increase the family's sensitivity to the effects of its own actions upon others.

Energy

Energy within families is easily discerned but is difficult to measure objectively. It can be observed in interactions among members through such variables as spontaneity of communication, attentiveness, and directness of eye contact. For instance, energy often is seen in the interactions of newly engaged couples. This same phenomenon can be seen in couples who have lived together for many years. The energy observed in the latter case frequently is more quiet and less intense than in the interaction of the newly engaged. However, it could be speculated that it is a steadier, less fluctuating energy level. Certain changes in energy levels can be detected when a family member becomes ill. The affection between the ill member and the others does not change, but the amount of energy displayed in their interaction often diminishes. This can become quite distressing to both the ill member and the other family members, since they are not used to operating at a diminished energy level. Considerable research remains to be done on this important concept as it relates to family relationships; however, there are impressionistic ways in which changes in energy levels within the family system can be noted.

Tension, which is a type of energy, exists in varying forms and degrees in all family systems. Sources of tension lie both inside and outside the system. Internally, the natural differences in components and the imperfect integration of these differences cause tension. Whenever autonomy is incomplete and the effective functioning of one component depends on relationships with others the inevitable result is a state of psychic tension. Changes in the components over time also necessitate adjustments, and the process of change produces tension in all the components. This is demonstrated when children leave the home setting and the distance and interactions among those who remain are readjusted. Externally, environmental factors such as peer group expectations, economic conditions, or political climate can cause disturbances in each of the components which ultimately affect the entire system. Tension which builds up among opposing factors within the system or between the system and external environmental forces is expressed as conflict. Other, more productive, forms of tension within families result from strong positive emotions such as love and caring for one another. Conflict results only when these positive feelings are disturbed by both internal and external forces which disrupt and fragment the balance within and between family boundaries.

Tension in families can be used to generate healthy changes in family living. Increases or decreases in tension provide clues for evaluating dynamic interactions among members. Positive changes in interactions can be obtained by manipulating or altering the relationships within the system as well as through responses to conditions outside the system.

SUPRASYSTEMS

There is an interchange between the family system and many other larger systems or suprasystems. Examples of suprasystems with whom the family commonly interacts include school systems and religious, political, and occupational systems. These interrelationships are illustrated in Figure 1-4. The lines surrounding the systems are semipermeable boundaries which regulate the degree of exchange between the systems. The family is a

Figure 1-4 The family system and suprasystems.

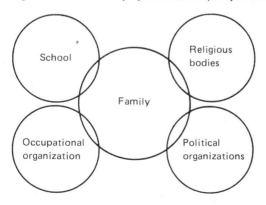

dynamic system in that it can regulate its degree of openness or receptivity to its environment. If a family is constantly reactive or receptive to changes initiated in the environment, disorganized turmoil or chaos is likely to result. Similarly a family system that is overly resistant to input from its environment will experience decreased efficiency.

CLINICAL EXAMPLE: FAMILY INTERACTION IN AN ACUTE SETTING

Mr. Johnson, age 40 years, married, and the father of two daughters aged 18 and 16 and one 12-year-old son, has been in the hospital with a myocardial infarction for 2 weeks. All physical symptoms have subsided and preparations are being made for his return home. Mr. Johnson has been advised that he will have to limit his physical activity and decrease stress in his executive position at work. He has also been advised to curtail his activities at home. During the 2-week hospitalization, Mr. Johnson had difficulty refraining from giving detailed instructions to his wife about tasks he wished her to do at home in his absence (*Structure*). The three children showed no adverse reaction to their father's absence, since they saw little of him under normal circumstances (*Structure*). They talked freely and easily to one another (*Sibling subsystem)* but interactions between them and their father were characterized by long silences and a sense of unease (*Function*). Interactions between Mr. and Mrs. Johnson around details and events of hospitalization and home management often resulted in small misunderstandings (*Function*). Mr. Johnson's nurse commented on this, but the couple said they had frequent arguments and disagreements at home, too (*Feedback*). They were concerned, however, that there wasn't the usual "life" in their relationship since Mr. Johnson had become ill (*Energy*). Much of their conversation centered on how they were going to afford the costs of a college education for their children should Mr. Johnson have to take a lower-paying job (*Goals*). During the hospitalization, relatives and friends visited Mr. Johnson and brought food to the home. The family frequently mentioned their gratefulness for outside assistance (*Boundaries*). They said that their friends in the church they attended were particularly helpful (*Suprasystem*).

Assessment

Structure   Strain was caused in this family by the dominance of Mr. Johnson over his wife. There was a lack of patterned relationships between the father and his children. The family boundaries were open to outside assistance.

Function   There was a lack of clarity in communication between the husband and wife and between the father and his children. Feedback within the family was varied; the siblings provided feedback to one another, but there was little feedback from the father to his children. Feedback between Mr. and Mrs. Johnson in the hospital setting was normal for them. The energy level of the family was lower than usual.

Intervention

The family structure was adjusted so that leadership could be shared by both mother and father. The clarity of communication was increased among all family members. The family was helped to accept lower energy levels during Mr. Johnson's recovery period.

SUMMARY

The usefulness of systems theory for health professionals who deal with families lies in the concepts which relate to total family functioning. A tendency in the health professions is to treat individual patients for specific physical and psychological problems as if these existed in isolation from families. Frequently, physical and psychological problems are alleviated by medication, surgery, or psychosocial support, but the root cause of the problem within the family system remains untouched. Each of the concepts discussed can be used to detect specific problems in the relationships between individuals comprising the family. As family-related problems are discerned, health professionals will have to decide whether to use a family-oriented approach or a limited individual one. If the first approach is chosen, these professionals can turn to established theoretical frameworks in which propositions have been developed to help in the understanding of the relationships between family variables. Some of the main theories which augment systems theory in the study of families will be discussed in Chapter 3.

The family is viewed in this chapter as a social system defined as a structural complex of elements in which there are patterned relations among the elements. The family is characterized by wholeness, nonsummativity, and equifinality. All families have goals which may be determined consciously or unconsciously. Specific goals lie within the general areas of biological, psychological, economic, and social goals. Family structure or organization refers to the patterned relationships among family members, and can be observed through family subsystems such as the parent-child subsystem. Permeable boundaries around the family system and its subsystems regulate the amount of input into the system. Input refers to variables such as information and people. Function is the process by which the family operates to achieve its goals. Analysis of the process should include a description of family communication, environment, and resources.

Feedback is the process whereby the family determines how its present level of functioning in a particular area is related to its usual level of functioning. When adjustments are made to bring family functioning to its usual level, this is called negative feedback. Often health professionals help the family set new levels of functioning through positive feedback. Energy in the family is a necessary component for effective functioning and can have healthy as well as unhealthy effects on system interaction. Finally, the family is a small system in the midst of many larger systems or suprasystems with which there is a constant interchange. The concepts which describe family systems also can be used to describe suprasystems such as religious, educational, economic, and political systems.

REFERENCES

Chin, R. The mobility of system models and developmental models for practitioners. In W. G. Bennis, K. D. Benne, & R. Chin (Eds.), *The planning of change.* (2nd ed.) New York: Holt, Rinehart and Winston, 1969.

Ford, F. R., & Herrick, J. Family rules: Family life styles. *American Journal of Orthopsychiatry,* 1974, **44**(1), 61–69.

Glennin, C. Formulation of standards of nursing practice using a nursing model. In J. P. Riehl & C. Roy (Eds.), *Conceptual models for nursing practice.* New York: Appleton-Century-Crofts, 1974.

von Bertalanffy, L. *General systems theory.* New York: George Braziller, 1968.

Yura, H. *The nursing process: Assessing, planning, implementing, evaluating.* (2nd ed.) New York: Appleton-Century-Crofts, 1973.

Chapter 2

Historical Perspectives on the Family

Susanne J. McNally

HISTORICAL OVERVIEW

Knowledge of the nature of family life in previous centuries provides three important insights for students of the contemporary family. First, present family realities are always more comprehensible when viewed in terms of the past because they are largely influenced by the past. No family exists in isolation from its environment, nor can it remain untouched by changing external forces. Second, reviewing the historical chronicle of the human family dispels automatic preferences for family forms which are personally familiar. It heightens sophistication and objectivity about the whole institution of the family. Finally, the examination of the historical process which produced the modern family is an appropriate introduction to the analytical approach of this book, which sees the family as an active and responsive subsystem within the whole society. While the form and structure of the family can vary greatly, certain functions, or tasks, remain constant (Winch, 1968). Historical perspectives demonstrate clearly that this is so and also provide concrete examples of how deeply and reciprocally the family is embedded in the social order. Attention will be given in succeeding chapters to events and patterns within the family system which affect the health and welfare of all members. In this chapter the family is presented as both cause and consequence of social change, in order to provide a coherent introduction to the phenomenon of structural and functional variation within the family system. It will become apparent that the structural-functional relationship is a powerful analytical tool when used to organize concrete information about specific situations.

A conscientious health professional usually begins the assessment process with extensive history taking and a searching appraisal of specific external signs. In a sense the tools of the historian can be used to accomplish a similar task. Historical perspectives alone are insufficient for a complete understanding of family theory, but they constitute a good beginning.

Prehistoric Origins

The origins of the human family must be sought in times which preceded the appearance of written historical sources. Archeologists and anthropologists have found evidence from earliest prehistory of this enduring institution whose place was usually at the center of individual and community life (Ogburn, 1968). Regardless of their form, the larger systemic arrangements of the community in terms of economics, politics, and religions intersected at the level of the family (Hareven, 1971). For millennia the economic skills needed by the social order were acquired in a familial context, and present-day families still shape career aspirations and plans. It has been the family which has taught basic political responses to its members, according to its own authoritarian or egalitarian, conservative or innovative patterns. Through the family, individuals continue to acquire sometimes inarticulate but profound concepts concerning the self and its relation to the natural, social, and moral aspects of life. As economic, political, and religious systems changed through time, so too did the family arrangements which supported them. Thus, the existence of a close relationship between the functional tasks of the family and its structure and values is widely accepted as a key to understanding family alteration and adaptation, and many analyses of this relationship have been made.

Murdock postulated that, as the prevailing form and the basic unit from which more complex forms develop, the nuclear family exists as a distinct and functional group in every society. The nuclear family performs four functions fundamental to human life, namely, sexual, economic, reproductive, and educational functions (Murdock, 1949). Levy and Fallers (1968) noted that two of these four universal functions, reproduction and regulation of sexual activity, were not primary, but rather secondary to the educational-socialization task, and that the economic function of the family existed on still another level, distinct and separate from the other three. There has been a tendency on the part of some theorists to consider socialization of members as the basic task of the family, since communities require families not merely to replace lost members but to replace them with persons acceptable to the social order (Winch, 1971). In accomplishing the task of socialization, the family has become the carrier of cultural as well as biological inheritance. Culture has been defined as the aspect of human life which is derived from membership in a particular group, and which is shared by others. It is composed of learned values and attitudes that allow us to behave in a predictable fashion and to predict the behavior of others, and it can be described as a social rather than a biological inheritance (Kluckhohn & Strodtbeck, 1961).

In the earliest era of human prehistory, family structure and function were probably expedient responses to everyday needs. As communities grew in size, family structure and function became institutionalized with associated obligations. It is important to note that, beyond abstract speculation, there is little detailed knowledge of the prehistoric family. Also, one must avoid an unwarranted equation of the prehistoric family with the "natural" family. The "natural" family is an idea which has no referent that one can point to in the real world. Conscientious historians are coming to realize that the coherence of premodern and prehistoric social organizations cannot be equated with similarity or uniformity among them. The earlier the historical moment, the greater the isolation and diversity of human social groupings. It is modern life, despite its complexity, which unifies and homogenizes, through communication, exchange, science, and technology, countless communities which were once heterogeneous (Goode, 1963). In the absence of modern influences, one must view skeptically any theories of family characteristics which claim universal applicability or formulate stages through which the early human family proceeded in lockstep fashion. The universalistic assertions of such nineteenth century theorists as Marx and Bachofen are rich sources of insight, but what they reveal in historical as opposed to theoretical terms is largely the nineteenth century European family's relationship to the realities of its own time (Bachofen, 1973; Marx, 1972). Such relationships are not necessarily applicable to a "natural" or prehistoric form of family organization.

Still, a limited number of inferences can be made about the human family in prehistoric times using the structure/function approach. It seems that, from a very early era, human matings tended toward permanence and monogamy. The unit formed by a pair plus their offspring is thought to be the oldest and most tenacious social unit. In it can be recognized the nuclear family which has come to dominate the modern experience. To state that the conjugal group was the oldest family structure does not imply that early families lived in isolation, for there is evidence that even prehumans lived in communities of conjugal units. Such an organization of nuclear families into small communities would fulfill several obvious functions. Biologically the human species can produce offspring every 12 to 18 months, but the offspring require a period of dependency for food and nurture which lasts nearly a decade. Prolonged ties between mother and child were essential to the survival of the child. A female therefore needed long-term dependable assistance so that several young children could be fed and guarded until maturity (Linton, 1959).

This functional requirement, encountered throughout human prehistory, did not dictate any particular family structure, only that the function be carried out. The most common response was to arrange some kind of long-term economic pairing of males and females in addition to the reproductive pairing. This was necessary because under premodern conditions a variety of skills was needed for survival, and no single person could perform all the required functions. With male and female forming a working unit, sex role differentiation of tasks evolved (Murdock, 1949). Eventually even communal activities came to be organized by gender, with the women hoeing, for example, and the men hunting. The work pair was not necessarily congruent with the reproductive pair. There have always been some societies (usually matrilineal) where male and female siblings are the economic unit, though in face of prevailing incest taboos siblings are almost never the reproductive unit.

In the majority of human societies in the past, the basic work pair was indeed the reproductive pair, and the simple biological function of nurturing offspring merged smoothly into economic arrangements, into sex role differentiation, and ultimately into socialization. All these activities were in turn highly influential in early religiosity, which was preoccupied with fertility and virility. So the chain of interconnected family functions turned back on itself, finally shaping with cultural mores the expression of innate biological impulses. In this example, the relationship between family structure and function was complex, with the family defining its functions in response to its own needs, joining with other families to create a community, and responding and mediating pressures from the community even as it integrated itself into the community.

As small groups of conjugal families adjusted delicately to local climate and perpetuated particularistic identities through language, custom, and esthetics, there was a tendency for simple communities to become more complicated. It is beyond the scope of this chapter to describe the modes by which families formed increasingly complex social orders, but it can be said that the process of complication affected the definition of family, so that the socially defined family expanded spatially to include individuals whose blood relationship was more distant than that of the nuclear unit. The family also extended itself in a temporal sense as blood relationships transcended generational boundaries. Family relationships in the extended family were based on consanguinity, and these relationships assumed various forms and importance throughout the world. In some cases the consanguine affiliation was so emphasized that membership in the nuclear family became trivial. The individual then found him- or herself in a larger network which included most of the persons living in proximity, and also extended backward and forward chronologically so that ancestors and descendents were perceived as persons whose reality was immediately felt (Linton, 1959).

The Historical Period

A sizable number of peoples throughout the world entered their respective historical eras with social organizations which emphasized consanguinity. While consanguinity did not assume its greatest strength in Europe, it remained active and influential throughout much of European history, and characteristics derived from it remain.

There is a tendency in nonnuclear family systems for marriages to be controlled by authority concentrated in a few individuals at the top of a hierarchical structure (Linton, 1959). The link between family authoritarianism and the existence of inheritable private property has been the subject of much speculation. Engels (1942) presented an extreme but persuasive view of the influence of property upon internal family structure, suggesting that the power to bequeath such precious resources as land was the foundation of patriarchal subjugation of women and children, and that the desire of a man to leave property to his own heirs was the motive for controlling his wife. The concept of property transformed the family from a cooperative, egalitarian institution to an authoritarian, coercive one. Not only was the father able to control his family through the monopoly of resources necessary to survival, but he came to regard women and children as analogous to resources, treating them as property as well as dominating them through property.

Whatever the accuracy of Engels's analysis, economic functions did influence the internal structure of the moderate consanguine family systems characteristic of traditional Europe. Strict control over women and children was associated with the rise of kingdoms which ruled over settled agricultural populations (Stephens, 1963). Marriages were occasions for mutual exchange and alliance without much regard for the preferences of the young couple. Such control could not be exerted suddenly, and patriarchal childrearing practices were a means of ensuring obedience at this crucial moment in the economic fortunes of the extended family. Again, these economically determined marriage contracts demonstrate how the deepest psychological processes of individual members can be affected by the family's relationship to an external system.

In a patricentric extended family, for example, the emotional bonds between a couple whose marriage had been arranged were unlikely to be very strong. The new bride joined the household of her father-in-law and often she entered marriage with severe feelings of isolation. This led her to develop close attachments to her children, especially her sons, since she realized her daughters were fated to leave her at an early age for marriages of their own. Often, elaborate coalitions would form between a woman and her sons against the authority of the father, and these would be increasingly successful as the sons matured. Upon the marriage of a son, the mother was likely to view her daughter-in-law with extreme rivalry and hostility. She would go to great lengths to prevent the growth of affection between the couple, thus exacerbating the loneliness which drove the daughter-in-law toward her own sons. The misery of the bride is a well-known motif in some European folk literature, and strong sanctions were invoked to keep her with her small children, who were considered to belong to the husband's family (Benedict, 1959). These sanctions involved monetary loss to the bride's natal family if she returned; as a result, most parents of daughters considered marriage in economic terms.

There was, of course, great variation among ancient and medieval European family systems, both temporally and geographically. Nevertheless, a patriarchal system of moderate consanguinity which recognized a kinship group larger than the nuclear family, preferred to transfer property in the male line, and treated marriage as a contract was typical of the European experience. This extended family structure persists in many peasant societies, and can still be found in Southern Europe and Latin America. The tensions generated by family migration from traditional agrarian societies to industrialized communities where old customs are no longer useful can be painful and disorienting to family members, whether young or old.

The Movement to Modernity

Until recently, the extended rural patriarchal family was thought to be characteristic of European society until the advent of industrialism in the late eighteenth and nineteenth centuries. Scholars as well as the general populace believed that this family system continued both in Europe and in North America with great stability until it was undermined by the Industrial Revolution, which appeared first in England about 1750 and spread during the next century to Western Europe and North America (Lazlett, 1973). The relation of the family to modernity and industrialism is now perceived as very complex. Not only has the family passed through more developmental stages than was previously thought, but it seems to have been actively involved in the shift to modernity rather than reacting passively to it. Industrialization seems to have been only the last of a long series of changes which have led to the modernization of the family. Industrialization is in no way a trivial phenomenon in its consequences for the family, but the most striking alterations in European and North American family structure and function occurred long before the Industrial Revolution and were perhaps prerequisites for it. These changes affected every aspect of family life—stability, mobility, authority patterns, even sexuality, and they represent a truly striking transformation of the central human institution.

Scholars are just beginning to grasp the dimensions of these changes. Their language reveals the magnitude of the drama seen in early modern family development. One writer speaks metaphorically of the family as a ship which, like other systems and institutions, was confined by a network of ancient custom and unquestioned precedent until the end of the Middle Ages. Then, from about 1500, a sweeping process of individuation, of heightened individual consciousness and assertion, began in Europe. This process of individuation appeared in the sphere of religion as the Reformation, in economics as commercial and agrarian capitalism, and in politics as the emergence of the nation state. At the same time the family began to gain self-consciousness and to sever the tissues holding it to an unchanging traditional order (Shorter, 1975). The same metaphor speaks of the modern nuclear family moving through heretofore uncharted seas of self-awareness and intense exploration undreamed of by medieval ancestors.

It is interesting to note the range of emotional response which scholars exhibit toward this momentous change. Some react very positively, emphasizing the possibility of higher levels of self-knowledge and human intimacy inherent in the new family system. Others mourn the passing of the world that was lost, perceiving the self-consciousness of modern individuals as intrinsically lonely and alienated, regardless of their efforts to touch and to communicate with each other. The cause of these general changes in European society are beyond the purview of this chapter, but it is possible to examine some basic family alterations in England, where change first occurred, and whose family system strongly influenced that of North America.

Size and Structure of the Modernizing Family   The size and structure of the English family no longer corresponded to those of the extended kinship organization at least a century and a half before the beginning of the Industrial Revolution. From the late sixteenth to the twentieth century the mean size of the average household remained rather constant at about 4.75 members (Lazlett, 1973). Variation in size was slight during those years and consisted almost entirely of adjustment in the number of servants rather than in the number of extended kinfolk. The structure of English families has been nuclear in form for 400 years, which refutes the popular idea that it was industrialization which produced the nuclear family. From this, it is evident that the family does not merely react to changes in the social order—it also initiates change. Indeed, the nuclear family may have been a precondition for the industrialization which proved to be the most significant event of modern history.

Authority Patterns Although its size remained relatively constant throughout the whole modernization process, the English family was changing markedly in other respects. Its importance to its own members grew as it became more independent of the traditional community. As the English economic system moved in the direction of modern capitalism, the whole feudal order of the Middle Ages was undermined. Opportunities for geographic and social mobility soared, so that by 1500 England was literally a nation on the move, with many villages losing as much as 90 percent of their populations over the space of a decade (Stone, 1975). Neither identification with a local region nor dependence on a large kinship group could be maintained under these conditions, which proved optimal for the rise of a new, centralized monarchical power. Here we see the political system, the nascent state, benefiting from decline in allegiance to blood kinship, as kings sought to secure for themselves the free-floating loyalty which had previously belonged to the extended family. In pursuit of this goal, the state began to provide through public and semipublic agencies the services which had once been performed by private, familial systems.

The mutual attraction between public state power and the nuclear family was as evident as the mutual tensions between the state and extended families (Kyrk, 1953). This was shown especially in the sixteenth century, when the state buttressed the nuclear family through explicit augmentation of the legal and economic power of its head by freeing him from the customary feudal constraints which had limited his authority. In return, the state received a measure of patriotism and social control that it had not previously attained. This affiliation between the state and the nuclear family meant the ascendence of the most extreme patriarchalism in English family history, in which the rights of women and minors were minimal and child-rearing practices were very harsh (Stone, 1975).

Another support for the rise of patriarchalism rested in the strength of Protestantism in sixteenth century England. The Protestant emphasis on the pious household as the repository of virtue enhanced the power of the household's head. This represented considerable revision of the semipublic guardianship of morality and salvation which had been the goal of medieval Catholicism. Answerable to God for the spiritual welfare of his dependents, the father assumed control commensurate with his responsibility, and demanded absolute subservience from his family.

Eventually the individualism inherent in Protestantism came to militate against extreme patriarchalism. By the seventeenth century there were those who believed that family life should be based on harmonious order rather than power. Couples did not expect to feel love at the time of marriage, but considered it desirable that they might foresee the growth of emotional attachment (Stone, 1975). By the end of the eighteenth century, English family life was more companionable. This recognition of some individual preferences was an important reversal of the authority concentrated in the father. The emergence of more numerous economic alternatives further diminished patriarchal power. As the father's monopoly of access to resources and status lessened, so did his coercive power over his offspring.

In historical terms the waxing of patriarchalism was short-lived, but it left a legacy of beliefs and values which continue to provoke tensions in contemporary life. The belief that children are possessed of an innate and dangerous willfulness which responsible parents must suppress through discipline had a long subsequent history both in Europe and in North America. Parental obligation to punish children by imposing physical or psychological pain became especially troublesome in the New World where it coexisted confusingly with a contradictory perception of the child as an unmarked and natural being who should be permitted to develop with as little constraint as possible (Rapson, 1973).

Women also continued to endure vestiges of the patriarchalism which was prevalent in the colonies in which mainstream American culture began. European families had been patriarchal for centuries, and women had been expected to obey their husbands and fathers. Before the sixteenth century, however, obedience had not been connected to any expectation of love (Stone, 1975). The introduction of love into the definition of wifely duty and womanhood proved a powerful force in limiting female activity. The conflict has not yet been resolved, for even now women wrestle to separate the attainment of love and womanhood from the necessity of submission.

Men as well as women must struggle with unrealistic role expectations bequeathed by patriarchal family life. In the modern world few men can sensibly assume complete responsibility for the spiritual and economic welfare of their families. Yet many men feel themselves less than adequate for failing to do this. This phenomenon takes some toll even of middle-class males, whose ability to provide for and direct their families is as great as modern life permits (Sennett, 1970). It becomes devastating for underprivileged men whose control over their family's future is minimal, yet who measure themselves against traditional European standards of paternal authority and power.

Sexuality   Another area of family life which underwent profound change during the move to modernity was sexuality. One scholar described the "melting iceberg" of social habit and constraint which permitted a new mode of sexuality to appear in Europe (Shorter, 1973). As part of the growing individuation which accompanied modernization, common people in the eighteenth century began to treat sexuality as a means of self-expression and fulfillment rather than a means to other goals such as economic security through the marriage contract. The presence of the sex drive may be universal, but expression of the drive is subject to cultural conditioning. The eighteenth century witnessed an enormous rise in open manifestations of sexuality among persons who had previously internalized the restraints imposed by communities which valued stability more than personal gratification (Shorter, 1973).

The consequences for lower-class families of heightened eroticism, combined with the social dislocation characteristic of the Industrial Revolution, were enormous. Mobile populations abandoned time-honored courtship customs under which the bride might be pregnant but was rarely abandoned. Crowded into impoverished urban neighborhoods, the working-class family endured severe privations. Between 1790 and 1850, when social change was greatest, illegitimacy assumed gigantic proportions (Shorter, 1973). Only in the last quarter of the nineteenth century did working people attain conditions in which expressive sexuality could be integrated into a sound family structure which produced and socialized legitimate children. The sufferings of this difficult period were attenuated for middle-class families. Although they, too, eventually accepted expressive sexuality, bourgeois families remained relatively stable. Until recently they provided an example of strength and permanence in family systems.

THE FAMILY IN THE NEW WORLD

Many of the stages typical of the English family in its move to modernity were replicated in American history. There has been considerable variety in the experience of the American family. While it did not follow European models in all respects, there are many similarities (Lazlett, 1973). The migration to the new world was itself part of the historical movement which altered the family in Europe. In the early religious colonies, there existed paradoxical impulses toward expansiveness and interiority, which freed communities from old restraints and allegiances while fostering in individuals an urge toward self-consciousness and self-awareness. The American family responded quickly to the imperatives and challenges of modernity as these affected classic family task areas.

The effects of economic functions on family dynamics were seen clearly in North America where high levels of prosperity were attained and where economic activity became central in society. Europe was transformed by the rise of capitalism and industrialization, but America was created by the union of these forces. In the New World, older structures of habit or belief were not present to mitigate the economic forces of modernity. Thus American society and the American family were molded from their beginnings by economic logic.

The sixteenth century English patriarchalism which was transplanted to the earliest American settlements was not maintained in a pure form for long. A tendency toward less authoritarian family arrangements was soon observable, since the arduous and precarious existence of settlers living at the periphery of European civilization not only required the labor of all individuals, but also gave that labor new value because of its scarcity. As the edge of colonization moved westward in the next two centuries, these conditions were repeated, and they were not supportive of elaborate status distinctions between husband and wife. By the eighteenth century, status within the American family was more likely to be achieved status than ascribed status, which depended largely on role labeling (Rapson, 1973). The legacy of frontier respect for women can be seen in the history of female suffrage, which was attained earlier and more easily in states with recent pioneer experience than in the older-established states.

For the children as well, the new conditions of life weakened the rigid family hierarchy. Paternal monopoly of land and skills was undermined in the colonies. Customary economic skills became outmoded so that inventiveness and flexibility were as valued as mastery of ancient techniques. Geographic and social mobility made possible by the material abundance and the expanding economy of the New World reduced parental control over the young. Except for the groups condemned to low positions by racism, the usual expectation among European immigrants entering America was that their children's lives would be better than theirs. Although this goal was ardently desired, it produced unavoidable conflict and anxiety in both parents and children. The belief that offspring would occupy a different social niche meant that immigrant parents lacked the assurance of parents in other societies (Rapson, 1973). As the number of immigrant families rose, children learned to move confidently in the new environment, becoming, in effect, the guides and mentors of confused, unsecure parents. One result of this role displacement was that American families began to surrender to public agencies many of the socialization functions that were dominated elsewhere by the family.

Despite these conditions, the stresses of the generation gap did not appear in American life until the late nineteenth century. Until then most American families lived on farms or in rural areas, so that there was some continuity in the activities of parents and children. Furthermore, in rural areas introduction of children into the family production system started early and gradually. When large numbers began to move to the cities, the smooth process of turning boys into farmers and girls into farmers' wives, which merged economic and socialization functions, could not be sustained (Demos, 1973). Industrial economic dislocation proved more extreme than geographic change. Mobility had merely permitted children to become farmers in different places, but in cities children labored at tasks unrelated to parental occupations, and the authority they confronted at work was distinct from that of their parents.

As child labor became less common, adolescents gradually came to have few or no economic functions. This trend toward discontinuous maturation was augmented by the presence in cities of large numbers of peers, so that the adolescents' search for identity took place not among supportive elders but among others searching like themselves. The concept of adolescence as a developmental stage is recent, and its appearance followed the diversifying, socially ambitious urbanization of American life. Faced with difficult choices regarding career, morality, and life-style, seeing parental guidance as insufficient, adolescents retreated into institutionalized identification with their own subculture, with the result that the generation gap has become endemic in American families (Demos, 1973).

THE FAMILY TODAY

Turning to the modern family, one can perceive the continuing applicability of the systemic approach. The reciprocal nature of the relationship between the family and larger society is as enduring as the family itself. Those forces which impinge upon the family at present are as intense as any which were known previously. Furthermore, such forces appear to be largely negative, although due caution must be used with evaluative labels.

The habit of idealizing past family arrangements and decrying change from a mythic nostalgic norm is equally common among scholars and in the popular culture (Goode, 1963). In fact the family has often engaged in behaviors destructive to individuals and to other social institutions. Here the point is simply that the climate of modernity seems to be gradually diminishing the strength of the family by contracting its sphere of activity and lessening its ability to both influence and react to the direction of social change. If one believes that the family is an institution beneficial to individuals and society, one easily becomes apprehensive when the family's traditional tasks are co-opted by other institutions, many of which exert further strains upon the family even as they weaken it (Kay, 1972).

Surely one of the most striking transformations can be found in the family's economic relation to society. For much of recorded history the family, extended or nuclear, functioned as the primary working unit. In modern America, however, the individual is the basic unit involved in production. Production and distribution are located in gigantic economic systems far removed from the daily life or undertakings of the family. The economic system governs large parts of the worker's life, and therefore pervasively affects the family, but its connection to the family takes place only through the involvement of the individual worker and its demands are set by economic logic, not family welfare.

At present the geographic mobility exacted of the American work force exceeds anything heretofore experienced. People go where the work is, often commuting hundreds of miles a day between bifurcated work and living spaces or repeatedly uprooting the family and relocating thousands of miles from relatives, childhood friends, and familiar social modes. An economic reality such as this has multiple ramifications in family life. Deprived of spatial and temporal continuity, lacking security in extended human relations, family members turn to each other for the satisfaction of all needs. This promotes an intensity of familiar interaction and expectation which is difficult to maintain consistently and wholesomely. The intensity introduced into relationships between spouses and between parents and children can create painful frustration when unrealistic expectations fail to be met.

The economic system operating upon the family has caused other strains. As the family's task of production declined, it was superseded by another, namely, the task of ensuring consumption. The pressure in American life to purchase and consume, and to judge others by their ability to do the same, involves the manipulation of family relationships. Advertisements which exploit a parent's feeling for family in order to persuade him or her to buy commodities can be destructive to those who cannot afford to do so. Parents who measure themselves against media advertisements of perfect mothers or fathers caring for perfect children who never suffer colds or dental caries are unlikely to feel truly competent or fulfilled.

Commercial invasion into the family, through which people are manipulated for economic purposes, is only one way in which traditional family tasks can be distorted. Socialization of children has long been a universal task of the family, but this, too, is changing. To the proponents of American youth culture, whose influence often supplants that of the family, there must be added the influence of establishment and quasi-establishment figures who advocate contraceptive measures and abortion for teenagers, with or without parental consent. Just as the public domain once supported the emergence of the nuclear family structure, the state now encourages individual efforts to break free of the nuclear family context. The issue is not whether such practices are justifiable or necessary, but only that they represent infringement on the family's traditional domain.

In the areas of sexuality and reproduction the family has managed to retain little control, perhaps because the two functions are no longer interconnected. Modern contraception has altered an elementary fact of life in which the risk of pregnancy accompanied active sexual behavior. For the past two centuries the strong nuclear family has been supported by cultural approval of voluntary, enduring sexual pairing, and cultural disapproval of sex or propagation outside a legal relationship. With the development of dependable contraception has come the option of reproductionless sexuality. Few would hazard a prediction regarding the effect of this development on the long-term pairing which is the basis of family structure.

The list of pressures operating on the American family today could be extended almost indefinitely, and a coherent presentation of the modern family's complex relationship to its total systemic environment is a major purpose of subsequent chapters. It may be useful to note here that external forces, however great, are not likely to destroy this institution, which has shown infinite capacity to endure. Its form and structure may surely change, but as our primary institution, the family is part of what it means to be human.

SUMMARY

Historical alterations and adaptations in the family have been examined over time. The family was described as both cause and consequence of social change. Active participation of the family in the shift to modernity was discussed. The role of the state in supporting the legal and economic power of the nuclear family was described as a maneuver to decrease rivalry between the state and extended feudal families.

Introducing the concept of love into the definition of the marital relationship was seen as a potent force in limiting female activity. The precarious existence of settlers in the New World was a liberating influence for women whose contributions were valued and appreciated. The same conditions of life reduced rigid parental control over children. The climate of modernity seemed to diminish the family by contracting its functions and reducing its importance as a unit of production.

Exploitation of the family through the media caused the family to become a unit of consumption. As the public domain once encouraged the emergence of the nuclear family against the feudal family, so the individual is now being influenced to separate from the nuclear family. Geographic and upward social mobility are among forces operating to attenuate ties to the nuclear family. Despite external pressures and reciprocal adaptation, the form and structure of the family may change but the institution will survive.

REFERENCES

Bachofen, J. J. *Myth, religion and mother right.* R. Monheim (trans), Princeton: Princeton University Press, 1973.

Benedict, R. The family, genus americanum. In R. N. Ashen (Ed.), *The family, its function and destiny.* New York: Harper, 1959.

Coser, R. L. *The family, its structure and functions.* New York: St. Martin's Press, 1974.

Demos, J. V. Adolescence in historical perspective. In M. Gordon (Ed.), *The American family in social-historical perspective.* New York: St. Martin's Press, 1973.

Engels, F. *Origin of the family, private property, and the state.* New York: International Publishers, 1942.

Goode, W. J. *World revolution and family patterns.* New York: The Free Press, 1963.

Hareven, T. K. The history of the family as an interdisciplinary field. In T. K. Rabb & R. I. Rothberg (Eds.), *The family in history.* New York: Harper & Row, 1971.

Hutchison, J. *Paths of faith.* New York: McGraw-Hill, 1969.

Kay, F. G. *The family in transition: Its past, present, and future patterns.* New York: Halsted Press, 1972.

Kluckhohn, F. R., & Strodtbeck, F. L. *Variation in value orientations.* New York: Row & Petersen, 1961.

Kyrk, H. *The family in the American economy.* Chicago: University of Chicago Press, 1953.

Lazlett, P. The comparative history of household and family. In M. Gordon (Ed.), *The American family in social-historical perspective.* New York: St. Martin's Press, 1973.

Levy, M. F., & Fallers, L. A. The family: some comparative considerations. In M. A. Sussman (Ed.), *Source book of marriage and the family.* Boston: Houghton Mifflin, 1968.

Linton, R. The natural history of the family. In R. Anshen (Ed.), *The family, its function and destiny.* New York: Harper, 1959.

Marx, K. The German ideology. In R. Tucker (Ed.), *The Marx and Engels reader.* Princeton: Princeton University Press, 1972.

Murdock, G. P. *Social structure.* New York: Macmillan, 1949.

Ogburn, W. F. The changing functions of the family. In R. F. Winch & L. W. Goodman (Eds.), *Selected studies in marriage and the family* (3rd ed.). New York: Holt, Rinehart & Winston, 1968.

Rapson, R. L. The American child as seen by British travellers, 1845–1935. In M. Gordon (Ed.), *The American family in social-historical perspective.* New York: St. Martin's Press, 1973.

Sennett, R. *Families against the city: Middle class homes of industrial Chicago, 1872–1890.* Cambridge, Mass.: Harvard University Press, 1970.

Shorter, E. Illegitimacy, sexual revolution, and social change in modern Europe. In M. Gordon (Ed.), *The American family in social-historical perspective.* New York: St. Martin's Press, 1973.

Shorter, E. *The making of the modern family.* New York: Basic Books, 1975.

Stephens, W. N. *The family in cross cultural perspective.* New York: Holt, Rinehart & Winston, 1963.

Stone, L. The rise of the nuclear family in early modern England: The patriarchal stage. In C. R. Rosenberg (Ed.), *The family in history.* Philadelphia: University of Pennsylvania Press, 1975.

Winch, R. F. Structure and function: Their analytical utility in the sociology of the family. In R. F. Winch & L. W. Goodman (Eds.), *Selected studies in marriage and the family.* (3rd ed.). New York: Holt, Rinehart & Winston, 1968.

Winch, R. F. *The modern family.* (3rd ed.). New York: Holt, Rinehart & Winston, 1971.

Chapter 3

Theoretical Frameworks Applicable to Family Care

Lenore Bolling Phipps

Family therapy is more than a treatment modality. It is also a philosophical approach which embodies the principle that disturbance resides not within an individual, but within the family system. The family member, represented as the identified patient, expresses the conflicts within the family. Family members contribute to and are an essential part of the sequence of reciprocal interactions within the system. Therefore, assessment and intervention should be focused upon the interaction process in an effort to alter the dysfunctional sequence and encourage a growth-promoting outcome (Group for the Advancement of Psychiatry, 1970). Effective communication, clarification of roles, rules, and boundaries, and increased self-awareness for all family members are among the goals of family therapy.

The objectives of this chapter are fourfold:

1   To provide an overview of family therapy and its relevance for all families, using general systems theory
2   To identify the major contributing theories of family therapy, and related concepts

3 To compare and contrast these major theories
4 To demonstrate the application of the related concepts to a hypothetical troubled family

While the initial, and perhaps major, emphasis of family therapy concepts has been on mental illness (for example, studies of families with schizophrenic members) these concepts have been recognized as having relevance for all families. It is the degree and frequency of similar behaviors in all families which enable theory and practice to be extended to families that may be partially, temporarily, or chronically troubled, as well as to those in which mental illness is clearly defined.

RELATIONSHIP OF FAMILY THERAPY TO GENERAL SYSTEMS THEORY

Power, mutual expectations, repetitive and reciprocal patterns of behavior, roles, rules, communication, and boundaries are the essential components which maintain homeostasis in the family system. Homeostasis is a balance which provides stability, consistency, and security for survival; it resists alteration by reinforcing stereotyped responses to internal and external changes.

Difficulties arise in the therapeutic process because the troubled family knows only those patterns of behavior which are familiar, and which seem least threatening to its system. The goals of the practitioner are deliberately to disrupt homeostasis, and to decrease stereotyped responses by introducing new experiences which teach members new ways of relating to one another. This is accomplished by focusing on one or more components of the system.

Roles

Within a family system, roles function to determine tasks, influence relationships and communication, and define power. They may be characteristically rigid, flexible, vague, or conflicted; they may be changed or reversed. In addition, roles may be assigned or assumed. The "scapegoat" sometimes assumes the "sick role," revealing the dysfunction of the family and frequently becoming the identified patient. Often, as the identified patient improves and no longer assumes the scapegoat role, another family member will accept it. This process is seen, for example, in the seesaw decompensation of alcoholic spouses or in the substitution of a sibling for the battered child. Other roles which may be imposed and become habitual as the result of family anxiety and conflict include the "model child," "baby," "black sheep," "peacemaker," and "pressure cooker."

Rules

Rules reflect the norms or values of the family and determine the behaviors which influence interactions and relationships. Rules may or may not be defined, but violation brings punishment and subsequent conformity. The power of a particular rule can be determined by the consequences of non-conformity. While all members exert influence upon one another to comply to collective standards, the covert implicit rules within a family frequently trigger problematic situations. Troubled families characteristically use covert, excessive and/or ambivalent rules to maintain homeostasis.

Closely related to roles and rules are expectations. All families have expectations for members, and when a member fails to assume the expected role, either by choice or circumstance, this may be seen as a threat to the family's equilibrium. Perhaps one of the most poignant and difficult challenges is posed by the birth of a retarded or congenitally abnormal child. The parents and grandparents must make heroic efforts to adjust their expectations, which were for the birth of a "normal" child.

Communication

Communication provides the medium for all transactions within the family system. All the other system components are greatly dependent upon the clarity and congruence of communication. Communication is so critical to family functioning that an entire theoretical framework based on communication patterns has emerged within family therapy.

In assimilating the major frameworks which contribute to the theory and practice of family therapy, it is important that the reader consider that each family encountered in clinical practice is different, and may need any of several approaches. The practitioner should be wary of becoming a purist and attempting to force families into a particular method.

DEVELOPMENTAL THEORY

This approach considers the family as it evolves over time, constantly changing as it proceeds from one chronological stage to the next. Each stage presents unique tasks for family members, who resolve these tasks with varying degrees of success. The end products of these stages and tasks are then carried over into the next stage. Central to this framework is the premise that developmental tasks must be completed within a critical period of time if successive stages are to be favorably negotiated (Erikson, 1963). The natural growth and development of children is the propelling force in the family's sequential movement through its life cycle. Family development theory, with its longitudinal perspective, is built around the process of sequential and cyclical patterns of growth, development, and decline.

Integration with General Systems Theory

The developmental framework encompasses the system triad of interdependence, interrelatedness, and complexity of family process. With its focus on change and on propelling internal and external forces, it provides a broad perspective on the openness of a system and the process of maturation.

Interdependence may be seen in the sequential linkage of individual and family developmental tasks. It is also evident in the interaction of biological growth, cultural pressures, and individual aspirations, which provides the impetus for movement into a new stage.

Interrelatedness is demonstrated by the emergence of family developmental tasks, in which the needs of individual members activate the family to undertake the responsibilities of stage-specific tasks. Interrelatedness is also in evidence during the periods of conflict that appear when members' developmental needs are in opposition. It becomes more complex as the family expands, adding new members through birth, adoption, or marriage; the number of relationships increases markedly as individuals simultaneously occupy several roles. The complex and reciprocal nature of family development will become clear to the practitioner as he or she assesses the background of family composition, sociocultural position, and current individual and family developmental tasks. This process assumes predictable significance as it is fitted into the template of the family life cycle.

Individual Developmental Tasks

The emergence of an individual developmental task results from the convergence of three factors: (1) the individual's physical maturation; (2) sociocultural expectations with regard to assigned roles; and (3) the individual's idiosyncratic aspirations and values. While the major influences are generally internal, arising from the individual's maturation and aspirations, the assimilation of cultural demands may also play a big role. Whatever the mix of these factors, the individual sees the possibility and promise of change. The developmental task becomes an assumed responsibility for adaptation and growth. Duvall (1977) uses the term "teachable moment" to indicate the time frame in which the individual is most receptive and ready to assume a developmental task.

Complementary and Conflicting Family Member Tasks

Ideally, the family unit functions to provide a relatively safe and secure environment in which all members have the opportunity for maximum growth. During periods of calm, members channel their energies in the same direction, and are alternately able to support one another in meeting developmental tasks. One such example is the college-bound young person who needs and receives financial and emotional support from the entire family unit as he or she embarks on a new phase of life. Similarly, families may unite in short-term activities such as planning a vacation or buying a home. Such activities provide a unifying and directive device for the family (Duvall, 1977).

In any family there will be periods of conflict, alternating with periods of calm as family members negotiate their particular developmental tasks within the system. Conflict arises when family members' goals, needs, and developmental tasks are incompatible at critical periods of growth. At several stages during the family's life normal conflict is inevitable. It emerges frequently, for example, in families with adolescent children, when adolescent strivings for independence are opposed by parents' continued needs to occupy supervisory roles.

Family Developmental Tasks

The family system has developmental tasks of its own, which arise sequentially, and which ensure its well-being and continuity as a functioning unit. Just as an individual's tasks shift over a lifetime, so the family's growth responsibilities change during its life cycle. Family tasks are also interrelated, and accomplishment or failure in earlier phases affects the later phases.

A family task originates in the blending of the needs of one or more members with society's expectations. As individuals mature, they assimilate society's values, crystallize their own aspirations, and then exert pressure on the family system to change. At the same time, the family must negotiate external pressures to conform. These external pressures vary according to the family's socioeconomic status and its composition. The family responds to these internal and external challenges by evaluating its identity, reputation, and goals, and by mobilizing its resources. This is the process which propels the family into a new stage of development, with its accompanying stage-critical tasks.

Critical events such as marriage, parenthood, or launching children impose new responsibilities and necessitate new behaviors. For example, while a newly married couple is facing the challenge of forming a mutually satisfactory relationship, the parents of the couple are involved with the problems of reorganizing the family as a smaller unit, releasing grown children, and providing a supportive home base (Duvall, 1977).

Family Life Cycle

This concept as proposed by Duvall (1977) divides family life into eight successive stages, beginning with the married couple and ending with the death of the surviving spouse. There is a predictability about the family life cycle

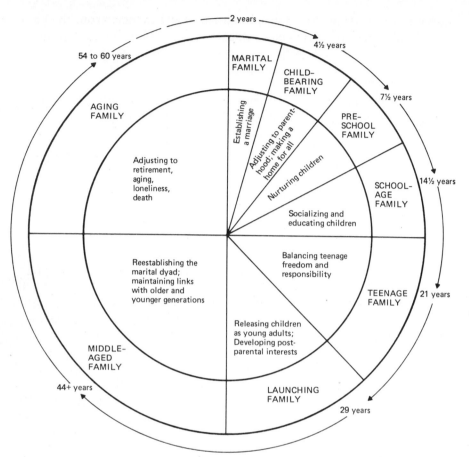

Figure 3-1 Stage-critical tasks in the family life cycle. (*Source: Adapted from Duvall, 1977, Table 7-3, p. 144.*)

in terms of expected patterns of behavior, developmental tasks, and duration. Based on census data, it is possible to estimate the time that a "typical" family will need to progress through each of the eight stages of the cycle. Contrary to media messages and popular opinion, the childbearing and child-rearing stages represent less than half of the entire cycle. Today's American woman lives more than one-half of her married life after her children have left home.

The family cycle becomes multigenerational as the family launches children who marry and begin new cycles. This continuous spinning off is termed the *generational spiral,* and may include two or three generations. As each new member is added, the number of possible relationships vastly increases. The following formula provides the number of interpersonal relationships within a family. x is equal to the number of relationships, and y is equal to the number of persons:

$$x = \frac{y^2 - y}{2}$$

Assessment and Intervention

All families experience stress and conflict from time to time as inevitable accompaniments to growth and change. The passage from one developmental stage to the next provides fertile ground for anxiety and tension within the family. However, growth and change can be constructively managed by dealing with issues and problems, rather than attacking with generalized and global accusations.

Assuming new roles and responsibilities brings hazards as well as rewards. Marital dissatisfaction and divorce peak during the early child-bearing and child-rearing years, attesting to the demands of financial pressure and role strain involved in this endeavor (Duvall, 1977). It is likely that the stress is most severe for the single-parent or low socioeconomic family.

In addition to the develomental crises and conflicts that all families face, there are unique situational crises which tax the system's resources, and threaten stability and integrity. A crisis may be described as any situation for which present coping skills are inadequate. A situational crisis may result from the addition or loss of a family member, especially in cases of illegitimacy, suicide, or divorce. One way of categorizing types of family crises is as follows: dismemberment (loss of a member), accession (addition of a member), demoralization (loss of status), and a combination of demoralization, plus dismemberment or accession (Duvall, 1977).

It is important to remember that crises typically occur not as isolated events, but within the context of an already existing family system, and are managed according to the resources available. Socioeconomic level, marital and familial relationships, and previously completed tasks are the variables which determine whether a crisis will strengthen or weaken the family. For instance, a financially stressed teenage couple that is socially isolated from extended family members may be expected to have excessive difficulty in dealing with the arrival of a congenitally impaired infant.

While the developmental approach does not provide cookbook techniques for identifying, assessing, and intervening with families in trouble, it does raise some provocative questions. The following list is by no means exhaustive, but it provides an introduction to assessment and intervention.

1 What is the composition of the family system?
2 What are its sociocultural characteristics?

  3 What are the stage-specific developmental tasks for the family? For the individual members?
  4 How are those tasks performed when conflict is present?
  5 What are the events surrounding the current crises?
  6 How is the crisis related to dismemberment, accession, and demoralization?
  7 What is the family's attitude toward the event?
  8 What are the family's tension-reducing aspirations?

The goal of the practitioner is to help families increase their success in surmounting developmental tasks. The developmental approach holds promise for primary prevention of mental illness and other stress-related diseases, and for anticipatory guidance in maternal-child health and community health. As the practitioner helps family members recognize and plan for developmental stages and their relevant tasks, individual and family resources will be strengthened.

STRUCTURAL THEORY

Structural theory envisions the family as an organization of patterned relationships enforced by the mutual expectations of family members and the power conferred by the roles which they assume. Therapeutic interventions are directed toward changing the organization, or structure, of the family in order to change its function. Altering the positions of family members transforms their experiences, and leads to changes in total family functioning (Minuchin, 1974).

Integration with General Systems Theory

This framework views the family as an open system composed of complex, interdependent parts defined as subsystems. A subsystem may consist of an individual, a marital or parental pair, or siblings. These subsystems provide experience and training in the process of self-definition and role enactment. Subsystems have boundaries (rules) which protect differentiation of function by defining the participants in a subsystem and regulating their behavior.
  An effectively functioning family system is able to reorganize to meet internal and external demands by using alternative transactional patterns. On the other hand, a dysfunctional or troubled family responds to stress by stereotyping its interactions. In the latter case, the practitioner attempts to modify the entire system by "joining" it, thereby deliberately disrupting the dysfunctional homeostasis.

Subsystems

Subsystems enable the family to differentiate and perform its various functions. Each subsystem has a different psychosocial territory and a specific function, and makes certain demands on its members. A system may be composed of dyads, triads, or subsystems having several members. Subsystems usually evolve according to sex, generation, or particular interests. Characteristically, in any family system, an individual belongs to a number of different subsystems. Membership within a particular subsystem influences a family member's power, influence, and even specific skills developed. A wife and mother who belongs simultaneously to spouse and parental subsystems may have varying ability to influence her husband's and son's behaviors. At the same time, she will need to learn and apply the skills required to perform the roles of both wife and mother. Because the family is in a constant process of development, subsystems tend to develop sequentially, most typically from spouse to parent. This process requires that members learn new skills and new ways of relating to other subsystems, again creating the possibility of conflict and adding internal stress to the system (Minuchin, 1974).

Boundaries

Boundaries that are clearly defined in terms of responsibility and authority reflect effective subsystem and family system functioning. Conversely, boundaries that are inappropriately rigid or diffuse often indicate maladaptive areas in the family. Minuchin (1974) saw boundary clarity as an effective parameter in assessment and intervention, and used the terms "disengagement" (rigid) and "enmeshment" (diffuse) to describe types of transactional styles which families develop.

Disengagement, at one end of a continuum, refers to inflexible, rigid boundaries which preserve separateness between subsystems and handicap communications and relatedness. Members tend to be emotionally isolated from one another, neither requesting nor responding to help. Only extreme stress will initiate interaction with others.

Enmeshment, at the opposite pole, is a style of diffuse, blurred boundaries and diminished differentiation of subsystems. Here members have a strong sense of belonging, but give up a measure of autonomy and mastery skills. Any stress on the enmeshed family system produces rapid, intense overreaction, frequently expressed by excessive concern and involvement. Most families have subsystems which operate to some degree as enmeshed or disengaged, falling within the middle range of a transactional continuum. It is at the extreme points of the continuum that these styles become problematic.

Assessment and Intervention

The goal of the structural approach is to seek alternative patterns in family transactions. The practitioner accomplishes this by "joining" the family system, by analyzing the current structural arrangements, and by implementing changes designed to restructure family organization (Minuchin,

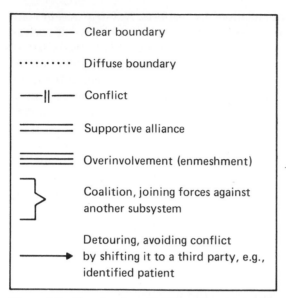

Figure 3-2 Mapping legend. *(After Minuchin, 1974.)*

1974). In joining the family, the practitioner accommodates to family norms and transactional patterns, at the same time maintaining a position of leadership which allows her or him to introduce change. Even though this appears to be an impossible stance, it can be accomplished by an initial acknowledgment of those members who wield power and by a temporary acceptance of existing subsystems. The practitioner endeavors to expand and clarify verbal and nonverbal communication, often imitating the family interactional style. This process requires the practitioner to enter the family but to maintain sufficient objectivity to ensure effective change. An analysis of the structural arrangement includes evaluation of (1) the clarity of subsystem boundaries and appropriate task performance, and (2) the sources of family stress and support (Minuchin, 1974).

The family map is a diagrammatic tool which organizes the data into a working hypothesis of family strengths and weaknesses, and therefore helps to determine therapeutic goals. A mapping legend provides symbols to depict typical interactional patterns, boundaries, and dysfunctional areas. The usefulness of mapping as a technique is depicted in the following situation. A family system is composed of mother, father, adolescent son, and two younger daughters. The father seems isolated and ineffective as he complains of his son's recent involvement with police regarding traffic violations. The mother condones and excuses her son's behavior. Mother and son both attack the father for his nonparticipation in family activities. The mother functions as the controlling executive of family life; she maintains distance from her husband and is overinvolved with her son. The two younger sisters have formed a separate sibling subsystem, which reduces their feelings of isolation from parents. The following is the family map of the current situation:

```
                Father
Mother  ═══════════  Son

 ──  ──  ──  ──  ──  ──  ──  ──

Daughter  ═══════════  Daughter
```

Therapeutic goals would include strengthening the spouse-parental subsystem by supporting the father's parental capabilities and disrupting the mother-son coalition, as shown in the following map:

```
Father  ═══════════  Mother

 ──  ──  ──  ──  ──  ──  ──

Daughters            Son
```

Restructuring Operations

Minuchin (1974) has suggested that members become willing to change their positions in the family if the practitioner appeals to their strengths and competence. This process involves various tactics: (1) clarification of self-system boundary, (2) alliance with the disenfranchised member, (3) support of age-appropriate independence, encouraging members to speak for themselves, and (4) support of subsystem interdependence (requesting that one member help the *other* to change, rather than change himself). These factors strengthen the system by encouraging the family's participation in its own healing and growth. The restructuring operations introduced by the practitioner are designed to precipitate disequilibrium and offer alternative experiences which may then be incorporated into the family coping repertoire.

Specific implementing techniques include reenacting a stressful family scene within a clinical session and assigning tasks to be accomplished at home. These interventions bring new experiences into the daily routine of family life.

Theorists have noted that family members tend to position themselves according to alliances, coalitions, and power. This spatial arrangement may provide an additional medium for restructuring operations. The practitioner may manipulate space, using self, family members, furniture, or the room to reinforce appropriate messages. The dimension of space can be used to encourage adaptive communication, disrupt maladaptive coalitions, or clarify diffuse boundaries (Minuchin, 1974).

COMMUNICATION THEORY

Communication theorists use communication as the primary assessment and therapeutic tool in working with families. They focus on observing the transaction and interaction patterns which infuence and define a particular family system. The process by which messages are sent, perceived, and verified is critically important; so is the degree of clarity and congruence of messages. Therefore, the therapeutic goal focuses upon improvement of communication, so that it becomes clear, accurate, and meaningful (Satir, 1967).

Integration with General Systems Theory

The influence of general systems theory may be seen in communication theory, which views the family as an ongoing, interactional system. Established communication patterns, implicit and explicit rules governing messages and participants, and corrective negative feedback are actions which maintain homeostasis in the system. Regardless of the conditions in which the family's interactions occur, the communication patterns will be the same. Therefore, a sampling assessment of the family's communication patterns permits the practitioner some understanding of its typical format.

Several accepted principles support the communication theoretical framework. It is impossible not to communicate, since any verbal or nonverbal behavior becomes a message; even silence may communicate an emotional or cognitive state (Foley, 1974). Communication is multifaceted in terms of content, affect, and context. The denotative level provides information on the literal content of the message, while the connotative level includes metacommunication which qualifies the content and implies the degree of intimacy, conflict, or power inherent in the dyad relationship (Foley, 1974). Metacommunication is "a message about a message," and may be expressed verbally or nonverbally (Satir, 1967). When the two levels reinforce each other, the message becomes congruent and functional.

Communication implies a reciprocal exchange of information. Within a family system, these interactions become sequential and circular patterns. Once a pattern of exchange develops, it is maintained. For example, if Dad usually talks to his son through his wife, the appropriate intervention would encourage direct communication between father and son, with the mother no longer an intermediary. It should be remembered that, despite precautions, the message that is sent is not always the one that is received. The communication process is subject to potentially distorting variables, such as context, feedback, and perception.

Theorists disagree as to the major influences upon communication. Much has been said about thought, feeling, or the struggle for power as modifying factors. For Jackson (1968), communication expresses what one thinks, whereas Satir (1967) sees it expressing self-esteem. Haley (1971) views communication as greatly influenced by the struggle for control. Nevertheless, these theorists share a common belief that dysfunction in a family system is the result of dysfunctional communication between members.

Examples of dysfunctional communication include acting on assumptions without validation, omitting connections between ideas, using stereotyped phrases such as "always" or "never," and sending mixed, or double-binding messages. The resultant lack of clarity and congruency produces confusion and anxiety in the recipient of the message.

Double-bind Messages

This concept was initially implicated as a contributing element in the etiology of schizophrenia; now it is believed to have ramifications for all dysfunctional communication. The double bind is a form of communication whereby a primary negative injunction is followed by a conflicting injunction; both injunctions are enforced by threatening punishment. In addition, the less powerful of the dyad (the victim) is not able to escape from the situation. The double-bind message is grossly incongruent and is reinforced by repetition. The victim is unable to grasp the meaning of the message, nor can he or she comment on it, since feedback is not tolerated (Bateson, 1956).

Rules

Explicit and implicit rules refer to the types of messages permitted in a family. The rules function to stabilize relationships, but may also prohibit feelings. To a degree, they operate beyond the awareness of the persons governed by them. Implicit rules may be determined by observing family decision making and identifying who speaks for whom, who gives credit to whom, and who attributes what to whom.

In dysfunctional families, the prevailing rules and patterns of communication discourage individualization and uniqueness (Satir, Stachowiak, & Taschman, 1977). There appears to be great pressure to conform, with decision making governed by power rather than by negotiations.

Self-Esteem

Self-esteem influences one's perception of the world, the transmission and reception of messages, and interactional patterns. People function according to their degree of self-worth, and learn various patterns of functioning as a result of early parental influence and modeling. During stressful situations that contribute to low self-esteem, one or more "stress postures" may be assumed: placating to assure acceptance by others, blaming to ensure power, or being "superreasonable" to deny feelings. These stances are growth-inhibiting and prevent the individual from making choices (Satir et al., 1977).

A more adaptive stance is congruency, in which feelings and verbal and nonverbal communication are all in agreement with the situation. Congruency involves awareness and acceptance of one's own thoughts, feelings, and behavior and facilitates clarity over ambiguity. A sense of self-esteem requires freedom to comment and to provide reality-based feedback. These are the communication elements that enable people to grow. Maturity is a state in which one assumes responsibility for one's behavior, and makes decisions as the result of reality-based perceptions of self and others.

Assessment and Intervention

The therapeutic focus involves changing the rules governing family communication to encourage growth for all members. The practitioner does not enter into the family system, but acts as a corrective feedback mechanism to disturb the present dysfunctional communication. Assessment involves seeking answers to the following questions: (1) Who labeled what behavior as a symptom? (2) What does the symptom indicate about the family's prohibition of growth for the "symptom bearer?" (3) How does the restriction of growth maintain homeostasis for the family system?

Satir et al. (1977) endorse the use of self-awareness as a vehicle for change. Role playing of various stress stances, together with discussion and sharing of members' thoughts and feelings, is often effective. Another method is sculpting, which uses spatial relationships to recreate problem situations. A third is parent-child role reversal, which enables individuals to experience "smallness" and "bigness" in relation to height and feelings of self-esteem. These exercises should be attempted only after the practitioner has become a trusted figure, and the family is ready to risk new experiences which promote reality and creativity.

Corrective feedback can be used to clarify and validate transactions. The practitioner serves as a role model for the family, commenting on stereotyped words such as "always" or "never" and diminishing the perception of feedback as a threat. "This is how I see you" becomes an objective observation when used by a trusted practitioner.

Clarification of rules defines whether it is "OK" or "not OK" to express feelings within the family or to be different from other members. Replacing implicit communication with explicit communication utilizes the idea that what cannot be said hurts and inhibits congruency and growth.

Relabeling is a method by which a negatively labeled motivation is replaced by one which is positive. For example, a mother who angrily criticizes a youngster for disobeying a curfew may be described as expressing her concern for the child's safety. The teenager who defies and challenges authority may be depicted by the practitioner as an adolescent in search of individuation and identity.

PSYCHOANALYTIC THEORY

Basic to the psychoanalytic framework is the conflict between the individuals' need to relate to the family group and their need to separate from it in order to establish self-identity. The person who is functioning effectively is able to balance these needs, and to relate to others and not lose self-identity. The family as a social organization is a major influence in strengthening or weakening that identity.

In families in which individuality is seen as a threat to survival, identity is "given up" for the sake of family cohesiveness. The term *pseudomutuality* describes a process by which family roles assume a rigidity that maintains homeostasis. Any family may become locked into rigid and inescapable roles. According to Foley (1974), the more pathological the family the more inflexible the roles.

Freud, while devoting most of his attention to individual, intrapsychic processes, also formulated some ideas about the significance of the family. He postulated that the family is a natural group which shares a collective emotional life. Feelings, attitudes, and values are transmitted from one generation to the next through an unconscious process of assimilation, thus creating an intergenerational continuity of emotional life (Anthony, 1971). Bowen (1976) has elaborated on this idea with his concept of intergenerational progression. The psychoanalytic approach is concerned with intrapsychic phenomena and family transactions, past and present, which shape patterns of behavior. Of all the family theories, this one is most likely to use the medical model as a frame of reference, often adopting a nosological classification for the purpose of diagnosis and treatment.

Integration with General Systems Theory

The psychoanalytic framework is compatible with a systems approach in which the wholeness of the family is seen to be reflected in the sharing of a collective emotional life. The interrelationships contribute to a dense network of transferences (parent, child, siblings) which, in turn, influences the relationships. Transferences also contribute to the formulation of family roles and family myths. In this manner, behavior patterns become increasingly complex and circular.

Interrelatedness can be seen in the dynamics of pseudomutuality and pseudohostility, in which family members become so enmeshed that individuation and separation of individuals are quite difficult. Psychoanalytic theory also provides the example of the "rubber fence," an illogical feedback process which maintains dysfunctional homeostasis.

Pseudomutuality

Wynne, Ryckoff, Day and Hirsch (1958) describe a type of family relationship in which members are totally enmeshed with one another. This emotional enmeshment prohibits the growth and development of self-identity, and any deviation is seen as a threat to the family system. Pseudomutuality is characterized by insistence on rigid role expectations, preoccupation with harmony, and an absence of spontaneity, humor, and enthusiasm. Pseudomutuality is an extreme family defense against individualization.

Rubber fence is the term used to describe how the family ensures its central focus. This is done by stretching family boundaries to include only compatible activities and ideas, and contracting them to exclude incompatible ones. When the boundaries contract and expand indiscriminately and illogically, the individual finds that he cannot trust his own perceptions of reality. This rubber fence process is similar to double-bind communication, where constantly changing rules and lack of structure contribute to confusion and anxiety in family members. Wynne et al. believe that pseudomutuality, with its rigid role expectations, affects all family members. Parents and children become caught in a web of reciprocal scapegoating and rescuing, with little hope of escape.

Pseudohostility

Wynne et al. use this term to characterize families in which quarreling and hostility express unconscious patterns of denial and defense against affection and the need to be close. Pseudomutuality and pseudohostility are both dysfunctional attempts to manage the basic conflict between relating to and separating from others (Foley, 1974).

Transferences and Family Myths

Each person carries with him an "internal family" composed of feelings, events, and attitudes. This intrapsychic family is the result of early perceptions which have been internalized and recorded unconsciously, and which influence what occurs in a current interaction. When the perceptions are projected externally to real persons, the phenomenon of transference occurs (Anthony, 1971).

Subjective distortions, or transferences, originate within the family context, and shape patterns of behavior that are repeated inappropriately in nonfamily interactions. Transference may be positive, negative, or ambivalent. Countertransference is the practitioner's (therapist's) subjective and distorted reaction to the client. If the presence of countertransference is not recognized, it may become an obstacle to treatment.

Transferences become patterns within the family and contribute to the development and maintenance of family myths. Family myths have a homeostatic function, providing a framework for the acceptance of behaviors and relationships within the family. Myths provide support for blaming and pardoning, and for anchoring members in roles. They exist as an attempt to make sense of the family's basic nature, relatedness, history, and current situation (Stierlin, 1975).

In treatment, the troubled family attempts to sell the myth to the practitioner. To the extent that this is successful, the perpetuated myth becomes a stumbling block to growth. Transferences and myths are deeply ingrained in the family history, and the practitioner who attempts to intervene here must be prepared to deal with the intransigent family system which opposes change (Anthony, 1971).

Assessment and Intervention

The psychoanalytic approach requires specialized training and broad knowledge of intrapsychic processes. However, practitioners may distill some of this framework and apply it to a variety of clinical situations when interacting with troubled families. Recognizing one's subjective distorted reactions to clients (countertransference) increases one's self-awareness and helps remove obstacles to effective practice. There are times when clients create frustration, anger, and anxiety in professional care takers. To the extent that one acknowledges and accepts this phenomenon, one opens oneself to therapeutic responsiveness rather than to emotional reactivity. Professionals tend to distort responses which reflect their earlier difficulties in separating and individuating from their own families of origin. This human predilection is shared by practitioners and clients alike.

Assessment involves identifying the roles that family members assume, whether scapegoat, victim, oppressor, or peacemaker. Consideration of ways in which the symptoms of the identified patient may help or hurt the family provides understanding of the myths which maintain dysfunctional homeostasis.

Countertransference presents some problematic issues in family intervention. For example, the young practitioner who identifies with a protesting generation, either by dress or manner, may have difficulty establishing a relationship with the parents of a rebellious teenage diabetic. Or, if the practitioner overidentifies with "victimized" parents and displaces his or her anger on the adolescent, trust is also jeopardized.

Working with families of adolescent children requires the practitioner to support the nurturing and caring characteristics of parents, and to avoid competing with them in order to be the rescuer of the child. Similarly, the male practitioner is cautioned to be sensitive to a father's need for self-esteem, and to avoid replacing father in the eyes of the child, thus escalating the father's feelings of inadequacy (Stierlin, 1975).

BOWEN THEORY

Bowen conceptualizes the family as an automatic emotional system, which establishes, maintains, and balances member relationships. The response to emotional stimuli within the family system determines the degree to which members are able to function. The ability to distinguish between a subjective feeling response and an objective thinking response allows the individual to develop a sense of identity and greater flexibility in coping with life's stresses. If one member learns to respond with objectivity, this will encourage change in the significant other's response because of the reciprocal nature of family interactions. Movement toward a rational, cognitive means of relating rather than reliance on emotionalism provides opportunities for improved relationships between all family members.

Integration with General Systems Theory

The Bowen Theory is composed of eight interlocking concepts, developed as a result of clinical research over the past 30 years. Although Bowen originally referred to his approach as a systems theory (1971), he has more recently clarified the distinction between his theory and general systems theory. He views any relationship with balancing forces and counterforces as an operating system which permits assessment of the complex balance in family life (Bowen, 1976).

The general systems concept of unity is implied in Bowen's term "emotional oneness" of the family system. Bowen also subscribes to the concept of the interrelatedness of subsystems and to equifinality. Although he denies that these concepts evolved from general systems theory, or are synonomous with it, Bowen's theory is nevertheless compatible with the conceptual framework of general systems theory.

Differentiation of Self

This is a central concept that refers to the degree of separation between emotional and intellectual functioning. Bowen (1971) postulates that this universal characteristic may be plotted on a continuum entitled the "differentiation-of-self scale." Further discussion of this concept can be found in Chapter 6.

Triangles

Triangles are basic, interrelated units in an emotional system. The triadic relationships may be formed by three members, or by two members plus an issue or component which assumes the significance of a third member. During relatively tranquil periods, the triangle is composed of a close dyad and a less close third person. When tension increases in the dyad, an available third member or issue is "triangled in" to maintain distance between the two original members. A troubled dyad thus becomes a triangle. The member of the dyad who feels the most tension is the one who initiates an alliance with a third party, seeking to create a new equilibrium. This third member forms a new close dyad with one of the members, reducing tension and restabilizing the triangle. The emotional forces within triangles are discussed in more detail in Chapter 6.

Nuclear Family Emotional System

Bowen's third concept describes the patterns of emotional functioning in a single-generation family. The life-style and level of self-differentiation that each spouse brings to the marriage influence the pattern of emotional functioning. Each spouse tends to replay the adaptive or dominant role learned in the family of origin. Mate selection involves a tendency to choose a partner at the same level of differentiation. The more undifferentiated the self, the greater the risk of emotional fusion. Fusion of self creates anxiety in one or both partners and may be expressed in several ways: emotional distancing, marital conflict, dysfunction-overfunction, or projection to children.

When both partners assume a dominant position, marital conflict occurs. Each is intensely fused with the other, and the relationship becomes a cyclical pattern of closeness and conflict. Bowen (1976) suggests that the conflicted marriage is not overly harmful to children as long as the conflict is not accompanied by transmission or projection of the problem to children.

Dysfunction-overfunction results when one partner chronically accommodates to the other and assumes an adaptive posture. As the dominant partner assumes major decision-making responsibility for the dyad, the adaptive person loses the capacity to function. One member overfunctions while the other is impaired. With any significant increase in stress, the adaptive partner may lapse into episodic or chronic physical or emotional illness.

Impairment of one or more children often occurs as a result of the projection of parental lack of self-differentiation onto the offspring. Two factors greatly influence symptomatology in these children: (1) the degree of emotional distance from extended families, and (2) the level of anxiety within the nuclear family. The greater the emotional distance from extended families and the higher the anxiety level of the nuclear family, the more severe are the symptoms.

Family Projection Process

The amount of undifferentiation in the parents resembles a commodity which may be transferred to a child. When the amount is too much for one child to absorb, it tends to be distributed to other children. If the child who has been the recipient of the projection process departs through physical separation or death, another child may be chosen as the repository of parental anxiety. The process begins with anxiety in the parent, which is transmitted to the child; however, the parent sees the problem as being limited to the child. She or he may assume a posture of overprotectiveness which further undermines the child's sense of self and ability to function with autonomy. Once this pattern is established, it is intensified by excessive anxiety in either parent or child or by the urgency of developmental tasks. The child then becomes a likely candidate for emotional impairment.

Bowen (1976) postulates that this chosen child develops a lower level of differentiation than the parents or siblings. After several generations of decreasing levels of differentiation, one generation ultimately produces a schizophrenic individual. Most families have one child who was the triangled candidate and whose life functioning was more impaired than that of his or her siblings. It is possible to follow this projection process through generations by gathering data regarding parent-sibling relationships and degree of life adjustments.

Emotional Cutoff

This concept was introduced by Bowen (1976) to describe the emotional process by which persons separate themselves from their families of origin in order to begin their own lives. All persons have some unresolved emotional linkage to their parents. The intensity of this attachment is greater at the lower end of the differentiation-of-self scale, and intense attachment indicates marked emotional dependency on the family of origin. Various cutoff patterns can be used; denial, isolation, or distancing may be attempts to resolve this issue. If emotional dependency on the family of origin is not resolved, it is perpetuated in the individual's own marriage and in future generations. The therapeutic goal is to reestablish emotional contact with extended families, encouraging the individual to assume an "I" position which ensures self-integrity. As each marital partner re-defines self in the respective family of origin, the level of anxiety and the symptoms diminish.

Multigenerational Transmission Process

This concept supports the idea that the family projection process may be transmitted through several generations. Bowen (1976) postulates that several generations are required for projection to create extremes of high or low self-differentiation and that the marital dyad is comprised of partners at very close points on the scale. Depending upon triangling sequences and projection processes, children in a family may progress or regress on the differentiation scale, or remain at about the same level.

Sibling Position

Toman (1961) originally conceptualized personality profiles of sibling position. These have been incorporated into Bowen's theory, and are discussed in more detail in Chapter 6.

Societal Regression

In another recently developed concept, Bowen (1976) postulates that society is an emotional system much like the family. The family system, subjected to continual chronic stress and anxiety, loses its ability to adapt to its environment in a rational-cognitive manner, and regresses to an emotional position, thereby expressing dysfunctional symptoms. Similarly, society, struggling with problems such as chronic pollution or food and energy shortages, makes legislative decisions which are emotionally based. Society unsuccessfully attempts to ameliorate the situation and propels itself further toward dysfunction.

Assessment and Intervention

Bowen emphasizes that family members benefit most from their individual efforts to learn how their family system functions. Change occurs only through attempts to respond cognitively rather than emotionally.

Three major interrelated therapeutic goals are explicit in Bowen's approach: (1) increase the degree of self-differentiation, (2) detriangle family members, and (3) rework the emotional cutoff with extended families. The accomplishment of these objectives requires a detailed assessment of the nuclear and extended families' symptomatic behavior over time. This assessment should include a definition of: (1) recent events in both nuclear and extended families, (2) relationship patterns between spouses, (3) circumstances surrounding birth of first child (the original triangle), and (4) the degree of closeness or distance with extended families (Foley, 1974).

Practitioners using the Bowen model strive to remain objective and detached from the family emotional system. They work primarily with the marital dyad, supporting their leadership positions in the family and focusing on their emotional reaction patterns. The premise is that, as the marital dyad grows in self-differentiation, the family system will change, enabling other members to grow. Bowen (1961) uses the terms "coach" or "teacher" to describe the role of the practitioner in this process.

The practitioner is encouraged to use the following goal-centered interventions to assist husband and wife to increase their level of self-differentiation (Bowen, 1971):

1 Assist spouses to define and clarify their relationship.

2 Ask for thoughts, rather than feelings, to increase cognitive awareness.

3 Comment on the process of the interaction to encourage observation and control of emotional reactiveness, and to enable members to understand the part each plays in family reaction patterns.

4 Encourage self-definition by demonstrating with phrases such as "I think" or "I believe."

5 Acknowledge and support members' attempts to remain calm and cognitively aware.

6 Encourage development of person-to-person relationships with families of origin to rework emotional cutoff and increase understanding of marital relationship.

Bowen (1971) emphasizes the need to rework unresolved emotional issues with extended families as a means of reducing anxiety and symptomatology. Working through the emotional cutoff from the original family enables the individual to avoid the classic dilemma of the adult in a family system—whether to stay and feel angry or to leave and feel guilty.

CLINICAL EXAMPLE: FAMILY RESPONSE
TO INJURY AND DEATH IN THE FAMILY

Ralph, an 18-year-old, was recovering in a rural general hospital from injuries sustained 2 weeks earlier during an automobile accident in which his 15-year-old brother, Tom, was killed. The extent of Ralph's injuries, while not life-threatening, jeopardized a college athletic scholarship for the coming year.

During hospitalization, Ralph did not openly grieve for his brother, but spent his time alternately watching television and criticizing hospital staff for their lack of concern for his discomfort and immobility (partial body cast). Because of his injuries he was unable to attend the funeral of his brother. During occasional visits from the family, Ralph's father blamed him for causing the accident.

Before the accident, Ralph and his mother had had a very close relationship. It was she who gave Ralph permission to take the car on the night of the accident. Ralph's father, a skilled laborer, had a similar special feeling for the dead son, Tom. As an avid sports enthusiast, he had invested much of his leisure time coaching the hockey team for which his sons played. Since the accident, Ralph's father spent increasing amounts of time away from home. The preference of each parent for one son over the other was not a source of stress before the accident. It was a recurrent joke that Tom could manipulate Dad and Ralph to obtain favors from Mom. The two younger girls formed a strong sibling subsystem which was mutually supportive. Loss of Ralph's scholarship funds introduced uncertainty into the girls' plans for attending a community college after high school. Conscious of the family crisis, the girls had not discussed their prospects except with each other. Ralph's accountability for the accident was another issue the girls did not discuss; their visits to Ralph were very infrequent.

The emphasis of family assessment and intervention varies according to the theoretical framework which is used. The main areas of assessment and intervention which would need to be investigated in the above example are illustrated through utilization of guidelines from the developmental, structural, communication, and psychoanalytic theories, and from Bowen's theory.

Developmental Framework

Assessment

1 Family faces crisis of dismemberment and demoralization, combined with financial and role strain inherent in family developmental stage (teenage).

2 Individual task of identity formulation is threatened by accident and probable loss of college funds.

3 Current stress and lack of intermember support are immobilizing family system.

Intervention

1 Support family as it deals with loss of son/brother (crisis intervention).

2 Encourage members to verbalize perception of the accident and redefine their goals and aspirations.

3 Assist members to recognize individual and family developmental tasks relevant to the teenage and launching stages.

Structural Framework

Assessment

1 Coalition between mother and son is disruptive to spouse subsystem boundary.

2 Recent death and accident has intensified disengagement process.

Intervention

1 Clarify and support spouse subsystem to encourage mutual leadership and shared grieving.

2 Strengthen teenage peer alliance and sibling subsystem.

Communication Framework

Assessment

1 Family is demonstrating dysfunctional communication pattern of blame, incongruency, and lack of feedback.

2 Members are not expressing affective concerns regarding loss and pain, causing increased emotional isolation.

Intervention

1 Increase members' awareness of their feelings of loss and pain.

2 Encourage them to verbalize feelings in a congruent manner.

3 Reduce blaming interactions by relabeling.

Psychoanalytic Framework

Assessment

1 Acting and behavior expresses unresolved adolescent conflict regarding authority and the need both to leave and to remain with the family.

2 Anger towards father is transferred to staff.

3 Grief work and anger concerning "lost" brother and "lost" opportunity have not been resolved.

4 Staff countertransference is implied in identification with parent role as result of acting-out behavior, plus own unresolved anxiety regarding issues of adolescence.

Intervention

1 Encourage patient/family to verbalize hostility concerning losses and authority.

2 Plan staff meeting to encourage verbalization concerning patient's behavior, and own adolescent memories. ("What was it like when . . . ?")

Bowen Framework

Assessment

1 Marital conflict is characterized by emotional distancing and triangle involving Ralph.

2 The crisis has crystallized the positions of the triangle, and increased the pattern of emotional reaction (blame and withdrawal) and the tension.

Intervention

1 Detriangle Ralph—work with marital dyad to strengthen "I" position.

2 Focus on a thinking response to situation.

3 Diminish blame. Include grandparents in family gatherings to reduce tension within nuclear family and provide support during grieving period.

SUMMARY

An overview of the developmental, structural, communication, psychoanalytic, and Bowen theory approaches to intervention in family systems was presented. Basic concepts which undergird these frameworks were described, and related to general systems theory. A summary of the focus, concepts, intervention methods, practitioner activities, strengths, and limitations of the five theoretical approaches discussed in this chapter are presented in Table 3-1 (pp. 56-57).

REFERENCES

Anthony, J. R. An introduction to family group therapy. In H. Kaplan & B. Sadock (Eds.), *Comprehensive group psychotherapy.* Baltimore: Williams & Wilkins, 1971.

Bateson, G. Towards a theory of schizophrenia. *Behavioral Science, 1956,* **1,** 251-264.

Bowen, M. The family as the unit of study and treatment. *American Journal of Orthopsychiatry,* 1961, **31,** 40-60.

Bowen, M. Family therapy and family group therapy. In H. Kaplan & B. Sadock (Eds.), *Comprehensive group psychotherapy.* Baltimore: Williams & Wilkins, 1971.

Bowen, M. Theory in the practice of psychotherapy. In P. Guerin, Jr. (Ed.), *Family therapy: Theory and practice.* New York: Gardner Press, 1976.

Duvall, E. M. *Marriage and family development.* (5th ed.) Philadelphia: Lippincott, 1977.

Erickson, E. *Childhood and society.* New York: Norton, 1963.

Foley, V. D. *An introduction to family therapy.* New York: Grune & Stratton, 1974.

Group for the Advancement of Psychiatry. *The field of family therapy,* 1970, **7**(Report No. 78.).

Haley, J. (Ed.) Changing families. New York: Grune & Stratton, 1971.

Jackson, D. (Ed.) Communication, family and marriage. Palo Alto, Calif.: Science & Behavior Books, 1968.

Janosik, E., & Miller, J. Theories of family development. In D. Hymovich & M. U. Barnard (Eds.), *Family health care.* (2nd ed.) New York: McGraw-Hill, 1979.

Minuchin, S. *Families and family therapy.* Cambridge, Mass.:Harvard University Press, 1974.

Satir, V. *Conjoint family therapy.* Palo Alto: Science & Behavior Books, 1967.

Satir, V., Stachowiak, J., & Taschman, H. *Helping families to change.* New York: Jason Aronson, 1977.

Stierling, H. Countertransference in family therapy with adolescents. In M. Sugar (Ed.), *The adolescent in group and family therapy.* New York: Brunner/Mazel, 1975.

Toman, W. *Family constellation.* New York: Springer, 1961.

Wynne, L., Ryckoff, I., Day, J., & Hirsch, S. Pseudomutuality in the family relations of schizophrenics. *Psychiatry,* May 1958, **21**(2), 205-220.

Table 3-1 Overview of Theoretical Frameworks

	Developmental	Structural	Communication	Bowen	Psychoanalytic
Focus	Process, change, predictable stages and roles.	Process, change position of members to change experience and function.	Process, growth, self-esteem, emphasis on verbal and nonverbal communication patterns.	Process, development of self identity. Fusion vs. autonomy. Differentiation of self. Triangles.	Process. Intrapsychic conflict between need to separate and need to belong.
Concepts	Longitudinal perspective, stage-specific individual and family developmental family life cycle with generation overlap. Children's growth mobilizes family's growth.	Subsystem, boundaries and autonomy. Roles. Disengagement vs. enmeshment. Current social context.	Double-bind. Functional vs. dysfunctional communication. Feedback, congruency, rules, tolerance of "differentness."	Nuclear family emotional system; family projection process. Emotional cutoff; multi-generation transmission process; sibling position; societal regression.	Transference phenomena; family myths; intergenerational collective emotional life; pseudohostility and pseudomutuality; "Rubber fence." Roles.
Method	Increase cognitive awareness, planning, and coping with developmental tasks. Anticipatory guidance. Crisis intervention.	Use restructuring operations. Do mapping assessment. Assign tasks, activities, alter spatial dimensions, alter coalition to strengthen subsystem and enhance roles.	Use exercises to increase feeling awareness. Relabel. Clarify transactions. Break up stereotypes. Increase tolerance for uniqueness of members. Increase congruency between feeling and communication.	Work with marital dyad; modify most important triangle; rework emotional cutoff; increase cognitive awareness to respond rather than react emotionally.	Delineate roles; decrease rigidity; decrease vagueness; use of transference phenomena; encourage expression of feelings associated with significant past and present events.

56

Practitioner activity	Not explicitly determined.	Very active, enters family system, comments, directs, supports, teaches.	Role model for communication. Active. Alleviates family anxiety.	Coach, teacher; remains emotionally detached from family system; becomes objective third point of triangle with marital dyad.	Less active; repository for family projections (transference).
Strengths	Dealing with grief/loss. Adding/losing family members. Anticipatory guidance, pediatric, obstetric, geriatric, community health and mental health nursing, medical-surgical nursing. All socioeconomic levels.	Assessment tool. Application to all clinical nursing specialties. Episodic and distributive care. All socioeconomic levels.	Application to all nursing specialties: clinical, administrative, education. All socioeconomic levels.	Assessment tool well-developed theory; clinical application with families of troubled children, adolescents; acute and chronic physical and emotional illness; anticipatory guidance; obstetric, pediatric nsg.	Increase practitioner awareness of subjective reactions; troubled families with adolescents, middle-upper socioeconomic level.
Limitations	Assessment tool not yet developed.	Requires supervised practice.	Need to overcome resistance to open communication.	May not be effective with lower socioeconomic levels; requires advanced education and supervised practice.	Requires advanced education and supervised practice.

Chapter 4

Variations in Ethnic Families

Ellen H. Janosik

During the last few decades the demands of minority groups for a share of economic and political power have dramatized to the public the meaning of ethnicity. In examining cultural influences on family life, it must be noted that ethnic membership need not be equated with minority status. The latter is usually considered a condition of economic neglect and political deprivation. Membership in a minority group implies lack of visibility and prestige, but ethnic membership is a positive term denoting shared interests and traditions. Ethnicity provides a frame of reference which gives families and individuals a sense of identity and continuity. At the same time ethnicity usually leaves room for the American dream of freedom and prosperity. Minority status, therefore, is regarded as a state of relative impotence and obscurity, while ethnic status is often seen as affirmative, particularly in recent years. The persistence of ethnicity as a cultural variable in American life was reported by Greeley (1974), who found correlations between attributes identified in various European family systems and in ethnic groups from those same systems in the United States three generations later. Since the American subjects were college students, the correlations survived changes in status as well as in geography.

Allegiance to an ethnic group results in certain structural and functional variations in family organization which are durable because they are valued. Aspects of family relatedness such as courting, mate selection, child rearing, and care of the elderly remain sensitive to ethnic influences despite the inroads of modern life. Family notions about propriety develop slowly over generations and do not readily disappear when transplanted to a new world. Indeed, many young people who abandoned the standards of their original family are surprised in later life to discover they carry within them the values they had challenged earlier.

Early in this century the ultimate disappearance of ethnic diversity was predicted, but more astute observers (Elkin, 1970; Queen and Habenstein, 1974) argued the contrary. In fact, forces urging assimilation continue to operate, but have lost much of their impetus. In contemporary life, apologetic acknowledgement of one's ethnic inheritance has been largely replaced by hopeful searching for family roots. This climate of ethnic assertiveness has imposed new demands on health practitioners. Since clients tend to be less defensive about their origins, care providers must extend their knowledge of cultural variables so they can consider families in the context of ethnicity. While ethnicity shapes family attitudes and behaviors, the practitioner who understands its significance can avoid offending, and utilize ethnic characteristics to restore or maintain family health.

Like all families, the ethnic family is involved in continuous transactions with the external environment. By means of boundaries families regulate input and output, differentiating between what is acceptable to the family and what is not. When family values differ markedly from those of the larger system, there is likelihood of conflict between the two systems. This may be reflected in conflict between family members which disrupts the family. Congruence between values of the ethnic family and the surrounding environment minimizes conflict. For ethnic families such congruence may be the exception rather than the rule. As a result, boundary maintenance may become problematic. Some family members may favor rigid boundaries which protect against unwelcome input, while other, less traditional, members may endorse permeable boundaries. Ethnic families which maintain defensive boundaries may succeed for a time in retaining the status quo, but deprive the family of input which is adaptive over time.

Families are not entirely dependent or independent of the systems around them. The preference of ethnic families to operate as closed systems must be moderated to maintain the integrity of the family. Ethnic families must adapt in order to satisfy members who wish to introduce new leadership styles and new role distribution. A traditional family member may require support in coping with input from the larger social system, which is perceived as threatening.

Human interactions have a complexity beyond the level of observable behavior, and this is especially true of encounters between persons of different backgrounds. Here the possibility of misinterpretation is unlimited. The destructive potential of ethnic misunderstanding can be explained by the theory of symbolic interaction (Mead, 1933). A fundamental assumption is that man lives in a symbolic as well as a physical environment, and that behavior reflects the meanings that we give to our own actions and to the actions of others. For ethnic Americans, as for all persons, interpretation depends on their perception of the immediate situation, which is affected by fears and expectations related to their cultural heritage. Through informed understanding of the diverse cultural factors present in the interaction, practitioners are better able to predict the needs and responses of clients, and to adjust interventions accordingly.

Theories of symbolic interaction have provided the term *generalized other,* meaning the composite representation of individuals and social groups whose values have been internalized by the individual. For ethnic Americans the generalized other is a mixture of traditional values that have never been renounced and new values that have been accepted. Older ethnic Americans may cling to a generalized other which rejects new values in favor of old ones. They then become embroiled in conflict with family members whose generalized other has discarded the old and embraced the new.

Ethnicity is an independent variable which affects the transplanted family in several ways. Variations in structure and function constitute

Figure 4-1   Position and role enactment.

		Position (ascribed role)	Enactment (achieved role)
Family structure (position)	**Coalition I**	**Mother** (instrumental leader)	Primary provider Manager Decision maker
		Oldest child	Surrogate manager and decision maker
Family Function Role enactment)	**Coalition II**	**Father** (expressive leader)	Secondary provider Nurturer Acceptor of decisions
		Younger children	Recipients of nurture Acceptors of decisions

dependent variables which are influenced by ethnicity and by the defensiveness and receptivity of family subsystems. Position indicates the location of the individual member in the family structure. Alternatively the term *ascribed role* may be used to indicate family position. *Achieved role* results from role enactment. This is the activist component of position, resulting from family norms and role expectations. *Norm* is used to describe a behavioral pattern shared by all or most of the family. In a hypothetical ethnic family, position (structure) and role enactment (function) may be diagrammed as shown in Figure 4-1. Ascribed roles are similar in all family structures. Achieved roles are the result of norms and role enactment, and are unique in every family system.

Many ethnic values are specific to certain groups, but a frequent result of the impact of a new environment on the ethnic family is conflict leading to disequilibrium of the family system. Role theory permits examination of structural and functional variations in ethnic families.

Three broad categories of ethnic families have been selected for discussion in this chapter. The categories show substantial differences and comprise sizable population segments in the United States. Every ethnic group has its own history to unfold, but for purposes of contrast the following distinctions have been made.

European Ethnic Families
The Irish-American family
The Italian-American family

Non-European Ethnic Families
The Puerto Rican family
The Mexican-American family

Ethnic Families of Color
The Afro-American family
The Asian-American family

EUROPEAN ETHNIC FAMILIES

The Irish-American Family

Structural Variations The Great Potato Famine, which lasted from 1847 to 1870, caused thousands of starving Irish peasants to immigrate to the United States. Most Irishmen who came to America before 1850 were craftsmen and farmers from Protestant North Ireland, which was closely linked to Great Britain. After 1850, the Irish immigrant was usually a farm worker from the Catholic South. Although the Irish economy was agricultural, the immigrants landed in American cities and remained there, transforming themselves from rural to urban dwellers.

Irish families living in the homeland had adopted a "stem" family structure. This structural organization resulted from the attempts of peasants to improve living conditions by stabilizing the size of their farms. The stem system meant that the family farm was managed by the parents until they became too old. At that point the farm was handed over undivided to a chosen son (or daughter) who was sometimes but not always the oldest. Unless the family was affluent, the heir was the only one able to marry and have a family. Elderly parents remained on the farm and became the responsibility of the heir. Often the brothers and sisters of the heir stayed on as workers, since their landlessness precluded marriage or separate homes. Regardless of their age, these unwed brothers and sisters were not considered full-fledged adults. Men well past middle age who worked but did not own the family farm continued to be referred to as "boys." While the stem family system was adaptive at the time, it was based on economic necessity, and sometimes became a cause of bitterness and dispute among family members (Greeley, 1974).

Another result of the stem family structure was that few Irish immigrated as intact families. Unchosen sons who were tired of their miserable existence on the family farm arrived singly or in pairs to work as stevedores, hod carriers, or bartenders. Unmarried Irish women without dowries or prospects came to find employment or husbands in America.

> Hours were long, pay was lower than for native born persons, work was wearing, and employers often unfriendly. The stability of the family was fragile when work was insecure. . . . Norms of rural family living and social forms such as drinking, argumentation, and visitation lost much of their meaning in the social context of high density urban living (Biddle, 1976, p. 98).

Irish immigrants whose religious affiliation was distrusted by the American Protestant majority drew strength from their church, which responded administratively by establishing parishes where a church building, convent, and parochial school were centrally located. These Irish Catholic neighborhoods resembled little villages in which people knew and trusted each other. Social norms were established by church and community. Even in these neighborhoods, however, there was some insistence on family privacy and reticence.

Hardships suffered in Ireland have made pragmatism an ingrained ethnic trait. Irish-American parents continue to hope that their children will marry a Catholic, preferably one with steady employment or some money laid aside. A man who is a good provider is respected by Irish women, many of whom work hard in their homes and hold outside jobs as well. Although the man is considered the household head, the Irish wife is energetic and influential in many ways. She is often the instrumental or task leader of the family, emotionally distant at times but prominent in the lives of husband

and children. Many writers of Irish origin, including James Joyce and Eugene O'Neill, have revealed in their works their ambivalence toward their mothers. Some Irish and Italian religious beliefs have been explained as reflections of national attitudes toward maternity. In Italy the Madonna is adored as a tender, loving mother figure, while in Ireland the Virgin Mother is venerated but seems more remote. Biddle (1976) wrote that the symbol of the Virgin Mother as conceptualized by the Irish was unlike that of the Italian religious vision. To the Irish, the Virgin Mother was a maternal deity with immense power in her own right, a personage to whom one could appeal directly in time of trouble. In the Italian mind, the Madonna functioned as a mediator whose power was derived from Father and Son. The implication is that in the Irish family the mother was a dominant individual who was subordinate to her husband only because she chose to be.

Greeley (1974) speculated that low self-esteem among the Irish may originate in the emotional climate of the family, contrasting the Jewish mother who controls by immersing her children in affection with the Irish mother who controls by alternately giving and witholding love. Greeley did not state that affection is lacking in the Irish family, but that it is not consistently expressed. Reluctance to show affection was explained by Wheeler (1971) as a fear of calling the devil's attention to the person being praised; this can be compared with the fear of the evil eye found in other ethnic groups.

In the immigrant Irish family, children were accepted as an inevitable outcome of marriage, and mothers generally showed partiality toward their sons. All children were disciplined firmly, but not always consistently. They were expected to know their place and to help when there was work to be done. Pride in children was felt but not shown, and greater decorum was asked of girls. The attitude of girls toward their brothers, and later toward their husband, was modeled after the mother's equivocal behavior toward the father.

Mattis (1974) found that the tendency of the Irish to delay marriage prevailed for a time in America. From 1855 until 1875, the average age for Irish bridegrooms in Buffalo, New York was 35 and for Irish brides 31. Among native Americans of the same era, the average age at marriage was 26 for males and 23 for females. A high proportion of Irish women chose spinsterhood over marriage. Delayed marriage and spinsterhood were explained in part as the pragmatic wish of the Irish to be economically secure before marrying.

The stem family structure with its inherent injustice made the Irish respect the extended family, but give priority to nuclear family obligations. In America the Irish family became nuclear in form, with aged parents sometimes included. Although they usually do not live under the same roof, adult siblings of Irish descent are emotionally close. After nuclear family obligations are met, help may be extended from one branch of the family to another. Help is sought only when it is really needed, and when it is given, there is an unspoken agreement that the helper expects the recipient to cancel the debt in some way at a future time. The nuclear family is expected to offer assistance first; later the extended family may be approached.

Functional Variations   There seems to be a paradox in the Irish character, which sometimes seems happy-go-lucky and sometimes moody and introverted. The Irish also combine rich and poetic language with understatement and biting wit. Greeley (1974) wrote that in many situations the Irishman uses indirect communication which provides "the flexibility that comes with ambiguity rather than the rigidity that comes with clarity" (p. 179). Direct statements and definitive answers tend to be avoided, perhaps to forestall commitment.

The Irish often expect the worst from life and do not seem over-whelmed when their expectations are realized. The defense mechanism of denial is sometimes used against hardship, for the Irish dislike giving fate the satisfaction of admitting difficulty. Irish wit is self-deprecating, and may be a form of denial of life's misfortunes. Denial in this context may be the functional equivalent of the Italian fondness for dramatization. Pessimism is so pervasive among the Irish that they often seem more at ease with sorrow than with joy. "Sing before breakfast, weep before supper" is a common admonition from an Irishman to a comrade guilty of rejoicing (Alfred, 1971).

Irish fondness for alcohol is reputed to have followed them to the United States. As early as 1840 an Irish priest wrote that "not only were our countrymen remarkable for their intemperate use of intoxicating liquors, but intemperance had already entered into and formed part of the national character" (Bales, 1946). A World War I survey of United States soldiers in treatment showed alcoholism among Irish Americans to be twenty times that of Jewish or Italian Americans. In World War II Irish Americans exceeded all other ethnic groups in numbers of draftees rejected for alcoholism (Chafetz and Demone, 1962). Bales attributed Irish alcoholism to three factors: (1) the belief that drinking was manly, (2) forbearance and tolerance of drunkenness, and (3) a consensus that the disquiet of women was met by religion and the disquiet of men by alcohol.

The working-class Irish-American family has deviated least from its immigrant past. Many of these families remain in their old neighborhoods where they have been joined by other blue collar ethnic groups. Looking for security, Irish Americans have entered government service as civil servants, policemen, or politicians. Most of them are proud of being Irish and are confused by, but loyal to their changing church. Middle-class Irish-American families show more diversity. Families of this class are less likely to send their children to Catholic schools and colleges, and are more integrated into American life. Changes instituted by the church seem more acceptable to them, and they may not follow restrictions against contraception, divorce, and even abortion. Sexual restraint among the unmarried has diminished, and the custom of delaying marriage has not continued in the face of economic opportunity.

The Irish-American family has found many of the values of American life congenial. Irish attention to economic security is compatible with the American value system. The hard-working Irish father, and the mother who works inside the home and outside as well, fit neatly into the American scene. Old-fashioned morality based on religion has been attenuated by American pluralism. Status and respectability remain important, even though children are allowed greater freedom in choosing mates and occupations. The ambivalence in Irish family relationships is still discernible. For example, the man is ostensibly treated as head of the household, but he is dependent on his wife in many areas. Boys are cherished by their mothers, but girls are brought up to be self-reliant, so that female capabilities are enhanced by the treatment given to girls. The Irish-American family is an ethnic group which is in some respects difficult to characterize, perhaps because of the contradictions and complexity of Irish family life.

CLINICAL EXAMPLE: TRIANGULATION AND TERRITORIALITY IN AN IRISH-AMERICAN FAMILY

Frank was a 44-year-old salesman whose commissions had dropped in recent years because of unreliability due to excessive drinking. He was an outgoing, energetic person who had been a top salesman. Only Frank's boss and family realized the extent of his drinking, which began at lunch and continued until he fell into a stuporous sleep at night. Frank's interest in his home was limited to the television screen and his next martini. His wife, Mary, and his two teenage sons had stopped trying to get any response from him and now ignored his existence as much as possible. After Frank had lost several sales because of missed appointments, his boss warned him he would be fired unless he obtained treatment. The medical work-up which Frank's boss insisted on showed moderate hypertension and liver damage. No one shielded Frank from the bad news. Because he was alarmed by the medical findings and because his boss was adamant, Frank entered a treatment program and stayed with it long enough to make a commitment. The program was effective to the extent that Frank remained sober for 5 months. He began to look, act, and feel like a new man.

On the job Frank felt happy and fulfilled, but at home the new Frank was hard for the family to accept. Frank's excessive drinking had been a problem for his family at first, but over the years they had adjusted to it. His wife and sons had rearranged their lives so that

Frank's involvement was not essential except as a wage earner. Sobriety made Frank want to have a more active role in family activities. His intrusion into family matters was hard for Mary, who had taken over the executive role in the family. She resented this strange, sober husband who wanted to become reacquainted with his family. Frank's sons, who had formed a collaborative relationship with their mother, found that their autonomy was reduced when Frank showed interest in their activities. New problems arose which had not been present when Frank was drinking every night. Mary tried to welcome Frank back but she felt that her freedom was being reduced. She had grown used to living without social or sexual interaction between herself and Frank. Her initial pleasure in his sobriety turned to anger at what she construed as interference. Realizing that this was unfair, she reacted by feeling guilty and depressed.

Tensions at home tempted Frank to resume drinking but he found the courage to talk to his counselor instead. The implications of the situation were seen by the alcoholism counselor who arranged for family sessions.

A goal of family treatment was to help the family adjust to Frank's sobriety as they had adjusted to his drinking. The life-threatening consequences for Frank if he continued to drink were re-emphasized. More importantly, the reluctance of Mary and the boys to accept Frank as a husband and father were pointed out. The adaptive strengths which had sustained the family when Frank was drinking now had to be mobilized on his behalf. The couselor explained that alcohol had been like another woman in the marriage of Frank and Mary. Alcohol had come between them, creating a precarious triangle out of the marital dyad. Mary and Frank had moved apart from each other. With alcohol removed, the couple could choose to draw closer or farther apart. Frank could again enter the family and begin to function differently only if Mary and the boys permitted it.

During the counseling sessions the family expressed fears of changing, but gradually realized that the system would be strengthened if Frank remained sober. The boys were beginning to think about leaving home in a few years, and saw that, with Frank active in the family, their separation from home and mother would be eased. Frank's new role enactment was understood as a stabilizing force in the family system, after reciprocal role adjustments were made. (Figure 4-2 shows triangulation in the family; Figure 4-3 shows the reorganized family structure.)

Assessment

Structure Triangulation of the marital dyad had resulted from the husband's abuse of alcohol. Mother and sons were excessively close, and had formed a coalition against the husband and father. The father was isolated and peripheral.

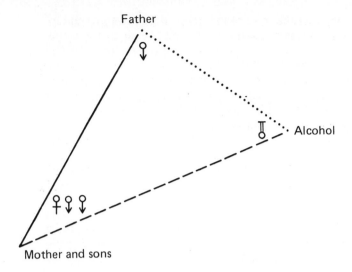

Key
····· Diffuse boundaries
— — Clear boundaries
——— Rigid boundaries

Figure 4-2　Irish-American family: triangulation.

Function　After alcoholism treatment the husband wished to reenter the family, and to interact with his wife and sons. Mother and sons reacted unfavorably to change. They were unwilling to alter their

Figure 4-3　Irish-American family: reorganization.

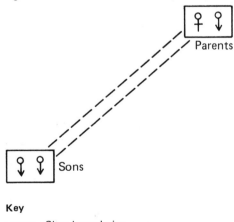

Key
— — Clear boundaries

☐　Subsystems

positions or ways of interacting in response to a positive change in one member. The family gave subtle messages that they preferred things as they had been.

Intervention

1 To encourage closeness between the husband and wife
2 To reassure the wife and children regarding their autonomy
3 To regulate the rate of change in the family
4 To persuade the family that the husband's sobriety would strengthen the family system
5 To establish new subsystems with primary alliance between the parents, secondary alliance between the siblings, tertiary alliance between parents and sons

The Italian-American Family

Structural Variations   The family system, extended and nuclear, has been called the only important institution in Italian society (Greeley, 1974). To the casual observer the Italian-American family, regardless of its local origin, has salient characteristics which are common to all Italians. In actuality Italian-Americans seldom consider themselves as simply Italian, but as subgroups, classified on the basis of regional derivation in the homeland.

For many centuries Italy was a divided land which was not unified until the 1860s. Even then, unification failed to produce substantial land reform. This failure disappointed the peasants and allowed continued exploitation by the landed gentry. Failure of land reform aggravated bitterness between the Italians in the northern part of the peninsula and their poorer brothers and sisters in the South. It also fostered immigration to the United States.

Earlier immigrants from Italy to the United States had come mostly from the north. After 1900 most Italian immigrants came from the impoverished south (Glazer & Moynihan, 1963). Immigration from Italy to the United States reached its height in the late nineteenth and early twentieth centuries. Southern Italian immigrants were people whose rough, humble ways embarrassed the Italians who had arrived earlier and were beginning to prosper. The peasant loyalties of immigrants from southern Italy caused them to find compatriots from their own or nearby villages, and to establish small enclaves of Italians from the same region. These enclaves reproduced the familiar customs which represented security. In pejorative terms such a neighborhood was called a "Little Italy," because it resisted assimilation. Within these Italian neighborhoods, as in the homeland, family reputations were the basis for judging individuals. Honor and dishonor were attributed to all persons sharing the same name.

Many Italians who came to the United States had suffered under exploitative landowners. They distrusted strangers and the world outside their villages. Blood relationships were of paramount importance, and it was only to the family that loyalty was owed. Almost as important as blood relatives were lifelong friends, and persons related to the family by marriage. The Italian nuclear family included godparents of the married pair and of their children (Greeley, 1974). Recognition was given to persons of higher status whose power was respected. Family loyalty extended outward in concentric circles, with greatest devotion given to blood relatives, then to in-laws and trusted associates, and finally to fellow villagers. The rest of the world was inhabited by strangers who were viewed with indifference or suspicion. The term *amoral familialism,* defined as absence of trust or concern for persons outside the family, has been applied to this pattern (Glazer & Moynihan, 1963).

The marriage arrangement gave the father the external trappings of authority. He was at the apex of the family structure, and the arbiter when important decisions were to be made. Nevertheless, the place of the Italian mother was not subordinate, for she was central to the household. Her adeptness at cooking, housekeeping, and child rearing was evaluated by the community. A family whose wife-mother performed her roles with skill was the envy of the village. The relative positions of husband and wife approached equality in subtle ways. Despite the apparent patriarchal structure of the family, the wife's contribution to household management was extensive. Gambino (1974) wrote: "Indeed the father was the formal chief executive of the family, but the actual power was shared by the mother in an intricate pattern of interactions" (p. 26).

There is marked territoriality in the Italian family. Male and female relationships are well defined, although this delineation has eroded as second- and third-generation Italian families have joined the American middle class. Gans (1962) observed what he called a "segregated conjugal pattern" in Italian-American families where women turned to female relatives for advice and support while men turned to relatives of their own sex. Such territoriality does not impair the high value placed on every family member regardless of age and sex. Cross-sex relationships are approached guardedly. Transactions between men and women are characterized as honorable or dishonorable, and casual, platonic friendships between men and women of the same age are exceptional.

Ascribed status, particularly of aging parents, is permanent even when role enactment is curtailed. A man remains head of the household after age or infirmity prevents his carrying out the accustomed duties of his role. There are strong mother-son bonds, but the father is respected and even feared. In most Italian-American families the parents exert control over adolescents. Order is maintained in the home neighborhood even if it is sometimes disturbed away from home (Suttles, 1968).

The structure of the Italian family is stable in several respects. The 1973 census showed that 87 percent of Italian-American families were headed by a husband-wife couple, only 10 percent by a woman. This last figure was the smallest of any comparable ethnic group. The Italian-American divorce rate is low, barely exceeding that of Irish Catholics who were the lowest-ranking group. Two trends have developed in recent years. First, although inter-marriage is less frequent among Italians than among many other ethnic groups, a rising educational level has been accompanied by decreased en-dogamy. Second, acculturation has produced rapid decline in the size of Italian-American families. Second-generation daughters of immigrant Italian women produce less than half the number of children born to their mothers, and even fewer children than native-born American women of non-Italian decent (Rosenwaike, 1973).

Functional Variations Italian immigrants flocked to cities in the northeastern part of the United States and competed for jobs with the Irish, who had arrived some decades earlier. In spite of their shared religion the two groups were not especially compatible. Aspects of the life-style and religious practices of the Italians were offensive to Irish Catholics, many of whom had advanced to prominent ecclesiastical positions (Feminella and Quadagno, 1976). Work was respected in the Italian immigrant family, and labor was considered to have an inherent dignity. Since many of the Italian immigrants were barely literate, they accepted the hard manual jobs which the Irish were beginning to relinquish. No job, however menial, was debas-ing for an Italian man struggling to feed a wife and family, or to amass the cost of steerage tickets to bring them to the United States.

Devotion to family is so entrenched among Italians that it has caused conflicts between family loyalty and personal ambition. Among Italian Americans, worldly success that does not separate the individual from the family is more welcome than success which takes the individual away from the family (Glazer & Moynihan, 1963). The same source noted that Jewish parents exult in the success of their children, but Italian parents rejoice only if they are included in it.

Among Italians, there is belief in a "natural" man and a "natural" woman. Males are expected to be sexually aggressive and to prefer pleasure over duty. Females are expected to cherish their children and to value hus-bands and marriage. There is also a sense of adhering to a "natural" law which opposes change. Since there is thought to be a limited amount of morality and material resources in the world, respecting "natural" laws protects the family and the individual (Suttles, 1968).

Italian fondness for histrionics has been noted by many social commentators. This tendency toward dramatization has been explained as a coping measure which serves the same purpose as stoic self-control for more inhibited groups. Barzini (1964) explained that for Italians dramatization was a compensatory device which helped them handle the vicissitudes of life. Through dramatization the Italian softens the harsh outline of reality and reduces feelings of powerlessness. Exaggeration of life's joys and sorrows enables the Italian to "get on in the world and obtain what he wants, solves many problems, lubricates the wheels of society, protects him from the envy of his neighbors and the arrogance of the mighty" (p. 104). Another explanation is that the expressiveness of Italians may be culturally determined behavior which discharges anxiety by releasing strong feelings that can be shared with others. It is possible that dramatization of events reduces their impact by desensitization through repetition.

Spontaneous expression of feelings is encouraged by the Italian family. Grief and joy are vicariously experienced by the entire group. The same is true of illness and pain, which are not solitary experiences, but the concern of all. A sympathetic account of the expansive Italian way of life has been offered by Novak (1972).

> The Italian has no worries about disease or being ill—these are future things. The only thing that worries him is the present pain which prevents enjoyment. . . . He couldn't care less about analysis, diagnosis, mechanics. The Italian hates "the knife" and "the needle." He likes personal things. His parents took such constant personal interest in him that he sees the world in almost wholly personal terms (p. 44).

Levels of tension within the Italian-American family may rise and fall, but the involvement of family members with one another is constant. Disengagement is rarely complete, if it occurs at all. At the same time the highly personalized life of Italian-American families reinforces suspicion of the unknown. The vitality of this ethnic group is sustained by emotional expressiveness, gregarious family life, and a long tradition of continuity.

Two aspects of the traditional Italian family structure are shown in Figures 4-4 and 4-5.

CLINICAL EXAMPLE: PREVENTION OF SCHOOL PHOBIA IN AN ASTHMATIC CHILD OF ITALIAN-AMERICAN DESCENT

Gina, the youngest child in an Italian-American family, was an asthmatic child whose symptoms increased when it became time for her to start first grade. Her older brother and sister were students in the same neighborhood school and were academically promising. Their father was the hardworking owner of a small shop. He was very

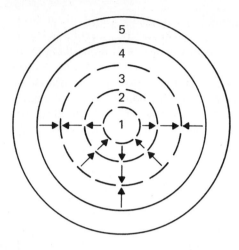

Key

1: Immediate family (including godparents)
2: Extended family related by blood
3: Extended family related by marriage
4: Trusted friends, associates, neighbors
5: Strangers and outsiders

Figure 4-4 Traditional Italian family showing its concentric interpersonal relationships.

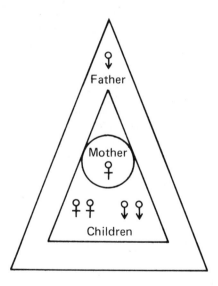

Figure 4-5 Traditional Italian family: pseudopatriarchical structure.

concerned for the welfare of his children but left most of the responsibility to his wife. Gina's mother did not work outside the home, devoting most of her time to home, husband, and children.

Confident that Gina was receiving adequate medical care, her teacher became concerned by the child's irregular attendance, and suggested that the school counselor make a home visit to try to correct this problem. Since the older siblings had expressed their fears to teachers about Gina, the counselor's second objective was to establish a positive relationship with Gina and her mother so as to alleviate their worries.

On the first visit Gina's mother was uncommunicative and guarded. She seemed defensive and reluctant to share information. Although the counselor felt like an intruder, she asked if she might return once or twice more so that Gina might get to know her better. On subsequent visits the counselor became aware of the closeness between mother and child, and of the mother's unconscious reluctance to part with her youngest child. Knowing that the family was closely knit, the counselor spoke of the good adjustment the older children had made at school. She also told Gina's mother about health services available at the school, and arranged for the mother to visit the health suite and meet the school nurse. The mother's concern for Gina was partly realistic, but her fears were aggravated by separation anxiety. Through communication with the counselor and the school nurse, Gina's mother learned that school personnel were attentive and caring. School personnel conveyed an indirect message that no one would take the mother's place with Gina, but that friendly, competent people were available to Gina if she became ill at school. Specific arrangements were made to deal with an asthmatic attack if it occurred. Gina's mother had been escorting her daughter to and from school; it was suggested that the three children walk to school together, without their mother. This arrangement enhanced the self-esteem of all three children. It strengthened the sibling subsystem by removing Gina from her closeness to her mother, and placed her nearer to the other siblings. In terminating her visits, the counselor promised to be available as a liaison between home and school. By this time school personnel were trusted by the mother, who was unaware that prompt intervention had averted a potential school phobia. Success was achieved because the counselor recognized separation anxiety in the mother, which was transmitted to Gina. These unconscious dynamics were not interpreted but were handled cognitively. The resistance of the mother was identified by the counselor and treated realistically.

Assessment

Structure Separation from her youngest child represented a loss for the mother. Her anxiety was transmitted to the child. As a result the child became reluctant to attend school. The asthmatic attacks enabled mother and child to avoid anxiety around separation.

Function Because she feared the loss of a valued role, Gina's mother assigned to her child the sick role. Mother and child used the asthmatic attacks to avoid separation anxiety. The frequent asthmatic attacks alarmed the mother and gave rise to realistic fears that Gina could not handle the school program.

Intervention

1 To ease the transition for mother and child by establishing a bridge between home and school
2 To utilize the excellent school adjustment of the older siblings as a model for Gina
3 To mitigate the closeness of the mother and Gina by strengthening the sibling subsystem
4 To indicate to the mother that control over Gina's regimen would remain with her, but that the school could provide adequate attention if Gina became ill at school
5 To help the mother see Gina's entry to school as an inevitable developmental progression
6 To stress the positive aspects of school life and the joy of daily reunion of mother and child

NON-EUROPEAN ETHNIC FAMILIES

The Puerto Rican Family

Structural Variations   Ethnic families who have arrived recently in the United States are susceptible to the disruptive effects of cultural dissonance. Sources of tension in Puerto Rican families can be traced to value discrepancies around positions (ascribed roles) and enactment (achieved roles). Role distribution, like role enactment, occurs in response to established norms. When family expectations are consensual, decision making is efficient and comfortable. But family consensus is an early casualty of ethnic migration or immigration, since it is altered by the new environment.

The Puerto Rican family can trace its lineage to three ancestral influences. The original natives were an Indian tribe of which little is known. Next came the Spanish heritage, from seafaring companions of Columbus who discovered the island in 1493. A third racial strain was introduced in 1511 when African slaves were imported. The island was under Spanish rule until 1898 when it was ceded to the United States, which granted citizenship to the islanders in 1917. Since Puerto Rico is a commonwealth, its people are migrants, not immigrants, and they have free access to the United States and to their own island.

Of the 1.5 million Puerto Ricans in the United States, about 60 percent live in New York State, mainly in New York City. Substantial numbers live in Connecticut, Ohio, Massachusetts, and Pennsylvania, locations that make travel to the island fairly easy. Living conditions for the average Puerto Rican family in the United States are far from utopian. Puerto Ricans rank lowest in income of all population groups in New York City. Many are on welfare and, because of poverty and racial mixture, they encounter considerable prejudice (Fitzpatrick, 1976).

An interesting result of the Spanish inheritance is the importance of lineage, which is evident in Puerto Rican customs related to surnames.

Puerto Ricans use a given name first, the father's surname second, and the family name of the mother in third place.

Many Puerto Ricans follow the Roman Catholic faith, but Protestant missions on the island have converted large numbers. Marriages are usually sanctified by religious ritual, but many unions are consensually made. As interpreted by Roman law, which prevails on the island, these consensual unions are not legally binding. Offspring of consensual unions are not legitimate, but they are rarely stigmatized. The descriptive term usually applied to children of consensual unions is "natural" children.

Nepotism strengthens the extended family system, even though kinfolk may live under separate roofs or be separated by migration. Frequent journeys between the mainland and the island prevent erosion of the extended family, although its strength has been attenuated by the rise of a prosperous and self-sufficient middle class. Even so, extended family structure persists, and the prevalence of consensual unions has created families in which children labeled "his," "hers," and "ours" live in the same household.

Family structure is patriarchal but an absentee father is not uncommon. Eighteen percent of the families on the island and twenty-eight percent of the families on the mainland are headed by a female. Intimate relationships within an extended kinship group provide a sense of pride and security. The inclusiveness and importance of the Puerto Rican family has been termed *familism,* and it is this value which causes the Puerto Rican to place family before community and self (Fitzpatrick, 1976).

Within the Puerto Rican family there is order based upon rank. The man of the household has extensive authority over his wife and children, even though Puerto Rican women may engage in role redefinition after coming to the mainland. Affection between parents and children is warm. Although the men are inclined toward authoritarianism, Puerto Rican women have been described as more assertive, outspoken, and even violent than their counterparts in Mexican-American families. However, there is probably a limit to female assertiveness based on the tolerance of the Puerto Rican husband.

Along with familism is found another value known as respect or *respeto.* This value implies that the Puerto Rican places emphasis on personal attributes such as dignity and self-esteem. The need for respect and dignity occasionally causes the Puerto Rican to behave in ways which are puzzling. Respeto can be defined as a high regard for hierarchical order and for self-worth. It is a reciprocal value which expects that one comport oneself appropriately and that one be treated by others with due respect. Because the family is an extension of the self, family obligations are essential to the maintenance of selfhood. The *machismo* associated with being male is partly linked with respeto. Machismo for the Puerto Rican man means authority within the family, along with influence and power over women; it takes the form of vigorous romanticism and possessiveness in relations with wife or sweetheart, or is expressed in premarital and extramarital relationships (Fitzpatrick, 1976).

Functional Variations Although the Puerto Rican husband has decision-making power, the wife has influence in the home, particularly as she advances in years. The exceptionally strong bonds which exist between the Puerto Rican mother and her sons cause a man to expect his wife to relate to him in a maternal as well as a conjugal fashion. Regarding the relative power of husband and wife in a family, Winch (1971) offered these formulations: (1) the larger the number of children and the younger the children, the greater the power of the husband in the family, and (2) the greater the economic contribution of the husband compared to that of the wife, the greater the power of the husband.

Contact with people of different cultures inevitably has repercussions inside and outside family boundaries. The Puerto Rican family arriving on the mainland experiences immediate culture shock. Most migrating families leave behind rural island homes which provided social supports even when living conditions were poor. Urban life is difficult and complicated for the Puerto Rican family, which suffers chronic economic insecurity and discrimination based on language and color. Dealing with a bureaucracy composed of impersonal social agencies is frightening to persons accustomed to personal transactions. As with many newly arrived families, Puerto Rican women find jobs more easily than the men. Economic independence and the pull of the major culture reduces the dependence of Puerto Rican women. Established role performance is soon questioned and role dissonance follows, with husbands resisting change and wives welcoming it.

As Puerto Rican children acquire the values of the prevailing culture, they challenge and often reject the authority of the parents. Young girls whose reputations were carefully guarded on the island begin to defy parental restraint. The phrase "cloister rebellion" has been used to describe this behavior of Puerto Rican girls (Stycos, 1955). Weakened loyalty to old values and a wish to display machismo by appearing tough and aggressive have contributed to adjustment problems among young Puerto Rican males.

A traditional custom which has not been relinquished is belief in spiritism, which is intermingled with the organized religions of Puerto Ricans. *Spiritism* is a mystical awareness that there is a world of powerful, invisible spirits, good and evil, with whom it is possible to communicate. Garrison (1977) wrote that spiritism did not compete with organized religions but represented a healing cult within the Catholic faith. Pain which is not alleviated by visiting a physician may be treated by a spiritist whose methods constitute a mental health resource for the Puerto Rican community. The effectiveness of spiritism in relieving symptoms and behaviors is considered comparable to the success rate of psychotherapy for the same population.

Many Puerto Ricans subscribe to the *hot-cold* etiology of illness and health. The hot-cold dichotomy was part of Spanish and Portuguese medicine over 300 years ago, and is still upheld. All ailments and physical conditions are considered to be either hot or cold, while foods and medicines may be either hot, cold, or cool. It follows from this that "cold" diseases must be counteracted with "hot" substances and vice versa. Thermal temperatures play a part in the classification, but not consistently. For example, a respiratory ailment is a cold ailment whether or not fever ensues. Therefore, it may not be treated with fruit juices, which are also cold. "Cool" foods are forbidden during menstruation and after childbirth. Since cool foods include fruits and vegetables which are rich in minerals and vitamins, this presents difficulties for a health practitioner attempting to teach principles of nutrition. During pregnancy a Puerto Rican woman is likely to avoid hot substances such as vitamin or iron supplements lest her child be born with a rash or red skin. The innovative practitioner who understands these requirements should be able to prescribe needed substances in forms which mask or neutralize hot-cold incompatibilities (Harwood, 1971).

Belief in spiritism and in folk medicine predisposes to distrust in Western medical science. The first recourse of a Puerto Rican who is physically or emotionally disturbed may be a native healer known as a *curandero* or *curandera*. Severe illness may induce the sufferer to consult a native healer in addition to a physician or other health professional, much as a member of another ethnic group might solicit a second opinion. The health professional working with Puerto Rican families must acknowledge these beliefs, and take account of them in the therapeutic regimen if compliance is to be achieved.

As noted earlier, a casualty of the migration of the Puerto Rican family to the mainland is consensus, which is threatened by the new environment. Role dissonance causes daily confrontation between husband and wife or between parents and children. The reactions of parents may be to isolate themselves from the new community in order to resist input which is frightening. Polarization occurs in the family when youngsters respond positively to external influences and parents do not. Ideally, adaptation takes the form of resolving marital and generational differences and reaching a compromise between the old and the new, but the process may be painful and prolonged.

During critical periods of confrontation, family tensions rise until a compromise or a breaking point is reached. At times, a compromise can be

negotiated, and revised behaviors are accepted by the whole system. The
health practitioner serving the family must assess which forces are operating
to maintain the status quo and which are restlessly seeking change. Beginning by appraising the strength of the impetus toward change, the practitioner then notes the locus of resistance to change, and introduces the family to processes of negotiation and accommodation. After assessing the
family, the practitioner may endeavor to restore family equilibrium by attending to the divergent but legitimate demands of everyone in the family.
Although essential to planning and intervention, assessment is not an activity which is accomplished once and for all. Assessment is the precurser of
planning and implementation, but it also accompanies these later steps.

Disequilibrium resulting from rising tension may be used to demonstrate to the family that coercion is not effective in producing change or in
maintaining the status quo. The practitioner can implement health
measures, physical and psychological, by assuring every family member
that he or she is being taken seriously and will be heard. Working to regain
family consensus is imperative whether the issue is birth control for the wife
or improved nutrition for the entire family. The process which the practitioner teaches by example is that of mediation and compromise, restoring
equilibrium of the system while allowing family members adequate time to
adapt to the input from larger systems that impinge on family boundaries.

The traditional Puerto Rican family is shown in Figure 4-6.

Figure 4-6   Traditional Puerto Rican family.

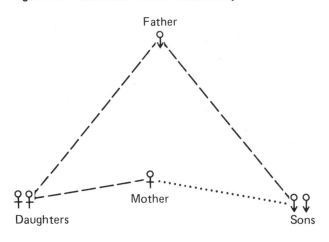

Key

— — Clear boundaries

• • • • • • Diffuse boundaries

CLINICAL EXAMPLE: MALFUNCTION IN A
MULTIPROBLEM PUERTO RICAN FAMILY

A Puerto Rican family who had been in the United States 1 year was living on welfare in a crowded urban apartment. The mother was pregnant with her sixth child but had not yet seen a physician. The father was ashamed of being jobless and resented the visits of a community nurse sent by the Health Department. His wife was homesick and frightened. Rosita, the oldest child, was burdened with housework and the care of the younger children. She was kept home from school to help because her mother felt ill and her father was inept, and reluctant to do "women's work." The three youngest children were not toilet-trained and were plagued with colds and earaches. This multiproblem family was anxious and defensive; the first objective of the community nurse was to win their trust. Since her first interventions were ignored, the nurse decided to set priorities and focus on the immediate problem.

Prenatal care for the mother seemed the most urgent need and this was an area where the mother was willing to accept help. A Puerto Rican homemaker employed by the Health Department was asked by the nurse to accompany the mother on her first visits to prenatal clinic. The homemaker also came several times a week to help with housework so Rosita could attend school. She was a middle-aged woman with grown children and the pregnant mother related well to her. In all interactions with the family the community nurse was friendly but unobtrusive and uncritical. She shared some of her unspoken observations with the homemaker in their weekly conferences. Both the nurse and the homemaker were deferential to the unemployed father, since his joblessness made him more sensitive to his position as head of the household.

At the suggestion of the nurse, the homemaker began to discuss toilet training for the youngest children. The two Puerto Rican women laughed at American insistence on early toilet training, but agreed it was bad to have so many children in diapers at one time. Eventually the mother asked the nurse for suggestions regarding toilet training. As a result the nurse was able to become more directly involved with the family. Within a few weeks her relationship with the family permitted her to make improvements in their nutrition. The nurse obtained vitamins for the children, explaining that their frequent colds were *fresca* conditions for which *caliente* substances like vitamins were helpful. She suggested that the mother's prescribed vitamins could be taken with "cold" substances like fruit juices, if this made the vitamins more acceptable.

Since the family resented the nurse's visits, she proceeded very slowly. She was able to win their trust by focusing on the most pressing need and the one for which the family was willing to accept her aid. The nurse began by offering concrete assistance, and the homemaker was carefully chosen and guided. In order to achieve long-term goals, the nurse deferred preventive measures until the suspiciousness of the family was dispelled.

Assessment

Structure   The position of the father as authority and provider was threatened by his inability to find work. Although he was worried about his family and his ability to support them, he was unwilling or unable to assume many of the household tasks that his wife was accustomed to handling. Overwhelmed by her pregnancy and family responsibilities, the mother delegated her functions to Rosita, who then became a parent-child.

Generational boundaries which were once clear in the family had become blurred. Neither mother nor father was functioning competently. Distance between husband and wife grew (see Figure 4-7).

Function   The family was apathetic and listless. Insufficient energy was being generated to perform necessary tasks. Family functioning and family interaction were at minimal levels. Each parent had needs that were not being met. Rosita was being asked to function in an inappropriate manner which exceeded her capacity.

Figure 4-7   Multiproblem Puerto Rican family.

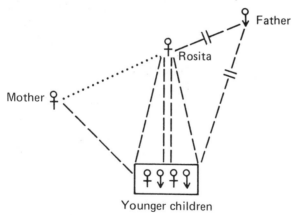

Younger children

Key

······ Diffuse boundaries

—||— Conflict

— — Clear boundaries

☐ Sibling subsystem

Intervention

1 To rank in order of priority the needs of the family
   a prenatal care for the mother
   b relief for the parent and child
   c personalization of professional services to increase family acceptance of help
2 To introduce long-range measures aimed at primary prevention after immediate needs were met
   a neonatal and post partum care
   b birth control methods acceptable to husband and wife
   c immunizations and continuous health care for all family members
   d improvement of family nutrition

The Mexican-American Family

Structural Variations Mexican Americans constitute the second largest ethnic group in the United States. A sizable number are illegal aliens who came in search of work. The total number of Mexican Americans legally or illegally in the United States is estimated to be between 10 and 12 million, most of whom congregate in the great Southwest near the Mexican border; states where large numbers of Mexican Americans live include Texas, Arizona, New Mexico, Colorado, and California.

The history of Mexico has been marked by violence and factionalism. Like Puerto Rico, Mexico was colonized and exploited by Spanish explorers who arrived in the sixteenth century and overcame the indigenous Indians. Spanish and Indian influences survive in the religion, diet, and folkways of Mexico. In 1821 Mexico obtained independence from Spain, and for some time afterwards encouraged European immigration. After 1821, Anglos, or non-Mexicans, entered the part of Mexico now known as Texas, in large numbers. By 1834 Mexicans were outnumbered by Anglos 6 to 1, and were a minority in their own country. Texas was annexed by the United States less than 10 years later, which led to the Mexican War. This war, which lasted two years, intensified bitterness between Anglos and Mexicans, and established an image of Mexican Americans as an inferior, troublesome minority group.

Immigration of Mexicans into the United States has continued since the turn of the century. The Rio Grande separating Mexico from Texas is traversed by thousands of impoverished Mexicans who risk discovery and deportation in order to work on the farms of the United States. Early efforts of Mexican workers to secure fair treatment from American employers were harshly quelled. Until World War II opportunities for Mexicans were limited, but wartime needs of industry and the armed services opened doors for Mexican workers. As confidence in their own ability grew, younger

Mexicans became less tolerant of injustice. The restless political climate of the sixties encouraged Chicano activists who demanded their rights. The submissiveness and fatalism of Mexicans were not eradicated, but a new attitude of self-help appeared among some of them.

There are commonalities between Mexican-American families and Puerto Rican families which can be attributed to their shared Spanish heritage. *Familism,* which has been described in the context of the Puerto Rican family, is characteristic of the Mexican-American family as well. The dominance of males and a hierarchical structure based on age and sex are other similarities. Reliance on support from an extended family structure enables Mexican Americans to engage in cooperative ventures. Several families may combine resources to cultivate land or help their men negotiate a border crossing. Combining resources allows elderly relatives to be cared for by many relatives rather than by one or two, and facilitates child rearing.

Mexican-American families are generally larger than Anglo families. Thirteen percent of Mexican-American families compared to four percent of American families have five or more children. Only 23 percent of Mexican-American families are without children under 18 years of age, compared to 45 percent for all American families (U.S. Census Bureau cited in Alvirez and Bean, 1976).

For the Mexican-American man, as for the Puerto Rican, machismo is a complicated value fraught with contradiction. Machismo may be expressed by sexuality and by infidelity; it may also be expressed in honor, courage, and devotion to the family. One aspect of machismo does not necessarily negate the other. The maternity of the Mexican-American woman complements the machismo of her husband. It also defines and affirms her own sense of self. In keeping with role complementarity, the girls in the family are given less freedom and more responsibility than their brothers. All children are taught discipline and respect for elders. Tasks necessary to the smooth operation of the household are assigned to children according to age and sex. With father in charge, the parental dyad forms the administrative component of the family, with the children as valued contributors. Clear boundaries and distance between parents and children make sibling subsystems important, with harmony maintained through subordination of female to male, and younger to older.

Functional Variations   After marriage it is not usual for Mexican-American women to enter the labor force on a permanent basis. Mexican-American males are as likely as Anglos to be in the labor market but this is less true of their wives. Alvirez and Bean (1976) attributed this to the following factors: (1) large numbers of small children in the family, (2) cultural preferences that women be homebound, and (3) educational disadvantages which severely limit employment opportunities for Mexican-American women.

The mutual suspicion that impeded relations between Anglos and Mexican-Americans in the Southwest created the *barrio,* which is the equivalent of the Afro-American urban ghetto. Life in the barrio offers the security of a familiar ethos for the Mexican American, but reiterates old values and opposes change. Spanish is the primary language spoken in the barrio, which means that Mexican-American children become bilingual while their parents must use the children as interpreters. As a consequence parents suffer the indignity of role reversal, and loss of parental authority. The barrio upholds traditional values, but prosperity causes aspiring families to leave the barrio for mixed neighborhoods with better housing. An upwardly oriented Mexican-American family leaving the barrio must resolve conflicts between stability and progress.

Children of Mexican Americans are discouraged from being assertive. They are taught to be unobtrusive and impassive, and to keep their thoughts to themselves. Resignation is transmitted from parents to children in significant ways. The message of submission to the dominant culture is, for Mexican-American parents, not unlike the explanation of sex given white middle-class children—an important and usually unforgettable moment (Coles, 1977). It goes without saying that the message is not equally accepted by all Mexican-American children, and that some do risk assertiveness and opposition to Anglo domination.

The Chicano movement which began in the sixties has been critical of stoicism, submission, and acceptance of poverty, which are behaviors permeating Mexican-American culture. Political activism and economic opportunity may gradually change the Mexican-American family, but the practitioner concerned with the health of this traditional group must work within the constraints of an established hierarchical system.

Stoicism in the Mexican-American family has contributed to a disregard of preventive health measures. If Mexican Americans are not in pain and can work, they believe themselves to be in good health. If they suffer ill health or misfortune in this world, they believe this will be corrected in the next. God tests man's courage and strength in adversity. One may as well submit to illness, since disease results from a sinful act or from unknown causes from which there is no escape. *Mal ojo,* or the evil eye, may fall upon an individual who has been guilty of arrogance or pride. A child who has been openly admired is susceptible to the withering effects of *mal ojo,* and the visitor who praises a child is a cause of uneasiness.

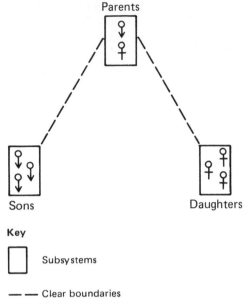

Parents

Sons

Daughters

Key

Subsystems

— — Clear boundaries

Figure 4-8 Traditional Mexican-American family.

Minor illnesses are ignored as much as possible. When the father is convinced of the seriousness of an ailment, or when a person is too sick to leave his or her bed, there is reluctance to seek outside help or to enter a hospital. Instead the family gathers round the patient, visiting constantly and trying one home remedy after another. Family members usually reject any precautions required by communicable illness, since it is thought that relatives and familiar household objects cannot transmit disease. Various medals and amulets are believed to have curative powers. An illness which can be treated within the family is not greatly feared, but a condition which requires separation from the family or the intervention of a health professional is ominous. In some Mexican-American families death may be less feared than the ministrations of a stranger (Murray & Zentner, 1975).

Figure 4-8 shows a traditional Mexican-American family.

CLINICAL EXAMPLE: COGNITIVE DISSONANCE
IN A MEXICAN-AMERICAN FAMILY

Maria, the 9-year-old daughter of a Mexican-American family living in Arizona, was discovered by the school health team to be suffering from a moderately severe case of scoliosis. A brief note to this effect was sent to Maria's mother, asking her to visit the school to talk over the problem with the school nurse practitioner and physician.

Although the note had been reassuring and friendly, there was no reply except that Maria and her brothers and sisters stopped coming to school. Their teachers and the nurse were perplexed by the absences, for the children had been happy at school, were well cared for, and attended regularly. None of Maria's little friends could explain the absences. After 2 weeks elapsed, the nurse decided to go to the barrio where Maria lived with her family. When the nurse asked Maria's best friend to show her the route, the child became upset, saying she couldn't because her mother didn't want her to go near Maria any more. Other barrio children were equally unhelpful. As an outsider, the nurse knew she was not quite trusted even by the children who loved her, so she decided to ask the Catholic priest in the barrio for help. Together the nurse and the priest visited Maria's house where they learned that it was the note which had produced the crisis. The note from the nurse had been written in English, which Maria's parents could not read. It had been translated by a neighbor woman who had interpreted the word "scoliosis" as "tuberculosis," a disease greatly feared by people in the barrio. Word that Maria had tuberculosis circulated, and from then on the family was virtually cast out of the community, except for relatives who continued to visit. Maria's parents knew only too well that other persons with tuberculosis had been taken to hospitals. Terrified by the prospect, they chose to keep their children at home where there was less danger that interfering school officials would take Maria away.

After a careful explanation of Maria's back problem, relatives and neighbors were invited in to hear the goods news from the priest, whose word was inviolate. In the scenes of relief which followed, plans for treating Maria were approved by her father, who regarded the whole misunderstanding as resulting from the folly of leaving important matters to women. In the father's opinion, Anglo women were apparently no wiser than Mexican women, but with his help and the priest's, Maria would be well. She was not really sick, anyhow. And God never sent more trouble than a family could bear.

Assessment

Structure The parental dyad distorted and rejected well-meaning input from the larger system. Afraid to ask for clarification, the parents confined their children within the home. The family closed ranks against the school and the community, keeping their problem within the system, and avoiding input which might have corrected distortion. Family boundaries became impermeable in order to protect against outside interference.

Function Parents did not seek help or clarification from outside sources. Cognitive dissonance due to misinterpretation of the letter caused them to exclude further input. They cut themselves off from the opportunity to correct cognitive distortion.

Intervention

    1 To ascertain the reason for the children's prolonged absence after a note was sent to the parents
    2 To enlist the help of a trusted advisor such as the priest who could interpret for the family and for the health professional
    3 To deal with fear, anger, distortion in the family and the community
    4 To clarify, reassure, and help plan treatment for Maria which her family would accept and understand

ETHNIC FAMILIES OF COLOR

The Afro-American Family

    Structural Variations The Afro-American family is the most conspicuous ethnic group in the United States, not only because of color but also because it is widely regarded as a system characterized by instability and malfunction. What is less accepted is that the black family is an adaptive system that has managed to endure in the harshest circumstances. Its adaptive ability sometimes causes the black family to be misunderstood, and to operate in ways which society finds irksome, but the black family has demonstrated a survival power which has enabled its members to wrest gratification from unpromising surroundings.

    Most ethnic families arrived in this country as immigrants or refugees, coming of their own volition even if alternatives were few. Black Americans came unwillingly, in chains, forcibly torn from their families. During years of enslavement their recollections of individual and tribal identity were discouraged by slaveowners, who hoped to erase treasured memories of native villages and kinship groups.

    The attitudes of white owners toward marital arrangements between slaves were insensitive and inconsistent. Breeding activities, especially between slaves on the same plantation, were encouraged since slave children were valuable commodities, but marriage was not permitted. A semblance of family life was allowed because domesticity was thought to make blacks more docile. Some slaves were permitted to share a cottage with a mate and children, but changes in the life of the owner often caused quasi-marital relationships to be disrupted and families disbanded.

    There are few indications that enslaved blacks took family commitments lightly. On the contrary, marriage and family were highly regarded by people whose lives lacked other personal meaning. Forbidden to enter legal contracts, slaves devised for themselves the marriage ceremony known as "jumping over the broom." This simple ritual, ludicrous to outsiders, was fraught with significance for blacks, and the choice of the broom as a symbol may have been due to its availability to the most humble. Regardless of the meaning of family life to blacks, it was the white owner who sanctioned slave marriages, controlled access to females, terminated relationships, and separated families.

After Emancipation, blacks strove to maintain intact families despite adverse conditions. One study of family records after 1860 showed the prevailing black family structure to be nuclear and headed by an adult male (Gutman, 1976). In the agrarian South this pattern continued, but migration to urban centers contributed to the fragmentation of family life. The economic difficulties that plagued the black family were aggravated by racial bias, which prevented the black man from competing equally in the job market. Domestic work, which was plentiful, and was unattractive to whites, was an avenue of employment for black women. Underpaid and exploited, they were still able to contribute to the support of the family. In addition, black women who were admitted to white households as cooks and nurses became trusted employees, and used these relationships to facilitate life for their families. A consequence of this was the creation of a family managerial role for black women. The competence of the woman has caused the black family to be labeled matriarchical. This has been refuted by Hill (1972) who distinguished between strong female role enactment and dominant female role enactment, stating that

> husbands in black families are actively involved in decision making and the household tasks expected of them. And most wives, while strong, are not dominant matriarchs but share with their husbands the making of family decisions— even in low income black families (p. 20).

Hill added that in 85 percent of low income black families the husband's income exceeded the wife's.

Staples (1976) wrote that the 1972 census showed that 30 percent of black households were headed by a woman, as opposed to 14 percent of white households. For black families this represented an increase of 38 percent in one decade. The trend continues, and more recent reports show that 36 percent of black households were headed by women compared to 11 percent of white households. The proportion of out-of-wedlock births was high, but fell in the same decade from 98.3 to 86.6 per 1000 unmarried women between the ages of 15 and 45 years. Nearly half the households headed by black women had incomes below the poverty level. As black family incomes increased, so did the number of households headed by an adult male. When the annual income reached $15,000 , there was no difference between blacks and whites in the number of families headed by an adult male. An obvious implication of these trends is that the structure of the black family is largely a reflection of socioeconomic class. When middle-class income levels were attained, black family structure approximated that of whites (Garrison, 1977).

The fact that 30 percent of black families are headed by a woman lends credence to the view that black families are matrifocal (Frazier, 1939) and not based on steadfast matrimony. Scanzoni (1971) wrote that in lower-class families several generations live together to form an enduring and cohesive group of related women who rely greatly on one another for comfort, support, and help. Among blacks the extended family structure provides the individual with a feeling of belonging, regardless of living arrangements. The extended black family is a structural norm favoring household arrangements where relatives of close or distant consanguinity live together for years or months. A feature of the extended black family has been its willingness to include nonblood relatives who are treated as kin (Staples, 1976). Child rearing and nurturing often transcend generations, as shown when the older black woman takes on the raising of her daughter's children partially or entirely.

That black women are ambivalent about marriage is implied by the findings of Lopata (1974), who studied a group of lower-income widows and found that black women were less likely than white women of comparable socioeconomic class to see marriage as a source of personal happiness. Fifty percent of the black women reported feeling sorry for married friends, and complained about excessive demands from adult children. The sample was a relatively small urban group in which a majority of the widowed black women were isolated from a close kinship structure.

The unemployment rate for blacks has been far greater than the 4 to 8 percent national unemployment rate in the United States since World War II. Therefore there may be little incentive for black women to tolerate long-term relationships with unemployed men who are financial liabilities. The original legislation introducing Aid for Dependent Children required the absence of an employable male from the home. This legislation was later amended to become Aid for Dependent Families, but its initial impact may have been to encourage deceit or separation of families from the father (Nye & Bernardo, 1973).

Slavery fostered a mother-centered family with tenuous bonds to the father, and social conditions which prevented black families from becoming self-sufficient have perpetuated this structure. The extended family remains, but this structural organization has been fragmented by geographical mobility and the pressures of the urban ghetto. A so-called matriarchical family may not be the family of choice for black men and women, but a compromise based on the realities of a tough existence. Structural variations which occur in black families are a consequence of events outside the family system and largely beyond its control. No longer enslaved, but not yet free of its past, the black family reacts adaptively as its capacities permit. Herzog and Lewis (1970) wrote that among black families the more desired norm was a stable marriage in which the male was the primary wage earner. This pattern prevails in the American ghetto just as it did on the African Gold Coast. Far from insisting on matriarchy, black women are very likely to resent the actions of men who do not function as breadwinners and household heads.

It is accurate to say that the black woman assumes major child-rearing responsibilities, but the same is true of most families regardless of social class. Herzog and Lewis criticized the habit of reporting proportions of fatherless homes by color rather than by socioeconomic class, and also attacked the stereotyping of inner city families, alleging that the aspiration of these mothers for their children is high, even though there may be great distance between aspiration and realistic expectation because of situational factors.

Functional Variations   In Western countries the mother is considered the most important figure in the life of the child. This is even more true of the 30 percent of all black families where the mother is the only visible parent. Ostracism from white society gave blacks freedom to develop a lifestyle with its own manners and customs. For example, the importance of the black woman as sole or collateral breadwinner has affected the socialization of black children in special ways (Epstein, 1974). As a rule, white children are exposed to the role model of the father as primary provider, even when the mother has a career of her own. Limited employment prospects for black men has caused preferential treatment within the family for girls with regard to educational advancement. Since behaviors which are unrewarded tend not to persist, lack of incentive may have caused male blacks to lose interest in education, self-denial, punctuality, and responsibility in performing tasks because reward for these virtues has been unpredictable (Nye & Berardo, 1973).

Failure of one family member to enact his or her ascribed role burdens others even when compelling explanations can be found. Conflict results from unequal role enactment between husband and wife based on the inability of many black men to equal the competence of the black woman. Problems attending blackness in a racially biased society undoubtedly have contributed to inadequate role performance among black men, decreased the importance of matrimony, and increased the divorce rate among blacks, which has risen 75 percent in the last decade. Staples (1976) wrote that dating behavior among blacks was accompanied by sexual activity unrelated to marriage, and was censured only when pregnancy resulted.

An interesting distinction can be made between: (1) individuals who see family roles as normatively defined and consistently try to enact these roles, but cannot do so because of limited opportunity or ability, and (2) individuals who do not perceive their family roles normatively and make no effort to enact them. Society is less concerned with the former even when minimal subsistence levels exist in families whose health and psychological needs are ill-attended. The marginal family, in which role enactment is attempted but not completed, receives less attention from the community because this family is less disruptive. A disorganized family receives disproportionate aid because the deviancy is blatant, often accompanied by alcoholism, drug addiction, and criminality. Both types of families are malfunctioning systems which cause individual discontent and social disquiet, but the marginal family can be ignored more easily. Many lower-class black families, like lower-class white families, may be found in both categories (Nye & Berardo, 1973).

Functional variations in black families have been found to be significantly related to socioeconomic class. Tendencies of middle-class mothers to be less directive toward and to interact more with their children have been found in both black and white households. Differences between lower- and middle-class black mothers were observed; middle-class black mothers stressed feelings and motives, while lower-class black mothers were more restrictive toward their children and had greater role expectations. White middle-class mothers were more cooperative with their children and black middle-class mothers were more inconsistent. In behavioral ways the black middle-class mothers resembled lower-class white mothers, but in verbal behavior they were more like middle-class white mothers. It was suggested that the inconsistent maternal behavior might be attributed to the upward aspirations of black mothers still in the process of integrating middle-class values (Zegiob & Forehand, 1975). Tendencies of middle-class mothers to be relatively nondirective and to interact with their children is probably true of all mothers of the same social class. Lower-class mothers, regardless of race, may be more directive and restrictive because of heavier responsibilities. Many of them are single parents who must combine child rearing with wage earning.

Research on the effects of children growing up in fatherless homes produced no firm evidence that father absence was a direct cause of juvenile delinquency, poor school achievement, or conflicted sex identity. A frequent conclusion of such studies was that family discord contributed more to juvenile delinquency than father absence. Delinquency was found more often in children living with unbroken but discordant families than in children living with harmonious one-parent families. In discussing behavioral styles of black families it can be argued that breadwinning and child rearing are not the only life activities of family black women. In some other areas such as sexual relationships, black women may not be dominant or even managerial (Herzog & Lewis, 1970).

The extended black family has been able to operate protectively for its members, who often live in conditions of external stress. Close affiliation between various family members has allowed work to be shared and companionship to be available. However, unclear role delineation and ambiguity around authority have sometimes caused the extended black family to become dysfunctional. In some extended black families role confusion has occurred when siblings were pushed into parenting roles or when young people were impeded from moving into new roles. A frequent effect of blurred generational boundaries is dissension due to role or boundary confusion.

CLINICAL EXAMPLE: ROLE CONFUSION IN A THREE-GENERATIONAL FAMILY OF AFRO-AMERICAN DESCENT

Charmayne, a black teenage mother, chose not to marry her child's father but to remain at home with her original family. In order to return to high school, Charmayne relinquished her child-care obligations to her 35-year-old mother, Becky. The older woman willingly agreed to this. She, in fact, related to Charmayne and the new baby much as she related to her own younger children. Even though Charmayne had wanted to return to school and enjoyed her freedom, she had mixed feelings about handing her baby over to her mother. Becky made all the decisions about the baby, and Charmayne felt she had no say at all. Her ambivalence was compounded by the fact that Charmayne had expected motherhood to release her from dependence on her mother. So a struggle began around child rearing which obscured the real issues, which were Charmayne's ambivalence and the unwillingness of the older woman to move into the grandmother role and to relate to Charmayne as a new mother with rights and authority of her own.

Based on general systems theory, an appropriate strategy was devised which increased the confidence of Charmayne in mothering her baby, but supported the contribution of the grandmother as resource and helper. The wisdom and experience of Becky were acknowledged, but the need to encourage Charmayne to mature was also suggested. A goal of therapeutic intervention was to resist Becky's wish to incorporate Charmayne and the baby as additional children in the family system. There was no thought of removing Charmayne and the baby from the family; the goal was merely to clarify and redefine roles. Figure 4-9 shows the family structure before and after intervention.

Assessment

Structure Among family members, there was no agreement on positions and status in the family after the birth of the baby. The grandmother assumed the position of mother toward her daughter and her new granddaughter. Generational boundaries were unclear. The teenage mother became conflicted; she enjoyed her freedom but wanted some of the rewards of motherhood. Grandmother and the new baby were joined in a close maternal relationship which excluded the young mother.

   Function   There was conflict in the system due to ambiguity around role distribution and role enactment. Tension was high and energy was dissipated in conflict. The price exacted by the grandmother for helping Charmayne was control of the baby. Charmayne needed help in raising her child but thought that the cost was very high.

Figure 4-9   Role confusion in a three-generational family.

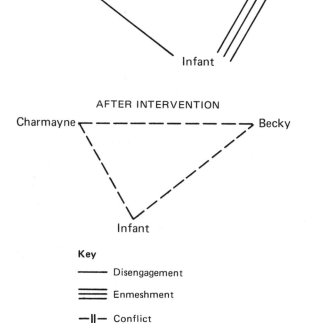

BEFORE INTERVENTION

Charmayne ⎯⎯⎯ ‖ ⎯⎯⎯ Becky

Infant

AFTER INTERVENTION

Charmayne ⟵ — — — — — — — ⟶ Becky

Infant

Key

⎯⎯⎯ Disengagement

≡≡≡ Enmeshment

⎯‖⎯ Conflict

— — Clear boundaries

Intervention

    1   To redefine role distribution and role enactment in the family
    2   To reduce the enmeshment of mother, infant, and grandmother, setting limits and assigning tasks so as to reduce sources of conflict
    3   To help the grandmother assume a valuable role as teacher and resource person for the young mother
    4   To encourage the young mother to perform tasks of mothering, with guidance and approval from grandmother

The Asian-American Family

The history of Asian immigration to the United States is a long and complicated one and it is important for those dealing with Asian families to realize that there is considerable diversity among people who appear at first glance to be similar. Asia is an enormous area encompassing many ancient and distinguished cultures whose national identity is now well developed. It is offensive to Japanese, Koreans, Chinese, and Vietnamese to be casually lumped together in one group by Caucasian Americans whose ignorance of Asian history and culture prevents their distinguishing among nationalities.

    In addition to national differences, we also find variations that are correlated with the arrival date of particular families. Asian immigration was heavy in the nineteenth century, and then nearly closed in the early twentieth century when severe restrictions were set on Asian immigration (Hsu, 1971; Kitano, 1964). These barriers were, of course, part of a general isolationism which also reduced the flow of Europeans into the United States; but the quotas set for Asians were stricter than for any other groups. Asian Americans whose families had been peaceful and industrious members of American society for generations accurately perceived these measures as racist. These quotas and other incidents, such as the internment of Japanese Americans during World War II, have undeniably left deep impressions in the psyches of individuals and in group memory of Asian communities (Kitano, 1964). Asian Americans are often simultaneously proud of their heritage, aware of their reputation as exemplary workers and citizens, and apprehensive about the security of their position in American society (Hsu, 1971). Resentment toward discriminatory laws and practices has united many Asians in cooperative action opposing inequity.

    Structural Variations   The complexity of the social composition of Asian communities has increased greatly since World War II as political upheaval throughout Asia has produced a new wave of refugees and immigrants. Many of these recent arrivals are not poverty-stricken farmers or laborers but highly trained professionals. Although these people have severe adjustment problems regarding status, language, and employment, they are often sophisticated and cosmopolitan individuals whose values are far less conservative than those of third- or fourth-generation descendants of Asian peasants who came to the United States 100 years ago. Again the health care professional is warned to investigate carefully the kind of Asian family being considered. The difference between the psychological experience of a 40-year-old Japanese American who was interned in Arizona in his youth and the scion of a Chinese scholarly family can hardly be overestimated, although both may adopt defensive withdrawal tactics. In spite of this diversity, the fact remains that all Asian Americans trace their origins to one of the traditional agrarian civilizations which have dominated that part of the world for thousands of years. Whether Chinese, Japanese, Korean, Vietnamese or Indian, such civilizations bear certain common traits which can be discussed as a whole.

Functional Variations   It is convenient for our purposes that perhaps the single most striking characteristic of Asian societies that differentiates them from American societies is the strength of the family. Until very recently, when industrialism and nationalism took hold in Asia, the family carried out all basic economic, social, religious, and even political functions (Welty, 1976). Family membership was necessary for an individual to participate in these activities. Because the family institution monopolized the distribution of nearly every benefit from food to status, the family was able to achieve extreme dominance over the lives of its members. The techniques by which this control was achieved were exceedingly efficacious and have proved to be resilient and durable even when transplanted to another continent (Hsu, 1971).

Asian family structure is strongly hierarchical and marked by very clear role differentiation. Equalitarianism and camaraderie are not valued; rather the proper performance of father, mother, son, and daughter roles are stressed. The duties and obligations of individuals to one another are far more important than their rights and are prescribed in detailed and specific ways. Fathers are honored through hard work and obedience; mothers are kinder and act as intermediaries with fathers; oldest sons are loved and privileged, daughters are docile and submissive. Role differentiation is rigid and traditional, although within the family individual characteristics of various members permit some role specialization. The person at the top of the pyramid is almost invariably the father, though very occasionally an old and experienced grandmother will assume this role. At first glance, it seems that the other family members exist for the benefit of the father. Certainly it is true that he expects and still is granted a degree of obedience and deference from other members which seems remarkable. Asian American children have been endlessly praised for their good manners in public and their industry in school (Hsu, 1970). Asian adolescents have markedly lower delinquency, drug addiction, and illegitimacy rates than any other minority (Kitano, 1964). Social aggressiveness is not valued, but academic and professional activities are. While marriages are now initiated by the young couple, parental permission is still deemed necessary (Wong, 1971) and the marriages are extremely stable. When queried about these "virtues," the explanation is almost invariably articulated in terms of respect for the father, appreciation for his strict moral training, and reluctance to shame him with any form of improper behavior (Hsu, 1971; Kitano, 1964).

Yet the purpose of family life is not ultimately to satisfy the father. Rather the family is its reason for being. The real goal of all family members is to perpetuate and bring praise upon the family; and the father is as much caught up in this as anyone else. The father is most responsible for ensuring that the family complete the next cycle of its life and he has, therefore, power commensurate with his responsibility. But ideally the goal of his effort is not his own gratification but to ensure that he leaves the family as vital and virtuous as he received it.

The attainment of this goal generates intrafamilial attitudes and practices very different from those of mainstream American culture although, as we have seen, the external behaviors of industry, responsibility, and achievement in Asian-American families fit into the wider society very easily. The crucial difference is that the Asian family does not seek to produce independence and autonomy in its offspring (Solomon, 1971). Competence and excellence are desirable because they bring material and status rewards to the family. But a constant effort is made to control these qualities because excessive competitiveness might generate a break from the family, whose future would then be in doubt. Parents whose whole personal identity is formed around that role stress the importance of family continuity and cohesion. The "best" offspring is one who is highly disciplined, ambitious, and confident but who is still basically dependent on parents for approval and personal happiness.

This different aspect of Asian family life produces fascinating nuances in the meaning of the word "role." While the continuance of the family is thought to depend on proper performance of clear familial roles, the cyclical nature of family life inevitably produces role reversals and confusions, especially between sons and parents. Because both father and son are acutely aware that the son is being prepared eventually to assume the role of father, the symbiotic fusion of their identities is very strong. It can be stated fairly that Korean males get a sense of strength and manhood from the presence of their fathers, not by revolting against them. Chinese proverbs have recognized the merging of the two identities: "First 30 years, one looks at the father and respects the son; second 30 years, one looks at the son and respects the father.'' The words suggest that as far as achievement and social status are concerned, the two are virtually one (Hsu, 1971).

Symbiosis is furthered by the fact that one never stops being a son, even when one has become a father. As long as one's parents live, one relates to them as a son. As parents reach old age, the ideal of filial treatment is to recreate for them again at the end of their lives the ease and indulgence of childhood. Thus the adult son repays parents for the years of his own early childhood when he was given unrestrained oral gratification through food and chatter (Solomon, 1971).

At age 5, boys begin to be initiated into the adult world of work, self-restraint, and proper harmonious social behavior; but the early years are the most pleasurable ones for the child. The son offers similar ease to his parents as a natural phase of the family life cycle. The psychological pain of elderly Asians whose offspring do not adhere to the old ideals is acute (Hsu, 1971).

The Asian woman is regarded as a temporary and less crucial member of the family. When she marries, her allegiance must be transferred completely to her husband's family, and she grows up with this expectation. Asian women face many problems specific to their background. For centuries women in Asia have been relegated to positions of inferiority. They are often raised with constant reminders of the higher worth of their brothers, ranging from inequitable allocation of food or educational resources to the most brutal laments against their very existence. When they leave home or become successful in school or business, they willingly abandon the previous constraints placed on their behavior, and find their parents puzzled and outraged by their conduct (Wong, 1971).

Among the problems facing Asian Americans are the influences which induce young people to depart from traditional values. Their predicament is greater because, on one hand, the energy and vigor they use to advance economically are highly regarded by the family, but, on the other hand, independence and competitiveness are expected to be left outside the Asian household. Submission to elders and dependency must be resumed as one returns to the family. Since much interaction in Asian families is governed by unchanging values, expectation of role enactment is implicit but clear. Manipulation and indirection are preferred to confrontation and struggle, but powerful forces exist to exact compliance. Contradiction between what is permissible outside the family and what is permissible within the family places excessive demands on Asian Americans.

In spite of the contradictions and demands of Asian family life, of which some are compatible with American values and others are not, the Asian-American family system has displayed great ability to produce stable, productive individuals. The family may take its toll, but sustains its members in countless ways. The incidence of marital discord, reported mental disturbance, and suicide among Asian Americans is lower than for most other minority groups (Hsu, 1971).

CLINICAL EXAMPLE: DISSONANCE BETWEEN HOME AND SCHOOL VALUES FOR A CHINESE AMERICAN

Hugo Chen was a bright but solemn Chinese-American boy who was friendless and unhappy in his first-grade class. An only child and the object of much parental solicitude, Hugo could not relate to the other first-graders. Invariably he was the target of their practical jokes. He was the last child to be chosen for games, and the first to be teased. Hugo's old world manners were very formal, and his deportment impeccable, but his teacher found that Hugo needed rescue from ridicule several times each day. He was only included in class activities when the teacher insisted, and her frequent interventions on his behalf alienated the other children even more. When his classmates baited Hugo by throwing his cap in the air or hiding his belongings, Hugo did not retaliate but watched in a forlorn way. Even in these instances his politeness did not desert him. Hugo's use of language was impressive but unchildlike, and his range of affective response was very constricted. He did not engage in spontaneous action, and indeed seemed fearful of behaving impulsively. Whenever he contemplated an action he announced verbally what he was thinking of doing, and this habit brought more derision from the other children.

As time went on Hugo became even more estranged from the others. Because of the mutual withdrawal behavior which she observed, Hugo's teacher asked his parents to attend a session or two in the classroom so they could observe firsthand the interaction between Hugo and his classmates. This was the first indication the parents had that Hugo was having problems.

In the conference which followed it became apparent that Hugo's father was very proud of his son's dignity and decorum, but he was able to understand the difficulty Hugo faced. The teacher explained gently that Hugo's formal manners were an oddity in an American classroom. While not wrong in themselves, the behaviors taught to Hugo by his parents were incongruent with those of his peers. The teacher suggested that Hugo's inhibited actions and his use of verbalized directions to himself were an effort to reimpose on himself the parental rules which were so hard to follow at school and which brought him ridicule.

On the basis of the teacher's suggestions, the parents agreed to reduce the formality they expected of Hugo, so that there was less disparity between standards set at home and those of the classroom.

His parents agreed to help Hugo become less pompous and more assertive at school. Realizing the burden they had placed on their son, they modified their guidelines. The father, in particular, who had strongly encouraged Hugo's verbal precocity, was helped to realize that intellectual progress could be achieved without making Hugo vastly different from his classmates. Important values could be upheld in the home, but setting priorities would reduce the problems of their conscientious little boy. Since Mr. and Mrs. Chen were devoted to their son, compromise on his behalf was something they were willing to try. Plans were made for the parents to attend a Home and School Association meeting with another couple, and to engage in related activities which would help them understand Hugo's life outside the home. They never became full participants, but even minimal involvement was helpful for Hugo and his parents.

Assessment

Structure   The 6-year-old Chinese-American boy was caught between his parents' insistence on deportment and the values of the dominant culture (see Figure 4-10). His mother and father were overinvolved emotionally with their son. Although Hugo's father was a successful business man, he had not been educated in the United States. Hugo's mother derived her sense of selfhood from being a wife and mother. She regarded her son as the major accomplishment of her life. Both parents had high aspirations for Hugo.

Function   The family maintained the traditional values of their homeland. Hugo's father dominated the household. He was a dignified man who was proud of his son but undemonstrative. Rough play, impulsivity, and emotional expressiveness were discouraged at home. As a result Hugo was dismayed by the antics of his classmates. Sensing his disapproval, his classmates retaliated by scapegoating Hugo. The protectiveness of the teacher further alienated Hugo from the companionship of his peers. Eventually Hugo's teacher sought help from the home in which the problem originated. She permitted the parents to observe for themselves the problems that were being created for Hugo.

Intervention

1 To demonstrate to the parents the dysfunctional interaction between Hugo and his classmates
2 To encourage parental compromise between traditional Asian values and those of the dominant culture
3 To foster ongoing communication between the parents and the school, so that Hugo would be released from the inhibited behavior which his parents fostered and his classmates abhorred

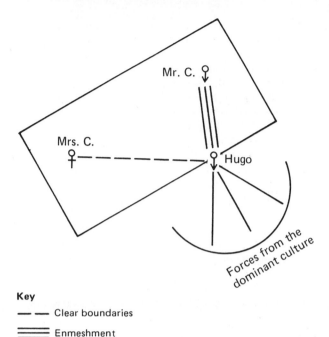

Key

— — Clear boundaries

≡≡≡ Enmeshment

Figure 4-10 Value incongruence in a Chinese-American family.

SUMMARY

Only a few of the variations in structure and function of ethnic families have been discussed in the preceding pages. The message of the chapter is that the clinician must work within the ethnic system, whatever it may be. Many folk beliefs concerning health and illness have been validated by generations of use. Even when the beliefs are erroneous, they are upheld by the tradition and prestige of the culture. The successful clinician is the one who shows respect for these values and who can offer a therapeutic regimen which is compatible with the life-style of the family.

Any chapter on ethnic differences suffers from reductionism. Nevertheless, a degree of simplification and generalization enables us to grasp differences which otherwise might be elusive. Stereotypes would probably not endure if there were no basic truth in them, but they must be evaluated carefully. Fifty years ago a warning was issued which remains true:

> What matters is the character of the stereotypes and the gullibility with which we employ them. . . . If our philosophy tells us that each man is only a small part of the world . . . then, when we use our stereotypes we tend to know that they are only stereotypes, to hold them lightly, to modify them gladly (Lippman cited in Herzog, 1968, pp. 19–20).

REFERENCES

Alfred, W. Pride and poverty: On Irish integrity. In T. C. Wheeler (Ed.), *The immigrant experience.* New York: Dial Press, 1971.

Alvirez, D., & Bean, F. D. The Mexican-American family. In C. H. Mendel & R. W. Habenstein (Eds.), *Ethnic families in America.* New York: Elsevier, 1976.

Bales, R. F. Cultural differences in the rate of alcoholism. *Quarterly Jr. for the Study of Alcohol,* March 1946, **6,** 400–449.

Barzini, L. *The Italians.* New York: Atheneum Press, 1964, p. 104.

Biddle, E. H. The American Irish-Catholic family. In C. H. Mendel & R. W. Habenstein (Eds.), *Ethnic families in America.* New York: Elsevier, 1976.

Chafetz, M. & Demone, H. *Alcoholism and society.* New York: Oxford University Press, 1962.

Coles, R. *Eskimos, Chicanos, Indians.* Boston: Little, Brown, 1977.

Elkin, F. *The family in Canada.* Ottawa: Vanier Institute of the Family, 1970.

Epstein, C. F. Successful black women. In J. Juber (Ed.), *Changing women in a changing society.* Chicago: University of Chicago Press, 1974.

Feminella, F. X., and Quadagno, J. S. The Italian American family. In C. H. Mindel & R. W. Habenstein (Eds.), *Ethnic families in America.* New York: Elsevier, 1976.

Fitzpatrick, J. P. The Puerto Rican family. In C. H. Mindel and R. W. Habenstein (Eds.), *Ethnic families in America.* New York: Elsevier, 1976.

Frazier, E. F. *The Negro family in the United States.* Nashville, Tenn.: Fisk Press, 1939.

Gambino, R. *Blood of my blood.* New York: Doubleday, 1974.

Gans, H. H. *The urban villages.* Glencoe, Ill.: Free Press, 1962.

Garrison, V. Spiritism in Harlem: Adjunct to religion. *New York Times,* November 6, 1977, p. 51, col. 1.

Glazer, N., & Moynihan, D. *Beyond the melting pot.* Cambridge: M.I.T. Press, 1963.

Greeley, A. M. *Ethnicity in the United States.* New York: Wiley, 1974.

Green, C. *Divided society: The ethnic experience in America.* New York: Basic Books, 1974.

Gutman, H. *The Negro family.* New York: Pantheon, 1976.

Harwood, A. The hot-cold theory of disease. *Journal of the American Medical Association,* 1971, **216**(7), 1153–1158.

Herzog, E., and Lewis, H. Children in poor families: Myths and realities. *American Journal of Orthopsychiatry,* 1970, **40**(3), 375–386.

Herzog, E. (Ed.) *About the poor.* Children's Bureau Publication, No. 451, 1968. pp. 19–20.

Hill, R. *The strengths of black families.* New York: Emerson Hall, 1972.

Hsu, F. L. K. *The challenge of the American dream: The Chinese in the U.S.* Belmont, Calif.: Wadsworth, 1971.

Kitano, H. H. L. *Japanese Americans: The evolution of a subculture.* Englewood Cliffs, N.J.: Prentice Hall, 1974.

Lewis, O. *La vida: A Puerto Rican family in the culture of poverty—San Juan and New York.* New York: Random House, 1965.

Lopata, H. Z. Social relations of black and white widowed women in a northern metropolis. In J. Huber (Ed.), *Changing women in a changing society.* Chicago: University of Chicago Press, 1974.

Mattis, M. C. Irish family in Buffalo, N.Y. 1855–1875. Unpublished dissertation, St. Louis: Washington University, cited by E. H. Biddle, 1976.

Mead, G. H. *Mind, self, and society.* Chicago: University of Chicago Press, 1933.

Minuchin, S. *Families and family therapy.* Cambridge, Mass.: Harvard University Press, 1974.

Murray R., & Zentner, J. *Nursing concepts for health promotion.* Englewood Cliffs, N.J.: Prentice-Hall, 1975.

Novak, M. *Rise of the unmeltable ethnics.* New York: Macmillan, 1972. p. 44.

Nye, I. F., & Bernardo, F. *The family: Its structure and interaction.* New York: Macmillan, 1973.

Queen, S., & Habenstein, R. W. (Eds.) *The family in various cultures.* (4th ed.) Philadelphia: Lippincott, 1974.

Rosenwaike, I. Two generations of Italians in America: Their futility experience. *International Migration Review,* Fall 1973, *7,* 271–282.

Scanzoni, J. *The black family in modern society.* Boston: Allyn and Bacon, 1971.

Solomon, R. H. *Mao's revolution and the Chinese political culture.* Berkeley, Calif.: University of California Press, 1971.

Staples, R. *Introduction to black sociology.* New York: McGraw-Hill, 1976.

Stycos, J. M. *Family and fertility in Puerto Rico.* Champaign-Urbana: University of Illinois Press, 1955.

Suttles, G. *The social order of the slums.* Chicago: University of Chicago Press, 1968.

Welty, P. T. *The Asians: Their heritage and destiny.* (5th ed.). Philadelphia: Lippincott, 1976.

Wheeler, T. C. (Ed.) *The immigrant experience.* New York: Dial Press, 1971.

White, E. H. Care of minority patients. *Nursing Clinics of North America,* 1977, **12**(1), 27–40.

Winch, R. F. *The modern family.* New York: Holt, Rinehart & Winston, 1971.

Wong, J. S. Puritans from the orient. In T. C. Wheeler (Ed.), *The immigrant experience.* New York: Dial Press, 1971.

Zegiob, L. E., & Forehand, R. Maternal interactive behavior as a function of race, socio-economic status and sex of the child. *Child Development,* 1975, **46**(2), 564–568.

Chapter 5

Social-Class Influences on Family Structure and Function

Jean R. Miller
Ellen H. Janosik

Social-class differences which affect the values and life-style of families are important considerations in the formulation of a therapeutic approach. Major class distinctions in structure and function are discussed in this chapter in order to increase understanding between practitioner and families, and surmount barriers that impede progress. Emphasis is placed upon lower- and middle-class families, since research has dealt primarily with these groups. There is a paucity of information about upper-class family patterns, perhaps because this class is less accessible to the investigator. Although studies of the poor often employ ethnic or racial variables, such studies will not be discussed in this section, since ethnicity was considered in Chapter 4.

One of the dangers of assigning general characteristics to a large group of people is that within any category there is considerable variation. Even when a group has shared characteristics, individual differences exist within the prevailing modes of thoughts, feelings, and behaviors. Generalizations about normative behavior in various social classes can guide the practitioner, but stereotyped assumptions about families require ongoing verification. Families change as external conditions change. Social-class differences reported in studies of a decade ago may be the result of less homogeneous styles in American life. Despite the influence of middle-class values perpetuated by the media, there is little doubt that many families continue to think and act according to social-class norms.

It is difficult to consign families to a particular social class because no single definition exists which truly encompasses the diversity and intricacy of the concept of social class. Social-class divisions are often arbitrary; nevertheless, it seems clear that there are stratified groups of people whose lives and aspirations are shaped by the class to which they belong. Families in the same social strata share similar occupational orientations, life experiences, educational accomplishments, and economic resources. It is therefore not feasible for a practitioner to ignore class distinctions, for to do so constitutes a form of denial.

While a number of indicators have been used to determine social class, education, occupation, and income are the most frequently employed. These indicators have been segmented at different points thus making it difficult for the practitioner to adhere to exact definitions. Absolute dividing points are less useful than relative ones, since the locality of a family's home or the stage of a family's life cycle influence the meaning of belonging to a designated social class. Families living on the same income in Appalachia and in New York City would have vastly different forms of existence. Given the same income, affluence in Appalachia may be equated with poverty in New York City. A young couple struggling to finish college may have the same income as an elderly couple, but the upward vision of the younger couple and the downward view of the older one may cause each to experience life totally differently. In many cases the family's perception of their social class is more important than precise considerations of occupation or income.

Social class may be divided into a large number of levels; however, for the purposes of the practitioner, four class groupings should prove sufficient. These are the upper, middle, working (blue collar), and poverty classes. The classification of a family into one of these categories is based on the interaction of occupation, income, and education. Families belonging to the upper and middle classes are likely to have household heads who are professionals, business managers, officials, or proprietors. Occupations of lower social prestige are, in descending order, clerical and sales workers, skilled workers, and semiskilled or unskilled workers. Income levels generally, but not always, correspond to occupational levels. Sometimes a plumber earns more than a college professor or a clergyman, but it is commonly accepted that the more years of schooling attained by the household head, the higher the social class of the family.

A few examples will illustrate some of the factors that contribute to social class distinctions. A family is classified as upper-class if the household head is in high-level management and has a bachelor's degree, and the total annual family income is $100,000. A middle-class family may have a household head who is a professional with a graduate degree and a combined (husband and wife) income of $28,000. Another example of a middle-class family is one with a single female parent who is an executive secretary with business training and earns a salary of $15,000 yearly. The working-class family is usually headed by an unskilled or semiskilled worker who may have graduated from high school but lacks additional education. The yearly salary of the blue-collar worker approximates $10,000 per year. Families in the poverty class have household heads who move in and out of the labor market, earning yearly incomes which seldom exceed $5,000. Educational attainment in poor families is usually at the grammar school level. The foregoing examples have been presented to supply general guidelines for classification according to social strata. Other salient details about status and class indicators can be found in Otto (1975).

STRUCTURAL DIFFERENCES

Family structure may be viewed in terms of size, positions of members, and accompanying status and roles. According to 1970 census data, families living in poverty are more likely to be large. Often babies are born to young, unmarried mothers and births are often close together. Members of poor families state that they believe in family planning, but they are less likely to use contraceptives. Attributed reasons for failure of the poor to practice contraception include ignorance, feelings of fatalism and alienation, poor communication between husband and wife, and the inaccessibility of family planning services (Chilman, 1975).

In low-income families nearly half the homes are fatherless and headed by a female. There is evidence that separation, desertion, and divorce vary in inverse proportion to income. Children are usually the responsibility of the mother, who must cope with severe financial stringency. Most lower-class women lack education and marketable skills, which makes it difficult for them to obtain jobs. If they do find employment outside the home, child care becomes a serious problem. Furthermore, the amount of income lower-class mothers can earn is less than that available to males. In these circumstances poverty becomes a vicious cycle which is difficult to break.

Children and young people are overrepresented in poverty-stricken families. In low-income families 25 percent of the members are under 14 years of age. Another 16 percent are between the ages of 14 and 24 years (Chilman, 1975). The likelihood of growing up in a female-headed household increased for black youngsters between 1959 and 1971, but this did not hold true for white children. Even with the proportion of female-headed, white households stabilized, almost half the children in poor families were raised in homes without fathers. Although the adverse effects of father absence have been disputed, it cannot be construed as a desirable arrangement.

Roles and positions in American households have been drastically altered by the great numbers of wives and mothers working outside the home. However, working-class families continue on the whole to emphasize the provider role for the husband and the nurturer/housekeeper role for the wife, despite the growing employment of women. Nevertheless, some role flexibility has been achieved, largely through the withdrawal of rewards and favors by the wife (Slocomb & Nye, 1976). Upper-middle-class families engage in androgynous task sharing, although most working mothers tend to view their jobs as supplementary rather than primary. Working wives, however, accept joint responsibility for enacting the provider role when their husbands occupy low-paying jobs. This may reflect the higher standards of living which the working wife of the low-status male enables the family to enjoy (Slocomb & Nye, 1976).

Men with a high school education or over are more likely to help with housework, and wives with college degrees are more likely to request that household tasks be shared. In families with three or four children there is shared enactment of household roles. With five or more children in the home there is less role sharing, but also less involvement of mothers outside the home (Slocomb & Nye, 1976).

FUNCTIONAL DIFFERENCES

In spite of the norms presented by the mass media for acceptable family behavior, differences continue to exist between classes. However, recent studies in the areas of family communication and child rearing reveal that the differences may not be as pronounced as earlier studies indicated. Nevertheless, practitioners need to consider even slight differences when assessing family functioning and planning goals of intervention with a family.

American couples have been moving over the years toward companionate marriage and person-oriented relationships rather than patterned role relationships. This has allowed for more flexibility in the ways couples interact with one another. Hawkins, Weisberg, and Ray (1977) found that better educated couples engaged in more open communication in situations which promoted emotional arousal. The marital communication style of less educated couples varied in the degree to which they maintained open communication but not in the way in which they communicated. Marital pairs in all classes valued talking things over calmly and detested controlled and inhibited verbalization of thoughts and feelings. All couples, regardless of class, desired a respectful confrontation of feelings in marital communications. The value placed on open communication can serve as a motivator for spouses who are having trouble expressing themselves to one another.

Differences exist between the classes in regard to parent-child interactive patterns, but again these differences seem to be of degree rather than of kind. Zegiob and Forehand (1975) observed that middle-class mothers were less directive and displayed more verbal interchange with their children than lower-class mothers. Kogan and Wimberger (1969) found that disadvantaged mothers and children were more detached from each other and less engaged in active social exchange than culturally advantaged mother-child pairs. Mothers in both classes, however, behaved similarly when they exerted control (ordering, prohibiting, restraining), exhibited expertise (teaching, explaining, demonstrating), or displayed assertiveness (demanding, contradicting, snatching). Likewise there was little difference between the classes in exhibiting or seeking warmth, love, friendliness, or personal interest.

When the practitioner is helping a parent with child-rearing methods, the educational background of that parent must be taken into consideration. The values and expectations of the parent who has the most sustained contact with the children usually prevail. A family may appear to be working-class, but if the mother has had a college education, the health professional may expect the mother's child-rearing practices to be more typical of middle- than of lower-class families.

Since the end of World War II, middle-class families have become increasingly permissive with their children; this is less true of lower-class parents (Gecas, 1976). White-collar parents tend to stress the development of internal standards in their children and to discipline on the basis of their interpretation of a child's motives for a particular act. Blue-collar parents, on the other hand, are likely to react on the basis of the consequences of the child's behavior (Gecas & Nye, 1974).

Early studies on child-rearing practices by class reported that lower-class parents were apt to use physical punishment while middle-class parents were more likely to use psychological techniques of punishment. More recent studies indicate that the magnitude of class differences is not as great as was found previously (Erlander, 1974). Punishment in the lower class now may take the form either of physical punishment or of deprivation of pleasures, for example, keeping the child alone or not permitting the child to watch television for a specified time. Nevertheless, lower-class children seem to be punished more often then children in classes above them. The consequences are that lower-class children learn to control much of their behavior out of fear. They expect others to control them with punishment, which does not give them opportunities to become self-directing. This results in rage, which usually cannot be expressed against parents or other important sources of the rage. Aggressive acts must therefore be turned toward others of whom they are less afraid. The satisfaction gained from ''getting away with it'' and taking advantage of another person comes to be valued. Such behavior is based on fear without guilt (Piuck, 1975).

Families may function with difficulty when the parents have originated from different classes or when they are moving as a couple from one class to another. The different values and behavioral expectations associated with the different classes may stimulate conflict over how the chidren should be disciplined or the degree to which problems should be discussed. Upwardly and downwardly mobile couples may experience loneliness and confusion when their values differ from those with whom they have frequent contact. These couples need to determine which values and behaviors are important for their families in light of past and present experiences.

PRACTITIONER GUIDELINES

When practitioners work with families from classes other than their own, it is important that they recognize and eliminate stereotypes and prejudice. Negative attitudes make it difficult to identify with a family and its problems. Furthermore, families quickly sense the practitioner's feelings and tend to turn away when they feel the practitioner does not understand them and their situation.

Practitioners need to be alert to nonverbal as well as verbal cues in communication. This is important for all classes, although it is especially important with lower-class families, who may have difficulty verbalizing their thoughts and feelings. Practitioners also should be aware of the nonverbal cues which they themselves emit, such as signs of disinterest or prejudice.

Families from all classes respond to accurate empathy, nonpossessive warmth, and genuineness (Ayers, 1970). Interaction with families should be characterized by an open expression of thoughts and feelings within the therapeutic limits. Lower-class families usually benefit from an action-oriented approach from which immediate results can be expected. Direct results are reinforcing for middle- and upper-class families also, although these groups generally are introspective as well as extrospective. In most instances a direct, practical approach is appreciated by families from all classes.

CLINICAL EXAMPLE: CLASS CONFLICT
IN AN UPWARD-BOUND FAMILY

Loretta and Floyd Ennis grew up in the same urban neighborhood and attended the same schools and church. Loretta was the oldest of eight children. Her father was a longshoreman, hard-working, hard-drinking, and the undisputed boss of the family. Loretta's mother worked in a small plastics factory, and it was Loretta's job to baby-sit, cook, and placate the uneven temper of her father in her mother's absence. The house was noisy, crowded, and disorganized despite Loretta's attempts to impose order.

Loretta was a very pretty girl, quiet and unassuming, and pre-occupied with her responsibilities at home. While in high school she began dating Floyd, whose home life was as orderly as Loretta's was disorganized. Floyd's mother had been a schoolteacher before marrying; his father was a bricklayer. As a union bricklayer, Floyd's father earned a good living; his wife did not work outside the home, but she was active in church affairs. Floyd's mother was a meticulous housekeeper. She also spent a great deal of time with Floyd, who was an only child. Even in grade school, Floyd showed academic promise, which his mother tried to cultivate. Both parents were very proud of Floyd and had high ambitions for him. They were disappointed when he began dating Loretta, particularly when Loretta dropped out of high school before graduating. During her senior year there was a long dock strike, so for weeks her father had earned no money. When union benefits were exhausted, the family accumulated many debts and sometimes even went hungry. The money earned by Loretta's mother was insufficient to support a large family. In desperation, Loretta dropped out of school and found work as a waitress. Six weeks later the dock strike was settled and Loretta's father returned to work. Encouraged by Floyd, she attempted to return to school, but was dissuaded by her teachers, who thought she had missed too much work to graduate. Loretta attended her high school prom with Floyd and she was his guest at graduation, along with his parents.

The friendship between Loretta and Floyd continued during his college years over the objections of his mother, who contended that he should marry a rich girl instead of wasting his time with "that dumb little waitress around the corner." Although influenced by his mother in many ways, Floyd showed no signs of giving up Loretta. They were married shortly after he finished college. At that point he had a fellowship for graduate work in physics and was self-supporting.

The years in graduate school were fulfilling for Floyd, but less so for Loretta. Since all their friends were poor, their own lack of affluence did not bother her. However, she was often at a loss for things to say to other wives or to girl friends. It was easier after her son was born, for then she had more in common with some of the other wives.

Being a mother made her feel more of a person, and less a pale reflection of Floyd.

Floyd moved easily from graduate school to the business world, where his abilities were soon recognized. Five years after the birth of her son, Loretta found herself in a suburban split-level home with four bedrooms, a manicured lawn, and no close friends. She remained very close to her mother and sisters whom she visited several times a week, taking her son with her to the old neighborhood. These visits were the only occasions on which Loretta felt relaxed and comfortable. Although she attended many company functions with Floyd—usually in a dress he had chosen for her—these were stressful events which often left her with a throbbing migraine headache.

The headaches were relieved only when Loretta retired to a darkened room while her husband or a baby-sitter cared for her son. Finally, at Floyd's insistence, Loretta visited an internist for an extensive medical work-up, which included a gynecological examination. Although Loretta had expressed concern that she was unable to become pregnant again, the medical report indicated no significant problems and no physiological reason for her infertility. Meanwhile the migraine attacks were becoming more severe and more incapacitating, and medication provided only minimal relief. Floyd gradually became impatient as Loretta became more dysfunctional. She was often unable to accompany him to various functions. Their sex life, which had been very gratifying, began to deteriorate. Floyd was also becoming concerned about the welfare of their little boy when Loretta was "out of it," as he described her episodes. Noting the strain in the couple's relationship, and unable to alleviate the intractable headaches, the internist suggested a psychiatric referral for Loretta. After an assessment of Loretta and a conjoint interview with both partners, family counseling was suggested by the psychiatric clinician. It was concluded that Loretta's problems originated in her insecure feelings about herself, her loneliness as a corporate wife, her inability to ask Floyd for emotional support, and her husband's immersion in his career.

Assessment

Structure The marital dyad consisted of two people who had begun life as members of working-class families. Floyd, however, came from a family with more stability and greater prosperity. As an only child, he was the object of much parental attention, particularly from his mother, who possessed many middle-class values. Through education Floyd had moved into the middle class and clearly identified with middle-class attitudes toward career and family. Loretta lived in a middle-class setting but retained her lower-class values. Remembering her dominating father, she was a passive wife and deferred to Floyd. She also repressed her hostility toward him for having taken her away from surroundings in which she was comfortable. Because Floyd loved her and was a good provider, Loretta felt guilty for being unhappy. All this turmoil exacerbated the migraine problem. Although the headaches were painful, they allowed Loretta to withdraw from the suburban activities that made her so anxious.

Because of his mother's problems, the 5-year-old boy was confused and uneasy. His mother's rules differed from those his playmates had to obey. The kindergarten he went to and the house he lived in were nicer than his mother's old home, yet his mother seemed happy when they visited there. Sometimes the child was not sure where he and his mother belonged.

Function   Loretta was perceived by the family counselor as a conscientious but very lonely woman who had allowed herself to be exploited by those she loved. She had been the parent-child for a large family, and had sacrificed her own aspirations for her family's needs. Like her in-laws, Loretta thought that Floyd had married beneath him. As a result she could not express negative feelings toward her husband. In the suburban world she inhabited, Loretta always felt alone. The permissive child-rearing practices of her neighbors appalled her. For example, when she discovered her little boy exhibiting himself to a playmate, she reacted fiercely. Her own son was spanked and his little friend sent home in disgrace. Loretta was shocked and surprised when the playmate's mother phoned to ask why Loretta was so upset. Other similar events had increased Loretta's feelings of alienation. Her recourse was to turn to her original family whose values she understood or to retreat to her darkened bedroom with an intractable headache.

Floyd was an energetic, competitive man who loved his wife and depended on her unfailing devotion. His attention to his career made him oblivious to Loretta's loneliness and sense of inadequacy. Floyd knew that Loretta's views on child rearing were at variance with those of their neighbors, but because of his own doting mother he tended not to interfere. In any case, he was too busy to be very concerned. Home and children were Loretta's domain, even if her strictness with their son worried him at times.

Intervention

The family problem was identified as conflict arising from Floyd's identification with and Loretta's resistance to middle-class values. The problem was compounded by Loretta's low self-esteem and Floyd's peripheral position in the family. The following goals were identified.

    1   Reduce the distance between Floyd and Loretta by encouraging Loretta to talk about her concerns, and by having Floyd listen.
    2   Help Loretta separate from her family of origin and become more comfortable with the values of the middle class to which she now belonged.
    3   Use the devotion both parents felt for their son to resolve the inconsistency of their behavior toward him. Unless the parents solved their social-class conflicts, the resultant ambiguity would be difficult for their son.
    4   Recognize the fact that there were valid reasons for Loretta's feelings of deprivation and inadequacy. With her only child ready for school, Loretta was in a position to remedy the deficiencies in her education and experience which made her feel inferior. With encouragement from Floyd, Loretta would be capable of undertaking a self-improvement program to increase her confidence and poise.
    5   Mobilize the deep affection between husband and wife to increase his understanding of her dilemma and her ability to communicate her needs to her husband.

Intervention and evaluation were based on these objectives.

SUMMARY

Social class has been operationalized in many ways with the main variables being income, education, and occupation. Research findings about class differences can provide a useful framework for the practitioner who is assessing family structure and function. However, practitioners are cautioned that within each class not all families are similar. Family values and expected behaviors are becoming more homogeneous as families spend increasing amounts of time watching television. Social-class differences appear to be a matter of degree rather than of kind in most areas of family structure and function. An accepting and direct approach benefits families from all classes.

REFERENCES

Ayers, G. E. The disadvantaged: An analysis of factors affecting the counseling relationship. *Rehabilitation Literature,* 1970, **31**(7), 194–199.

Chilman, C. S. Families in poverty in the early 1970's: Rates, associated factors, some implications. *Journal of Marriage and the Family,* 1975, **37**(1), 49–60.

Erlander, H. S. Social class and corporal punishment in childrearing: A reasseessment. *American Sociological Review,* February 1974, **39**, 68–85.

Gecas, V. The socialization and child care roles. In F. I. Nye (Ed.), *Role structure and analysis of the family* (Vol. 24). Beverly Hills: Sage Publications, 1976.

Gecas, V., & Nye, I. F. Sex and class differences in parent-child interacion: A test of Kohn's hypothesis. *Journal of Marriage and the Family,* 1974, **36**(4), 742–749.

Hawkins, J. L., Weisberg, C., & Ray, D. L. Marital communication style and social class. *Journal of Marriage and the Family,* 1977, **39**(3), 479–490.

Kogan, K. L., & Wimberger, H. C. Interaction patterns in disadvantaged families. *Journal of Clinical Psychology,* 1969, **25**(4), 347–352.

Otto, L. B. Class and status in family research. *Journal of Marriage and the Family,* 1975, **37**(2), 315–332.

Piuck, C. L. Child-rearing patterns of poverty. *American Journal of Psychotherapy,* 1975, **29**(4), 485–502.

Slocum, W. L., & Nye, I. F. Provider and housekeeper roles. In I. F. Nye (Ed.), *Role structure and analysis of the family* (Vol. 24). Beverly Hills: Sage Publications, 1976.

Zegiob, L. E., & Forehand, R. Maternal interactive behavior as a function of race, socio-economic status, and sex of the child. *Child Development,* 1975, **46**(2), 564–568.

Part Two

Family
Developments

Chapter 6

Assessment of Family Structure

Ann Cain

Professionals working with families do not know precisely what they should be looking for when they try to study individual families. Therefore, the emphasis should be upon making as wide a range of observations as possible, in order to include all dimensions.

A family can be viewed in a variety of ways. It can be viewed as a number of individuals, each with his or her own needs and expectations. It can be viewed as a primary group, usually small in size, which has considerable emotional involvement and shared goals. It can be considered a basic unit of society and therefore a medium for the transmission of societal values. It also can be viewed as a system in which the action of each individual family member has an effect on the family as a whole. Jackson and Lederer (1968) described the family as an interacting communications network in which every member influences the nature of the family system and is in turn influenced by the system. In order to develop a complete understanding of a family, it is necessary to take all these views into consideration.

Observation and analysis of family structure are essential to assessment. Every family develops systematic ways of being a family. These include communicating, problem solving, meeting family members' needs for affection and intimacy, resolving conflict, and dealing with loss and change. These systematic processes may be considered the structural components of the family's functioning. Structure refers to the family organization and the patterns of relationships among family members. In *Webster's New World Dictionary* (1976), the word *structure* is defined as a combination of interrelated parts forming a whole. This definition is similar to that of a system, and the structure of the family is in fact an interrelated system.

Another way to think about structure in terms of the family is to focus on the composition of family groups or the manner of family organization. The *nuclear family* is the center of development and consists of two parents and their children. An individual's nuclear family consists of his or her mother, father, and siblings. An individual's nuclear family is sometimes referred to as the *family of origin,* i.e., the family the individual was born into. In contrast to the family of origin, the term *family of procreation* refers to the family that an individual helps create. If an individual marries and has children, the new family is his or her family of procreation. *Extended family* refers to the larger family group consisting of parents, children, and all other relatives. This includes grandparents, aunts, uncles, cousins, and all other family members. Other types of family structure also influence interaction, among them the two-parent family, often called the intact family, the single-parent family, the family with no children, and the family with an extended family member living in the home. Each of these types has its own patterns and form.

A useful way of assessing the family structure is to collect meaningful data by taking a detailed family history. The family history is a valuable assessment tool, and it provides factual information about the overall functioning patterns of the family for at least three generations. The history taker asks many questions, and the more he or she learns about the family, the more the family learns about itself. It is important to obtain a factual picture and a description of events so that the family situation can be accurately assessed. A family diagram is an organized way of collecting family information which is represented pictorially (see Figure 6-1). This type of diagram has information about at least three generations of family life, and relationship and familial patterns are highlighted. The diagram includes names, birth dates, marriages, divorces, deaths, job and residence data, and illnesses. A pictorial family diagram is an extremely useful tool for assessing structure and for teaching families about family systems and how they function. If the diagram is used consistently in working with the family, it may assist family members to think in broader terms of the family system; many patterns—social, psychological and biological—can be traced through the generations. Once these patterns have been identified, family members can discover ways of changing their own behavior if they desire change.

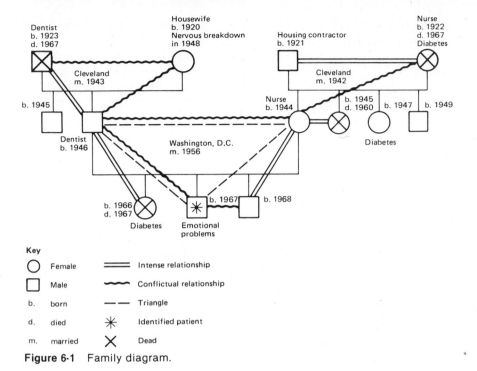

Figure 6-1 Family diagram.

The health professional who is more interested in physical factors might use a genogram, or family tree, to determine the incidence of familial illnesses such as diabetes or hypertension. A professional engaged in genetic counseling would find a genogram an effective way of diagramming and illustrating to families the potential risk for certain couples of having children. The responsibility of the genetic counselor is neither to persuade nor to dissuade families from propagation, merely to help them make decisions on the basis of knowledge. For example, the prevalence of malignancy or of heart disease in certain families, if known, becomes information which facilitates primary prevention.

GENERAL SYSTEMS THEORY: ITS APPLICATION TO STRUCTURE

General systems theory is a discipline whose subject matter is derived from principles which are valid for systems in general. A system is simply a set of interrelated elements that has a boundary. It is a set of persisting interrelationships between the parts of a whole. A boundary is something which separates a system from its environment and imposes a limit on the extent of its relationships. The environment can be defined as the setting in which the system exists. It is all that is outside the boundary of the system; within the boundary, all family members are part of the family system.

The concept of open and closed systems is useful to the discussion of family structure. However, it is only a relative concept, since no family systems are completely open or completely closed. All of them are open to some degree, but some are more so than others. To determine the degree of openness of a family system, the following questions are useful:

1 To what degree does the family system take in information from outside its own boundaries?
2 Can the family deal with new information flexibly and continue to maintain its equilibrium?
3 To what degree does the family relate to its environment?

A family with a greater degree of openness is able to take in more messages from its environment and to adapt to what it hears; it does not find it necessary to distort this information because of an inability to handle change. Some families tend to shut out or distort almost all information coming from their environment in order to avoid upsetting their equilibrium. These families would be examples of closed systems. Closed systems are like locked vaults—nothing can get in. A family with a relatively open system is able to take in outside information, respond to it flexibly, and continue to maintain its equilibrium.

Elements may be part of more than one system. The family is a member of other larger systems and also has various subsystems of its own. Systems function at all levels of efficiency, ranging from optimal functioning to total dysfunction. Functioning of any system is partly dependent upon the functioning of the larger systems of which it is a part.

The nuclear family is a part of a larger system, the extended family, and both nuclear and extended families are parts of still larger systems such as school, work, church, community, state, nation, and world. Each of these larger systems influences the family's functioning. Effective or ineffective alliances or coalitions (subsystems) within the family also alter family function. Examples of subsystems in the family include different combinations of members such as dyads consisting of husband and wife, or of mother and children. Triangles, resulting from a combination of three members, are also formed. Minuchin (1974) described these coalitions as situations in which two or more family members have a special bond or alliance that excludes or is different from other relationships within the family network. He wrote of the spouse, parental, and sibling subsystems in the family and also pointed out that "subsystems can be formed by generation, by sex, by interest, or by function" (Minuchin, 1974, p. 52). All these subsystems affect the family's structure and function.

Centralization is another term used to describe a system's structure. A centralized system is one in which one element or subsystem plays a major or dominant role in the operation of the system. A small change in this subsystem will have repercussions on the entire system.

In all systems, parts compensate for each other. In all family systems, family members compensate for each other. If one family member is underfunctioning in certain areas, another member will compensate by overfunctioning in those areas. Family members do not have to overfunction or underfunction entirely; they may overfunction in one area and underfunction in another. What is important is that the family system maintains an equilibrium or balance. The concept of overfunctioning and underfunctioning is an example of the reciprocal patterns that exist in all families.

Family members continually relate to each other in specific, reciprocal kinds of ways. Eventually mutual patterns of interaction evolve and these become predictable to family members. These patterns are the organizational structure of the family. The systems concepts presented are useful in determining that structure.

THE STRUCTURE OF THE FAMILY

Much of what has just been discussed has to do with the concept of boundaries. Minuchin believes that determining the clarity of boundaries within a family can provide a useful parameter for the evaluation of family functioning. He focuses in particular on three subsystems: the spouse, the parental, and the sibling subsystems. His conviction is that, without clear boundaries, the family system and its subsystems cannot function effectively. Minuchin maintains that subsystems must be able to function without the intrusion of other subsystems, but that at the same time they must maintain contact with each other. He sees boundary clarity as ranging from disengagement, where there are inappropriately rigid boundaries, to enmeshment, where boundaries are diffuse and blurred. In the middle is the "normal" range in which boundaries are clear but not rigid.

The concept of a range of boundary clarity can be used to describe patterns of interacting between subsystems. It does not necessarily refer to function or dysfunction, although possible areas of dysfunction can be hypothesized when subsystems are operating at either extreme of the range. In most families there are both enmeshed and disengaged subsystems. When interaction patterns are enmeshed, there is a lack of subsystem differentiation, boundaries are blurred, contact outside the system is minimal, and there is less room for autonomy.

The three subsystems most emphasized by Minuchin (1974, p. 56–59) are:

1 Spouse subsystem: This forms when two individuals marry. Patterns must be developed so that each spouse's functioning is supported by the other. Some separateness is yielded in order to belong, and there is an acceptance of the mutual interdependence. The boundaries of the spouse subsystem are important since, if they are very rigid, the subsystem will be isolated and if they are too diffuse, other subsystems may intrude.

2 Parental subsystem: This forms when the spouse subsystem differentiates to care for a child, while maintaining its mutual support system. It is important that the child have access to the parental subsystem but not to the spouse subsystem. The use of power and authority is absolutely necessary if the parents are to carry out their executive functions.

3 Sibling subsystem: In this system, children first learn to experiment with peer relationships. What they learn here will have great influence on their future relationships. Children require autonomy within this subsystem without undue interference from parents.

Figure 6-2   Family map. (Adapted from Minuchin, 1974.)

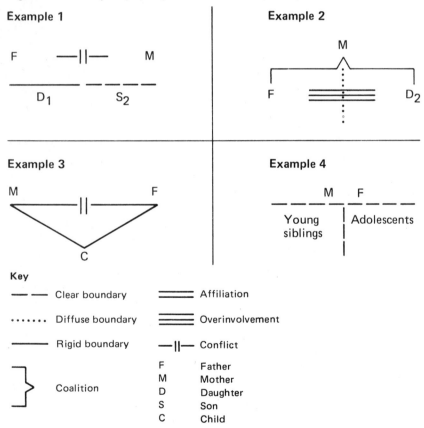

In depicting family boundaries and subsystems Minuchin (1974) used what he described as the family map (see Figure 6-2). Like the family diagram mentioned earlier, this map deals primarily with positions, relationships, and boundaries. Both the family diagram and the family map are used to collect and organize family data, identify functional and dysfunctional areas, and help determine therapeutic goals.

Family systems theory as presented by Bowen (1971) is a composite of eight interrelated and interdependent concepts which describe the emotional functioning (i.e., the structure) of a family system. The major concepts of the Bowen Theory are:

1   Nuclear family emotional system
2   Differentiation of self
3   Triangles
4   Family projection process
5   Multigenerational transmission process
6   Sibling position
7   Emotional cutoff
8   Societal regression

Only those concepts that apply specifically to structure will be discussed at length.

Nuclear Family Emotional System

The nuclear family emotional system may also be referred to as the *undifferentiated ego mass*. Both terms describe emotional fusion which may occur between members of a family system who do not see themselves as separate from one another. They are functioning on a dependent level and at a high emotional intensity. Fusion is a blending of self with others—when one's center of gravity lies in another. Highly fused individuals do not have a clear definition of their individual boundaries in close emotional relationships; they do not know where they leave off and others begin. This can be a precarious position. If people get too close to each other, they will seek distance to maintain self boundaries again. In all families members are connected to one another and they are also separate from one another. The degree of connectedness (fusion) and the degree of separateness are different in each family. Some families are highly fused, others are not, depending on the patterns learned in each spouse's family of origin.

Three major mechanisms exist for handling fusion or undifferentiation in the family (Bowen, 1971). Depending on the degree of fusion present, spouses may use one or a combination of the three to achieve distance in the relationship. The mechanisms are:

1 Marital conflict: The spouses engage in open conflict with each other after a period of intense closeness (fusion). This conflict results in a period of emotional distance before the spouses then reunite in their intense focus on each other. This is a cyclical and predictable pattern of relating that temporarily reduces the anxiety of fusion in the relationship.

2 Dysfunctional spouse: Large amounts of undifferentiation can be absorbed through physical, emotional, or social dysfunctions. This is a reciprocal relationship in which one spouse dominates the relationship, while the other is submissive and adaptive. The dysfunction of the spouse who has handed all responsibility over to the overfunctioning spouse may be manifested as drug or alcohol abuse, irresponsible behaviors, poor work history, psychiatric problems, chronic physical illness, or other conditions which seriously affect the individual's functioning.

3 Projection to one or more children: This mechanism is so important that it has been included as a separate concept in the theory—the family projection process. This is the basic process by which parental problems are projected to one or more of the children and can be observed in such child-related problems as learning difficulties, behavioral problems, psychiatric symptoms, delinquency, and physical illness. "The family projection process is universal in that it exists in all families to some degree" (Bowen, 1971, p. 398). There is less likelihood of impairment in the children if the focus is on several children rather than on one child.

Differentiation of Self

The nuclear family emotional system and differentiation of self are very closely related to each other. There is something similar to an inverse relationship between them, i.e., the more the nuclear family emotional system dominates the functioning of the family, the lower the levels of differentiation between family members. Another way to describe it is that the amount of fusion in a family is determined by the level of differentiation exhibited by family members.

Bowen (1971) wrote that the differentiation-of-self construct deals with the degree to which an individual is emotionally differentiated from the parent, with the amount of unresolved emotional attachment to parents equivalent to the degree of undifferentiation of self. In a later work Bowen (1976) equated the concept of differentiation of self with the ability to distinguish between the affective process and the intellectual process, stating that persons with the greatest fusion between thinking and feeling, function poorly and are prone to life problems (see Figure 6-3).

The concepts of solid self and pseudoself are also important to the understanding of differentiation. Solid self is made up of firmly held principles, beliefs, and convictions that are not negotiable. It is formed slowly and can be changed from within the self, but never through coercion or persuasion from others. It represents what a person truly believes.

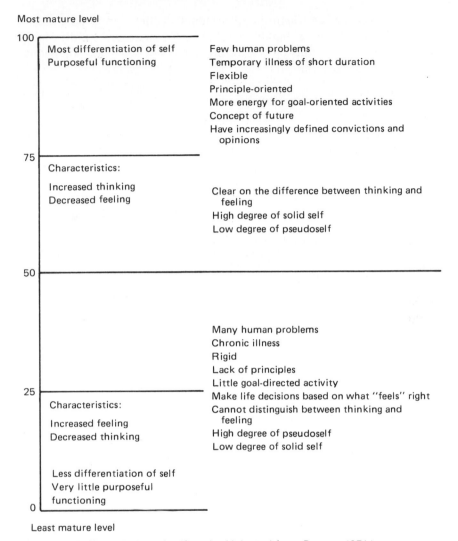

Most mature level

100	
	Most differentiation of self — Few human problems
	Purposeful functioning — Temporary illness of short duration

Figure 6-3 Differentiation-of-self scale. (*Adapted from Bowen, 1971.*)

Pseudoself is made up of knowledge incorporated by the intellect and of principles and beliefs acquired from others. It is negotiable in relationships and can be changed by emotional pressure or external influences. People who are less differentiated have more pseudoself, operate in an affective world, and experience more emotional fusion with others. People who are more differentiated have more solid self, are more autonomous, and experience less emotional fusion in their close relationships. They have more energy for goal-directed activity (Anonymous, 1972).

The assessment of whether an individual's actions are predominantly on a feeling level or on a thinking level provides an accurate indication of where that individual falls on the differentiation-of-self scale. Individuals whose actions are determined by their emotional system are concerned with togetherness, "we-ness," happiness, and love and approval from others. They disapprove of others who do not provide all these things for them. They make little distinction between what is their own responsibility in attaining their goals and what they can reasonably expect from others. They frequently blame others for their own unhappiness and they are almost totally relationship-oriented. In contrast to this, individuals who operate mainly from their thinking system can distinguish between their thoughts and their feelings, can state clearly what they believe without having to attack others who think differently, and do not find it necessary to try to change the other's mind to be in accord with their own thinking. Their self-appraisal is realistic and they are not dependent on others for approval. They can choose emotional closeness but do not hold the other person responsible for providing satisfaction from that closeness. Their goal-directed activity is not hindered by intense emotional involvement. It is important to realize that this assessment only has meaning when it is made over time and that it must reflect a total picture and not just what is happening at a particular moment. Thus, a complete family history serves as an assessment over time and can provide a good idea of the basic level of differentiation in a family or an individual. Once this assessment is made accurately, the goal of the helping person is to assist individual family members to rise out of the emotional togetherness that binds them together and to achieve higher levels of functioning.

Triangles

Another important concept of the Bowen Theory having to do with structure is the concept of triangles. The triangle has definite relationship patterns that predictably occur in periods of calm and stress. In periods of calm, the triangle is made up of a comfortable, close twosome and a less comfortable outsider. The favored position, then, is the inside position of togetherness. Each person in the triangle makes moves to achieve the inside position when tension is minimal.

In periods of stress, the outside position is the most comfortable and the most desirable. Each person in the triangle works to get the outside position to escape the tension of the twosome. Much of the time members of the triangle are able to move and shift within the triangle. When this is not possible, one of the original twosome will triangle in another person, leaving the former third person outside for reinvolvement later. The emotional forces duplicate the same patterns in this new triangle. Over time, in families, these emotional forces continue to move from one active triangle to another, finally remaining mostly in just one triangle, as long as the total system is calm. These patterns keep repeating themselves and the individuals who form the triangle come to have fixed roles in relation to each other (Bowen, 1971).

Another way of describing triangling is:

> In times of stress between two people, it becomes too uncomfortable for them to focus on their conflict. They will attempt to pull in a less involved third person, shift the focus to him, and in this way will relieve themselves of some of the intensity and pressure they feel. Triangling is always an attempt to reduce tension and to avoid dealing directly with a problem or an issue (Cain, 1976, p. 66).

Triangulation has been defined as the by-product of emotional reactivity in a system.

In periods of very high tension and when family triangles have been exhausted, the family system may triangle in outside persons or groups such as neighbors, schools, police, clinics, and social agencies. Family members use these to reduce their own tension. Once they transfer the anxiety to someone else, they are much calmer.

It is also important to realize that, although the third side of a triangle is usually filled by a person, it is not uncommon for an issue (alcoholism, discipline, money), an object (pet, car, boat), or a combination of two or more persons (in-laws, own parents) to form the third side of the triangle.

Family Projection Process

The classic example of a triangle is the one that occurs in the family projection process. The basic pattern involves a mother whose emotional system is directed more toward her children than toward her husband, and a father who recognizes his wife's anxiety and supports her emotional involvement with the children. The degree of the mother's fusion with the children varies with each child and there is usually one child with whom the fusion is more intense. This is the projected child. The triangle consists of the mother and this child as the close twosome and the father in the distant position. The end result of this process is the emotional impairment of the child.

Minuchin (1974) has spoken of coalitions and alliances. As stated previously, a coalition is a situation in which two or more family members have a special bond or alliance that excludes or is different from other relationships within the family network. A triangle is a specific type of coalitionary process that becomes a problem when there is a disturbance between two people that is handled by bringing in a third person or an issue to defuse the anxiety. Whenever a triangle is formed under these circumstances, there is less chance of the original problem being resolved and the disturbance will eventually intensify. Developing a sense of patterns in the family is the key to understanding family triangles and how they operate. Triangles are an extremely important part of family structure.

Sibling Position

The last Bowen Theory concept to be discussed in terms of family structure is the theory of sibling position. This theory was developed by Toman (1976) who has written extensively about his research results, particularly in his book *Family Constellation.*

Essentially, Toman's theory depends on the combination of only two things: the sex and age ranks of all the persons in one's immediate family. Toman believes in a duplication theorem, i.e., that the kinds of persons one chooses as spouses, friends, and partners of any kind will be determined by the kinds of persons one has lived with the longest and most intimately. He also believes that the more complete the duplication is, the greater the chance that the relationship will last and be happy. Family constellations are viewed as systems which are influenced by preceding generations and which interact with subsequent generations. The theory is based on the belief that the early family represents the most important context of life and that the family exerts its influence earlier, more regularly, and more extensively than any other cultural system.

Sibling positions are viewed as roles that a person has learned in the family and tends to assume in situations outside the family. On the basis of his research, Toman has found that sibling positions and family configurations imply certain behavior trends, personality traits, and social inclinations. He has developed eight basic sibling positions plus the position of the only child and twins. They are:

1 The oldest brother of brother(s)
2 The youngest brother of brother(s)
3 The oldest brother of sister(s)
4 The youngest brother of sister(s)
5 The oldest sister of sister(s)
6 The youngest sister of sister(s)
7 The oldest sister of brother(s)
8 The youngest sister of brother(s)

Each of these positions in the family carries a certain description of behavior characteristics. The profiles permit knowledge of any sibling, thereby giving the helping person a presumptive knowledge about various family members. Various family systems theorists have found that their observations of families have supported Toman's theory, with the reservation that it does not take the family projection process and strong triangles into consideration. The basic theory of sibling positions has been incorporated into Bowen's Theory and is considered among the eight basic concepts.

To arrive at a sibling-configuration analysis of a person, one establishes sibling position in terms of sex and rank. If Toman's descriptions do not fit, certain questions may be asked to explain the discrepancy. Some of these are:

1 Have you discounted any siblings who are either 6 years younger or older? More than 6 years difference is equivalent to an only child. The farther apart in age two siblings are, the more distant their relationship will be and the less influence they will have on one another.

2 Have you noted if the person's brothers and sisters formed subgroups? The more children there are in the family, the more likely they are to cluster in subgroups. The oldest and the youngest of these subgroups could have the traits of an oldest or youngest sibling in the family even though they are not in that position in the total family constellation.

3 Have you considered any special events that might make a difference, particularly separations and losses? Losses can be temporary losses or more severe permanent ones. Losing a parent when one is under 16 and losing a sibling when one is 6 years or older are both considered severe losses. Also the smaller the family, the greater the loss of a member is felt.

4 Have you inquired into the sibling positions and losses of the person's parents? Toman's configurations are based on patterns of identification with the same-sex parent and patterns of direct relationships with the opposite-sex parent.

Toman looks at certain attitudes in each basic sibling position such as attitudes toward work, property, same- and opposite-sex friends, children, politics, religion, philosophy, and losses. All this information is very useful when trying to obtain a complete picture of the entire family system, i.e., the structure of the family.

CLINICAL EXAMPLE: ENMESHMENT AND PROJECTION IN A CENTRALIZED FAMILY SYSTEM (Minuchin Structural Therapy)

Mrs. Verita Evans, aged 34 years, was a heavy-set but attractive black woman who had lived in a Northern city for about 10 years. She grew up in the rural South and married her only legal spouse when she was 16. John Evans, like Verita, was a teenager at the time of marriage. Within the space of 3 years they were the parents of Rosalinda, Marchon, and Ruby. The problems of providing for a wife, two daughters, and a son had been overwhelming for John, who had deserted them nearly 15 years earlier and had not been heard from since.

Because it was the only work available, Verita began working in the field, harvesting whatever was ripe for picking. When the children were old enough to help her, Verita joined a group of migrant farm workers who moved North or South following the crops. Her hard work enabled the family to survive, but the migrant life did not satisfy Verita, who wanted a better life for herself and her children. One year, instead of returning South for the winter, she decided to stay in the North and find work. Although uneducated, Verita had great reserves of determination and physical strength. There were many bad times, but eventually she obtained a job as short-order cook in a diner located in a factory district. Here her stamina and cooking skills were recognized. She found herself steadily employed at a job she enjoyed. Best of all, Verita was able to stay in one place and send her children to school every day. In time she acquired a male friend, but her work was not interrupted even by the birth of her youngest children, Anne and Elizabeth.

After the twin girls were born, Verita sent for her own mother who was still in the South. The grandmother moved in to help with the babies so Verita could continue working. Ambitious for herself, Verita was trying by sheer willpower to counteract the effects of a deteriorating neighborhood and of companions for her children who were less disciplined than they. None of her children had ever been in serious trouble, and Marchon sometimes said jokingly that he was more afraid of his mother than he was of the police.

The day her oldest child, Rosalinda, graduated from high school was the proudest of Verita's life. Although the girl hinted that she would like to work in a store or office, Verita decided that Rosalinda should take advantage of the educational opportunities which were opening for blacks and begin college in the fall. Rosalinda began college with a new wardrobe and with no enthusiasm. She was able to express some doubts and fears to her younger sister, Ruby, who advised that it was always better to do what Momma wanted. Both girls were somewhat apprehensive of their mother's moods, but were also aware of her protection through the years when she battled school and neighborhood on their behalf.

Before the first college semester was over Rosalinda began to suffer mysterious headaches. Her usual good humor gave way to long periods of silence. Attendance at college was interrupted by headaches that responded to no medication and for which no physical cause could be found. Rosalinda had been a family favorite, cheerful and fun-loving. Now she stayed in bed all day, refused to answer when spoken to, come to meals, or enter into any interaction with her mother, who became worried and angry. One evening when Verita entered her daughter's room, Rosalinda was lying in bed pulling wildly at her hair, and yelling incoherently about headaches that never went away and "things" that were always after her. Frightened, Verita held her daughter and stroked the girl until she calmed down. The next day Rosalinda could not recall the incident, but Verita stayed home from work to take her daughter to a neighborhood physician. The physician concurred with Verita's diagnosis that Rosalinda was having a nervous breakdown and referred them to a mental health clinic.

The clinic intake worker suggested that the whole family attend the first session. Noteworthy was the exceedingly good behavior of Anne and Elizabeth who sat quietly as the others talked. The older children, including Rosalinda, expressed the greatest devotion to Verita. Grandma joined the chorus of tributes, but toward the end of the meeting Marchon and Grandma criticized Rosalinda for bringing so much trouble to the family.

In subsequent sessions only Verita and the older children were asked to attend. The therapist began subtly to align with the identified patient, Rosalinda, without undermining the tremendous accomplishments of Verita. It was apparent that through somatization and hysterical behaviors Rosalinda was enacting a process of differentiation from her mother, in which Marchon and Ruby would also need to engage. The goal of therapy was to introduce changes into a system which had been historically appropriate but was now threatened by the centralizing force which previously sustained it. The dominance of Verita had to be reduced in the lives of the older children without diminishing the regard in which she was held and which she needed.

Much attention was paid to the rapid progress the family had made in one short generation. Verita's upward aspirations were praised, but it was also suggested that attending college was not what Rosalinda wanted. With support from the therapist Rosalinda was able to talk about some of the awkward experiences she encountered in the strange environment of the college campus. Going to college was not devalued as a goal, but Verita was helped to understand that it would not be Rosalinda who would fulfill this dream. The mother was asked to listen to the hopes and feelings of the children without imposing her own ambitions on them. As a result of the meetings Verita gradually became more willing to defer her goal of giving her children a college education until a child or grandchild showed a similar ambition.

Assessment

Structure   The family was a centralized system in which Verita played the major operational role. She was enmeshed in the lives of her children, projecting her hopes and ambitions upon them, particularly on her oldest daughter with whom she closely identified.

Function   Verita had succeeded in overcoming her impoverished background, and had learned values appropriate to the new environment where she lived. However, she had not totally separated from her own mother, and had arranged for her mother to join the family as soon as it was economically feasible. Even though Verita's family was prospering and the children were succeeding at school,

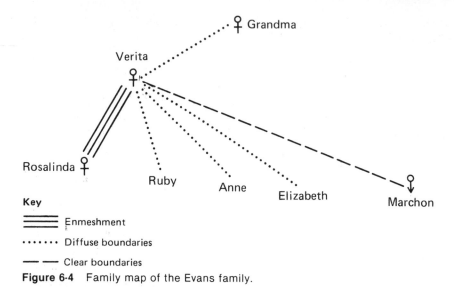

Figure 6-4   Family map of the Evans family.

the members did not see themselves as separate entities. All the daughters were fused to their mother, were excessively dependent on her, and functioned at a high level of tension (see Figure 6-4).

Intervention

Rosalinda's symptoms were an effort to communicate her distress in a way the family would accept. If she became physically or emotionally ill, then she might drop out of college without challenging her mother or disappointing the family. Therapeutic intervention consisted of establishing role-appropriate behaviors for the older children, encouraging them to express their feelings verbally, and enabling Verita to listen. The readiness of the children to assume mature, adult behaviors was interpreted as testimony of Verita's fine mothering. At the same time she was helped to see her adolescent children not as threats to her authority but as family resources that she had helped form and to whom she could now turn for support. Rosalinda withdrew from college with her mother's consent and began a short typing course which she felt competent to complete. Another result of the family meetings was the formation of a coalition between the three older children which had not previously existed because of massive sibling rivalry for Verita's favor.

SUMMARY

This chapter has presented concepts related to the assessment of structure in family systems. The need to observe a family closely for sustained periods of time was noted as essential to accurate assessment. The detailed family history, the family diagram, and the family map were described as useful tools in assessing family structure.

Some general systems theory concepts were directly applied to the family. The characteristics of systems in general and family systems in particular were discussed. Differences between open and closed systems were identified. Concepts from Minuchin's structural family theory were included, among them the family map, boundary clarity, family subsystems, coalitions, and alliances.

Concepts of the Bowen Theory of family structure were described. These included the nuclear family emotional system, differentiation of self, triangles, and family projection processes. The work of Toman as it enhances the Bowen Theory on the concept of sibling position was also discussed.

REFERENCES

Anonymous. Toward the differentiation of self in one's family of origin. In J. Framo (Ed.), *Family interaction.* New York: Springer, 1972.

Bowen, M. Theory in the practice of psychotherapy. In P. Guerin (Ed.), *Family therapy.* New York: Gardner Press, 1976.

Bowen, M. Family and family group psychotherapy. In H. I. Kaplan & B. J. Sadock (Eds)., *Comprehensive group psychotherapy.* Baltimore: Williams & Wilkins, 1971.

Bowen, M. Toward the differentiation of self in one's family of origin. In Andres & Lorio (Eds.), *Georgetown family symposia: a collection of selected papers.* (Vol. 1). Washington, D.C.: Georgetown University, 1974.

Cain, A. The role of the therapist in family systems therapy. *The family,* 1976, 3(2), 65-72.

Jackson, D., & Lederer, W. *The mirages of marriage.* New York: Norton, 1968.

Minuchin, S. *Families and family therapy.* Cambridge, Mass.: Harvard University Press, 1974.

Toman, W. *Family constellation.* New York: Springer, 1976.

Webster's new world dictionary. Cleveland: Collins & World, 1976.

Chapter 7

Assessment of
Family Function

Ellen H. Janosik
Jean R. Miller

Family theorists have drawn upon many disciplines to formulate useful concepts for the assessment of family systems. Anthropologists, historians,
sociologists, psychologists, and psychiatrists have made major contributions to the expanding body of family theory, and their contributions often
reveal commonalities in family life which transcend interdisciplinary bias. A
common denominator is that families are functioning systems; however, it
must be remembered that no family configuration exactly replicates a prototype. This means that each family's functioning is unique to that system,
reflecting idiosyncratic choices, struggles, and compromises.

For the purposes of the health practitioner is is probably more helpful
to explain differences in the ways individual families function than to
describe a prevailing cultural norm. The following considerations are relevant to the assessment of function in an individual family.

   1 Does the family function in conflict or harmony, and to what
extent?
   2 How attached, or bonded, are family members, and what are the
causes and effects of bonding?

3   How does the family reach decisions and allocate tasks, and to what extent?

4   Are family roles enacted adequately and family rules clearly defined?

5   How do family communication patterns affect family functioning?

Structural family concepts are less dynamic than concepts which apply to family functioning. When the foregoing questions are applied to assessment of function, they allow data to be organized in a coherent form while conveying some understanding that family function is not static (Burgess, 1976).

FAMILY CONFLICT AND FAMILY HARMONY

Family functioning may be accompanied by habitual conflict or habitual harmony. Family conflict differs from disagreement or opposition among family members. Conflict is marked by a wish to hurt the person holding opposing views, and the wish to hurt may be more compelling than the wish to reach agreement. Thus, conflict in families impairs decision making and effective negotiation. Paradoxically, conflict flares up most frequently between individuals who are bonded in some way and is rarely a problem between those who are indifferent to one another. Family conflicts arise from the desire to protect oneself from attack combined with the urge to undermine the self-esteem of the adversary. When conflict between family members escalates to the point at which bonds are threatened, there follows greater willingness to see value in the opposing viewpoint. Conflict resolution can then be achieved and the strength of bonding endures.

The resolution of conflict differs qualitatively from the resolution of disagreement, and sometimes assumes maladaptive forms. Disagreement resolution means that all debate is seriously considered, and that debate tends not to be tangential (Turner, 1970). Conflict resolution, on the other hand, may not include the negotiation of substantive issues. In conflict resolution there may be no agreement, but insults must nevertheless be discounted and accusations made in the heat of conflict must be dismissed. Greater rationality accompanies the resolution of disagreement, and issues are more often faced and decided than in the case of conflict resolution, which is not always marked by genuine agreement between the protagonists.

While it would be inaccurate to state that conflict behaviors are totally irrational, they are nevertheless characterized by high levels of emotional reactivity. Often there is adherence to a flight-fight pattern of behavior. Because of attachments between family members some degree of conflict is almost inevitable. In classifying family conflict, Turner (1970) employed the following typology.

1 *Chronic conflict* This is conflict which is recurrent in the family but which does not greatly alter or destroy relationships. In dealing with chronic conflict it is less important to investigate the precursors than to observe the consequences and aftermath.

2 *Episodic conflict* This type of conflict occurs over and over again, but alternates with periods of harmony during which family members live peaceably together. In dealing with episodic conflict, attention may justifiably be directed to precipitating events which repeatedly lead to conflict situations.

3 *Cumulative conflict* This type of conflict is very disruptive to the family. Since family bonds can deter conflict, cumulative conflict may signal tenuous bonding. Unlike chronic conflict, cumulative conflict is not followed by reconciliation or forgiveness, but continues unabated and uninterrupted.

Conflicts in families may be dealt with in several ways, but the practitioner must be aware of the family's preferred method of functioning. Some dysfunctional families manage accommodation between protagonists without ever solving the problem, except in respect to family equilibrium. In accommodation, conflict is abandoned without a resolution of the issues. Because they are unsuccessful in altering divergent views, the protagonists merely agree not to disagree.

Another form of conflict resolution involves conciliation between the participants. As in accommodation, there is no settlement of opposing views, but further attacks on other family members are discontinued. Apologies are offered and accepted. The participants do not change their opinions, but, for the good of the family, the conflictual behaviors of the protagonists are reinterpreted and explained away.

Observing and assessing family conflict patterns is not easy for the practitioner. There is an ever-present danger of being pulled into the family conflict, and of being persuaded to support one member at the expense of others. These hazards may be reduced if the practitioner recognizes habitual patterns of conflict resolution in the family. At the same time the practitioner may derive comfort from knowing that, while family bonds predispose to conflict, the same bonds may effect conflict resolution. When conflict reaches the stage of endangering family bonds, either conciliation or accommodation may be sought by the participants. If only accommodation is achieved, a reassessment of the contested issue may follow. One or another of the participants may engage in prolonged reexamination of the situation. There may be a reenactment in the imagination of the conflict or the issue may be raised again. Fantasized reenactment of the issue reduces the impetus toward realistic problem solving. A desire for reconciliation rather than for the solution of problems usually dominates the thinking of adversaries who engage in imaginative reenactment of the conflict (Turner, 1970).

CAUSES AND EFFECTS OF FAMILY BONDING

Family bonds are emotional ties or attachments which draw and hold families together. In the preceding discussion, family bonds were identified as both precipitants and ameliorators of conflict. Because bonding greatly affects the quality of family life, the assessment of family function necessitates some consideration of the nature and extent of bonding. Some types of family bonds seem to be especially vulnerable to the stresses of conflict, although it is quite possible for bonding and conflict to exist side by side. As has been stated, family bonds may predispose to conflict while simultaneously assisting in its resolution.

When conflict continues for extended periods of time, families become accustomed to and even dependent on it. Various members develop complementary roles in relation to conflict. A counterdependent member may learn to define his or her own strength through the weakness of other members. The shortcomings of one member may be frowned upon, even as they increase other members' feelings of virtue. Bonds may be taken for granted by family members, so that alterations in bonding are not always immediately apparent in the family. An observant practitioner will be attentive to such alterations, and a comprehensive assessment of family function will include historical and current attachments in the system.

Changes in family bonding are illustrated in the following example. A couple was drawn together through a shared interest in music, art, and drama, which led ultimately to marriage and to rewarding social and sexual gratification. In a year or so a child was born to the couple, and the advent of parenthood drastically changed the nature of family bonding. Confined at home with the child, the wife no longer had the time or the opportunity to pursue the artistic interests which had first established bonds between the partners. Immediately after the birth of the child, parenting became the major task of the wife, who felt restricted and neglected as a result. However, as the child became more active and appealing, the bonds between father and child strengthened. With the deepening of the father's interest in the child, different bonds were formed between husband and wife. Their shared interest in artistic endeavor was put aside temporarily to be replaced by new bonds between themselves as parents, and toward the child as a shared source of joy and responsibility. New parents often sense that their relationship has been altered, but do not attribute this to changes in bonding.

When family bonding is adaptive, shared values and family consensus are maintained. Although family members may not be consciously aware of bonding, the health practitioner is advised to include in the assessment extensive data related to family bonding over time. In family assessment one cannot safely ignore the dynamic nature of family bonding. Many bonds are transitory, especially those formed between the partners before or just after marriage. Even bonds between parents and children, while far from ephemeral, have variable tensile durability. Family bonds are sensitive to conflict, especially chronic or cumulative conflict. Attenuation of family bonds may continue even after conflict is resolved unless new bonds are established. The erosion of bonds without suitable replacement in the form of new attachments reduces a family's ability to resolve conflict, makes the children uneasy, and makes the marital partners more likely to search for alternative bonds outside the family system.

DECISION MAKING AND TASK ALLOCATION

Family function takes place at several levels, with interactive and reactive forces constantly at work. A critical element of family life is the functionality of the parental coalition, since this is the means through which the major needs of parents and children are met. If its decision making and task allocation deviate greatly from the mores of the surrounding community, a family may suffer maladjustment of one sort or another.

To appraise family functions, a health practitioner requires a theoretical structure that describes what is being observed. Jackson (1976) proposed that family transactions constitute one such framework, and that quid pro quo is a versatile construct to employ. *Quid pro quo* means that everyone receives something in return for something else, and that no one gets anything for nothing. Task allocation based on quid pro quo can apply to virtually every family transaction, prescribing the rights and duties of the persons who comprise the marital dyad and family subsystems. By means of quid pro quo a pattern is maintained which delineates the contributions of family members and distributes tasks.

Quid pro quo exchanges are often, but not always, adaptive. An example of adaptive quid pro quo may be found in a stable, traditional family which delegates instrumental leadership to the husband and expressive leadership to the wife. This use of quid pro quo preserves a balance which is culturally sanctioned and acceptable to all members of the family.

In dysfunctional families the quid pro quo process implies that there is collusion which perpetuates maladaptive behaviors. A typical example is the trade-off between abusive husbands and battered wives; both partners are debased, but the interaction is collaboratively maintained. Similarly, the protective but punitive attitudes of a nondrinking spouse may be part of a quid pro quo transaction. The nondrinking spouse enjoys social approbation and dominance, while the weakened but protected alcoholic continues drinking. A delinquent child who craves attention and acts out a parent's antisocial fantasies provides still another illustration of quid pro quo. In general, the assessment of family structure relies heavily on distinctions based on age, status, position, and gender. Many structural distinctions have become blurred in recent years. The quid pro quo construct is an excellent tool for assessing function in families in which role flexibility and role reversal go beyond structural boundaries. Having first observed the presence of quid pro quo in family transactions, the practitioner may begin to gauge the adaptiveness of the process and the wisdom of attempting to modify it.

When quid pro quo operates to the advantage of family members, the system is functioning well. Attention must be given to family equilibrium, particularly if the anxiety level of family members is not high or if there is little desire for change. Unless family members are somewhat motivated, a practitioner must weigh carefully the cost of intervention in systems which are in a state of equilibrium. If, on the other hand, the exchange is detrimental to any member, this is an inducement to intervene.

A literary example of disequilibrium that followed years of family adjustment can be found in Ibsen's play, *A Doll's House,* in which the quid pro quo rule is eventually challenged by the maturing heroine. Previously content, Nora, the doll wife, finally grows dissatisfied with her transactions with her bourgeois husband. There follows the transformation of Nora, the disillusionment of her husband, and the disruption of family equilibrium (Pittman & Flomenhaft, 1972).

To summarize, quid pro quo is a family arrangement in which the behaviors of family members are influenced by an unspoken bargain negotiated by the principals. The advantages of the construct are that (1) it helps the practitioner analyze family interactions in a meaningful way; (2) it enables the practitioner to identify and describe some rules of family relationships; and (3) it enhances the practitioner's ability to predict family interactional patterns (Jackson, 1976).

FAMILY ROLE ENACTMENT

Like any small group, a family has a normative system which governs its interactions. The normative system develops out of family rules and roles, becoming in effect a network of duties and expectations that support family functioning. Through the normative system, agreement concerning the obligations and rights of family members is sustained. As the primary group of society, families depend on roles and rules to maintain their operations. In assessing family operations through role enactment the following chronology may be helpful.

1   Bonds or attachments between members organize individuals into families, and help families to survive.
2   Family interactions, whether harmonious or conflicted, define and implement family decisions.
3   Family decisions and the way in which they are carried out form patterns of interaction which profoundly affect all family members.

4 Patterns formed by successive family interactions determine how roles are enacted and rules enforced.

Formal (*ascribed*) role enactment involves a cluster of activities normatively assigned to the role. Informal (*achieved*) role enactment includes acting as family peacemaker, aggressor, negotiator, cheerleader, or pessimist. Two concepts found in role theory are the differentiation of roles and the distribution of roles. *Role differentiation* arranges role activities into configurations which restrict what the enactor does or does not do. *Role allocation* or *distribution* designates particular persons for particular actions, thus creating role specialization.

Role enactment affects the way in which a family accomplishes necessary functions. Some families thoroughly articulate role enactment and operate with much efficiency and little hesitation. In other families, role enactment is accompanied by emotional outbursts of affection or of anger. Whether role enactment proceeds cognitively or affectively, with dispatch or procrastination, it influences the whole texture of family life.

Role inadequacy in a family member may cause disruption even when role conflict is not overt. Conversely, role adequacy may not always engender harmony, unless the adequacy is acceptable to the family system. A competent wife and mother whose role enactment is adequate may become frustrated if her role performance is unacknowledged or unmatched by a husband whose role performance is ineffectual. Or an ambitious, hard-driving father may be disappointed by the role enactment of an indolent wife, or that of children incapable of social or academic success.

Role consonance (or consensus) predisposes to family equilibrium because there is compatibility among family members. Compatibility means that parents agree about their respective roles and that the children do not unduly reject the values of the parents. A viable role system depends on consensus, role reciprocity, functional role enactment, and a normative system which is stable yet flexible. All these considerations are important in assessing the nature of family functioning.

Any group normatively defines role enactment but, within the group, members may have somewhat dissimilar role expectations. This causes a normative role system to coexist with a behavioral system which deviates from accepted norms. To the assessment of the normative system (what should be done and by whom), the practitioner must add an assessment of the behavioral system (what is being done, who does it, and how it is done) (Nye & Gegas, 1976).

A discrepancy between what is being done in the family and what should be done represents the difference between the family normative system and the behavioral system. Any such discrepancy is worth including in the assessment of family function because it is a potential source of dissension and disappointment within the system. A related factor in assessing function is the ratio of shared role enactment to segregated role enactment. Since a majority of wives and mothers now work outside the home, the father is no longer the only family provider. Working women increasingly expect husbands to assume a share of the nurturing and housework that were formerly the responsibility of the wife and mother. Because of changed social acceptability, shared role enactment is conducive to satisfactory levels of family functioning (Nye, 1976). Undoubtedly there is greater equality and sharing in some families than in others. LeMasters (1974) commented that parental role enactment resembles life in the armed forces in that some individuals volunteer for service while others must be drafted. Obviously, the voluntary aspect of shared role enactment is an important but hard-to-assess dimension.

Blood and Wolfe (1960) offered the "resource theory," which maintained that the dominance of one partner over another was a function of greater competence. This is an amplification of exchange theory, which speculates that the more one is rewarded by a partner, the more compliant one becomes. In this context the term *resource* describes any gratification that one spouse offers the other. The practitioner may wish to compare the relative competence of the partners in bestowing gratification so as to understand the locus of power in the family.

Basic to resource theory is the idea that competent role enactment by one partner gratifies the other. Role competence may therefore be a valid indicator of marital satisfaction. Bernard (1973) states that for each couple there are two marriages, one as experienced by the husband and a second as experienced by the wife. Even with this cautionary note, exchange theory, with its cost-reward ratio, can be adapted for the purpose of appraising family function.

COMMUNICATION

The processes of bonding, conflict/harmony, decision making, task allocation, role enactment, and rule delineation are accomplished through family communication. Families are ongoing interactional systems in which information is transferred between members and between the family and other systems. When barriers to the transfer of information exist, problems are likely to occur in the above processes.

Problems in family functioning can be detected by observing family interaction. Opportunities for observing natural interaction patterns unobtrusively occur during hospital visiting hours or home visits. Ease of conversation is more difficult for persons under direct observation in clinical settings; however, patterns of interaction are likely to remain the same no matter what the setting. Regardless of the way observations are made, families seeking professional assistance can be helped to interact naturally through selected questions and tasks.

One way of assessing the various aspects of functioning, including interactional patterns, is to ask families to describe the chronological development of their problem(s). Questions such as the following can be introduced.

1 What is the sequence of events which led to the problem?
2 How did you feel at each of these times?
3 What might you have done differently?

All members should be encouraged to describe their perception of the problem so that assessments can be made of every feasible interaction pattern within the family. Equifinality in the family system should assure the practitioner that patterns of interaction remain the same regardless of the vantage point from which the problems are approached.

Another method of generating family interaction is through the *simulation of tasks,* which can then be categorized as problem-solving, decision-making, conflict-resolution, and naturalistic tasks. Tasks should be selected on the basis of their relevance to issues which typically occur in families. The more closely tasks simulate real life experiences, the more likely the elicited behavior will be typical of family interactions. Problem-solving tasks are least likely to elicit typical behavior because of the game aspect of the tasks. In addition, family members tend to respond to the situation posed by the task rather than to one another. Decision-making tasks have slightly more relevance to real problems, since the tasks force the family to reach decisions by working together. Conflict-resolution and naturalistic tasks have the highest relevance because they stimulate family reactions which resemble typical behavior under stress. Observing naturalistic tasks such as conversations at mealtime also provides excellent data, but this simulation is not often used for both practical and economic reasons.

Several methods can be used to obtain ideas for simulated tasks. The health professional might ask families for examples of conflicts they have had trouble resolving, and then ask the family to deal with the conflict in the clinical setting. Specific simulated tasks have been developed and tested by researchers; descriptions of the tasks, along with the validity and reliability of the measures, can be found in the literature. Cromwell, Olson, and Fournier (1976) have classified these according to the nature of the task and whether the tasks were designed for marital dyads, partial families, or whole families.

Clinical facilities often dictate the manner in which families can be observed performing tasks. The goal is to provide a setting in which the most typical interaction can occur. A practitioner may choose to remain in the periphery in the same room or to observe through a one-way glass. In many instances it is preferable to leave the family alone and to record their interactions by means of an audio tape recorder or video camera. Families initially are inhibited by these devices but in most instances adjust quickly and begin to interact naturally.

Analyzing family interactions is a complex process. One systematic approach is to study the interactional process of who does what to whom, with whom, and after whom. For example, the practitioner might ask the family to discuss how they reach routine decisions. This process could be observed by using a simulated decision-making task. The focus of observation would be on the interpersonal processes which impede or enhance the parts played by each member in fulfilling the requirements of the task. The flow of conversation during the process could be checked for logic and relevance.

Practitioners often find the content of interactions helpful in assessing family problems. The focus of conversation usually follows a primary theme in healthy families. In problematic families conversation may shift from primary to secondary themes or be wholly diffused. In other problematic families residual fragments of a common theme may emerge, so that the content of the present interaction is not addressed.

Style of communication refers to the manner in which families express their thoughts. This also is subject to analysis. The emotional tones or feelings that accompany verbal expression give the practitioner an estimate of family affective involvement. Style of communication should be assessed in light of a family's ethnic background, social-class norms, and the positions of individual family members.

Finally, a common method for analyzing family interaction is the use of *outcome scores*. This method is often used by researchers, since scores are obtained by counting the number of times family members interact in a certain way. Examples of variables that can be measured are the number of times that messages are unclear, and the number of times that spontaneous agreement, tension, or dominance can be observed. Decisions on the method to be used in assessing family interaction should be based on the purpose of the assessment, the nature of available facilities for observing families, and the skill of the practitioner in analyzing the data.

An evaluative review of family interaction research by Riskin and Faunce (1972) revealed differences in interactional patterns between normal and abnormal family functioning. Disturbed families are likely to show a high degree of fragmentation and a lack of clarity in their interactions with one another. This is particularly true in families with a schizophrenic member. Seriously troubled families seem chaotic in their cognitive and behavioral patterns. Role confusion and role reversal often occur in families under stress. Healthy families tend to laugh and use humor more often than troubled families. Family disagreement is not to be confused with family argument; disagreement is indicative of high stress levels while argument may be a stress-releasing mechanism which can be used to clarify issues or to negotiate differences.

CLINICAL EXAMPLE: DYSFUNCTIONAL
COMMUNICATION IN A FAMILY SYSTEM

The Sherwoods owned and operated a "mom and pop" grocery store in a middle-sized Ohio town. The store was fairly prosperous; the income from it had supported Dora, Ben, and their five children for many years. The children were Jim, Dave, Bess, Al, and Benjie, whose ages ranged from 10 to 18 years. The grocery store was open for business 14 hours a day, 6 days a week. These long hours demanded a great deal from Dora and Ben, but they were accustomed to hard work. For years the family had lived above the store and Dora would steal a few hours from the business to fix meals and take care of the home. Ben was a diabetic who required a restricted menu, and this took more of Dora's time.

When the children were growing up they loved to spend time in the store waiting on customers and putting stock away. In the evenings they would do their homework upstairs while Dora and Ben worked in the store. Some years before the referral, when Ben was 40, a large crate had fallen on his foot, crushing it severely. Because of his diabetes and his premature return to work, an infection set in which necessitated an amputation. During Ben's convalescence the family combined forces to keep the store open. The three older children got up early to open the store and arranged shifts to help Dora in the afternoons and evenings. This emergency period lasted 6 months, after which Ben returned to the store, functioning well for several years. During Ben's convalescence, Jim entered college, Dave and Bess were in high school, Al attended junior high, and Benjie was in elementary school.

The disengagement of the children from the business was so gradual that for a time Dora and Ben were not aware of change. At first they were only conscious of being more tired at night; then Ben began to complain of his throbbing stump. Because the Sherwood children were handsome and popular, they were much in demand. School activities became all-engrossing for the older three, and the store seemed dull by comparison. Before long Dora and Ben were getting little help, except from Benjie, who was willing to help out now and then. Ben, who had to endure the discomfort of a prosthesis, alternated between anger and bitterness. He had always been the decision maker in the family, proud of being bigger and stronger than his sons. Dora was the family placator, pleading the case for Ben when he was too hard on the children and making excuses for them when he was angry.

Ben was angry most of the time now. He raged at Dora when none of the children came in to the store to help, but was unable to admit to his sons that he could not do as much as he used to do. After one of Ben's outbursts, Dora would ask the children at supper to come and help the next day. This request invariably caused an argument among the three older children about who was the busiest and who should help. The argument never failed to enrage Ben, who would shout angrily that he didn't need any of them, whereupon Dora, the peace-maker, would explain that the store wasn't so busy right now and may-be they could manage without help. After the parents retired for the night, the older children would vent their feelings on each other and on "the damn store," which they were sick of hearing about. In the bedroom, as Dora attended to Ben's inflamed stump, her husband would berate her for producing such ungrateful children. The two youngest boys would huddle near the television set, trying to ignore the quarreling, feeling miserable and resolving never to be as selfish as their older brothers and sister.

Things went on like this for over a year. The only discernible change was that Ben stopped berating the children, and turned surly and taciturn in their presence. Dora's agitation increased as she moved between her popular, successful children and her bitter hus-band. Attending to Ben's bad leg was now a nightly ritual of bathing, massaging, and dressing the stump. She suggested once that they might shorten their work week but this set Ben off on a tirade against his lazy children and against Dora for spoiling them.

Ben had little faith in physicians. He followed his diabetic diet as prepared by Dora and depended on her to take care of his leg. In time, however, even her careful ministrations proved inadequate. The flesh around the stump broke down, becoming dark and odoriferous. Only then did Ben agree to see a physician. He was hospitalized for several weeks and for a time further amputation of his leg was contemplated. In conversations with their physician Dora and Ben revealed the dif-ficulties in the family. A referral was made to the family nurse-practi-tioner who would be assuming responsibility for Ben's primary care after discharge from the hospital. After meeting once with the couple, the nurse-practitioner suggested that family counseling might be helpful. All five children were invited, and were willing to attend.

Assessment

Structure   As a couple Dora and Ben were in the child-rearing stage with their younger sons and the launching stage with their older children. They had begun their married life during the depression and had been quite poor at first. Through the years their hard work in the store had made the family prosperous. The business had benefited from the contributions of the three older children, who had worked willingly beside their parents; now, however, they were involved in their own tasks of individuation and separation from the family. The youngest boys still helped the parents, but their efforts were not enough to compensate for Ben's disability and Dora's waning energy. As a result of these changes in the system, a family which had func-tioned well for years was now functioning poorly. The parents were isolated from each other and from their older children. The two sibling subsystems were separate: the three older children felt guilty and resentful while the two younger ones felt helpless.

Function Despite the problems in the family strong bonds existed between the members. Dora, who could not tolerate dissension, passively endured the recriminations of her husband and the indifference of her children. Ben wanted and needed help but never asked for it directly. There was no clear request to the children to work in the store for a stated number of hours, nor to distribute working hours equitably so that no one was seriously inconvenienced. What had happened was that, as the children matured, old rules were discarded but new rules were not clearly defined.

To Ben the store was a symbol of his role as provider and decision maker, and reducing business hours meant the erosion of his manhood, even though the family's financial condition no longer required such long hours. Seeing his sons mature made Ben feel old and helpless. He wanted to lean on his sons, but thought they should help without being asked. The children, engrossed in their own lives, feared being engulfed by the business. As a result, they manipulated in order to avoid helping in the store.

Intervention

1   Ben needed to separate his sense of identity from the business and to realize that it was no longer necessary to work himself and Dora into exhaustion. The first step in the family meetings was to reduce the business hours to a reasonable amount. All the children, particularly the older ones, were involved in this negotiation.

2   Ben's reward for reducing the store hours was a written commitment from each of the older children to give 8 hours a week to the store. The younger boys promised to work 5 hours a week. In addition, a part-time helper was to be employed on Saturdays, so that the children would be free on weekends.

3   Since schedule conflicts were bound to arise, the family was given the simulated task of looking for solutions in such situations. The following procedure was devised. When a child could not work a designated time in the store, that child was responsible for providing a substitute. A sibling might substitute, in which case the time given became a debt to be repaid later. The right of each member to have activities outside the home would be respected, and individual priorities given due consideration. However, the 8 hours promised to Ben was a primary obligation which could not be avoided or cancelled without renegotiation. Dora was not to be called upon to work extra hours to make up for the absence of any son or daughter. Ben was to deal directly with the children when he was dissatisfied with them, and not displace his resentment on Dora.

At the family meetings the changing needs of each member were emphasized. This emphasis helped the children see their parents as individuals deserving of consideration.

Communication guidelines were established in which directions were clearly given and rules clearly stated. Change was interpreted as an aspect of life which could be dealt with constructively if communication remained open and feelings were expressed. In this family many positive emotions were experienced but seldom expressed. Members were encouraged to show love and pride in each other's accomplishments and to be less withholding toward one another.

SUMMARY

In this chapter five basic processes were introduced to assess family functioning. These were: (1) family conflict or harmony, (2) bonding, (3) decision making and task allocation, (4) roles and rules, and (5) communication patterns. A typology of family conflict as conceptualized by Turner (1970) was presented, and the influence of each type of conflict on the family system was discussed. Bonding was described as a dynamic process of emotional attachment between family members, a process which is subject to change over time. In the discussion of decision making and task allocation, the concept of quid pro quo was presented. Family roles and family rules were explained as determinants of the family normative system, which supports family functioning.

Communication was explored as the means by which the five basic processes were accomplished, and some observational methods for analyzing family systems were identified. The importance of asking families to describe the chronological development of problems was emphasized. Simulated tasks were recommended as tools to produce family interactions that could be systematically observed by the practitioner.

REFERENCES

Bernard, J. My four revolutions. *American Journal of Sociology,* January 1973, **78**, 773–791.

Blood, R. O., Jr., & Wolfe, D. M. *Husband and wives: The dynamics of married living.* New York: Free Press, 1960.

Burgess, E. W. The family as a unity of interacting personalities. In G. D. Erickson & T. P. Hogan (Eds.), *Family theory: An introduction to theory and technique.* New York: Aaronson, 1976.

Cromwell, R. E., Olson, D. H. L., & Fournier, D. G. Tools and techniques for diagnosis and evaluation in marital and family therapy. *Family Process,* March 1976, **15**(1), 1–49.

Jackson, D. D. Family rules: Marital quid pro quo. In G. D. Erickson & T. P. Hogan (Eds.), *Family theory: An introduction to theory and technique.* New York: Aaronson, 1976.

LeMasters, E. E. *Parenthood in modern America.* Homewood, Ill.: Dorsey Press, 1974.

Nye, I. F., & Gecas, V. The role concept: Review and delineation. In I. F. Nye (Ed.), *Role structure and analysis of the family.* Beverly Hills, Calif.: Sage Publications, 1976.

Pittman, F. S., & Flomenhaft, K. Treating the doll's house marriage. In C. J. Sager & H. S. Kaplan (Eds.), *Progress in group and family therapy.* New York: Brunner/Mazel, 1972.

Riskin, J. & Faunce, E. E. An evaluative review of family interaction research. *Family Process,* December 1972, **11**(4), 365–455.

Turner, R. H. *Family interaction.* New York: Wiley, 1970.

Chapter 8

Establishment of a Family System

Kathleen Kuhn
Ellen H. Janosik

It is extremely important that the health professional assess the organization of the family system before attempting to offer care to any individual member. In order to provide optimum counseling and care, information relevant to the client's past and current life situation must be obtained. Areas of strength and weakness in the individual and in the family which constitutes the support system should be assessed before formulating a therapeutic plan.

The assessment process is not a simple one, because many variables operate simultaneously in the family system. All human beings are in part the products of their families of origin. Whether they elect to replicate the patterns of their original family or to adopt alternative arrangements, most persons have a preference for a particular family style. Despite the differences in family systems, many commonalities exist. This chapter explains some of the mechanisms involved in the establishment of family systems and presents parameters to be used in assessing families and in determining the goals of intervention.

Establishing a family system is usually viewed as the act of creating or founding a family through a sequential process of dating, courtship, and marriage. For the purposes of this chapter, families are defined as legal or extralegal systems with some degree of permanence, which are established through the commitment of members and based upon emotional attachment rather than legality or consanguinity. Any established family organization, whatever its structural components or functional variability, is subject to internal and external tensions, and therefore requires frequent assessment in a time of crisis. Tension in a family system largely results from attachments between its members or subsystems. A family without tensions is a system which is disengaged and usually dysfunctional. When a family is in a state of disequilibrium, levels of tension may become intolerable for the members.

General systems theory provides one framework for analyzing families. This conceptual framework considers all interactions as taking place within systems that have recognizable patterns and rules. Predictable operational patterns help the individual members of a system to maintain their integrity and to achieve certain goals. Systems theory outlines five components or standards by which a family system may be evaluated. These are: (1) structure (who is involved); (2) function (how they are involved); (3) boundaries (what rules govern function); (4) tension (what energy levels are involved); and (5) equilibrium (how the system maintains a steady state). While systems theory provides guidance for assessment, it does not indicate how families are established nor what forces hold individuals within the system.

FAMILY BONDING

The answer to what holds individuals in a family system lies to some extent in the concept of *bonding* (Turner, 1970). A bond exists between individuals or between groups when they have a shared value or a similarity of purpose. Bonds may be temporary and casual, as when a group is addressing a common task, or subtle and profound, as in a long-term dyadic relationship. Before examining family bonding in order to assess a system, the practitioner must comprehend the nature and diversity of the bonds that are present in the family. The practitioner should also realize that bonds, once made, are continually being adapted to the needs of the persons involved and to changes in the environment. Bonds possess the power to contract or expand in response to conditions within and surrounding the family.

The easiest bonds to identify are *membership gratification* bonds. Simply stated, these bonds give an individual a sense of esteem and validation merely through association with a particular group. Much has been written about peer group bonds and their crucial importance during adolescence and early adult life. In many communities, as individuals mature, youthful gratification bonds impel them toward marriage. Because young people observe that married couples are the most influential social group in adult society, most of them are drawn toward membership in this group, whether or not they are ready for marriage or child rearing. Knowledge of this powerful social pressure within the culture can be of great assistance to the practitioner advising a client who is considering marriage but seems doubtful or ambivalent for one reason or another.

A second consequence of membership gratification bonds is the emergence of objectives not directly related to the purposes of the group. For example, an individual may enter a profession not for the work involved, but for the social or monetary rewards associated with that profession. Or a striving young business executive whose company favors married men for promotion may decide to wed for reasons of career expedience, when he is actually unready for marriage.

A danger arises from the fact that membership gratification bonds may not be strong or compelling enough over time. The strength of these bonds depends upon the gratification derived from membership in the chosen group. Such bonds loosen or rupture when the gratification once enjoyed diminishes.

Task bonds are another type of bond which causes families to be established and to survive. These bonds enable individuals to accomplish goals which they might find difficult or impossible to achieve alone. Bonding tasks of families are many and diverse; they include mundane activities such as fixing the evening meal, taking care of the car, or making the social engagements. Sharing such tasks bonds individuals into viable family systems. Less specific tasks with greater emotional overlay also create bonds. Sexual gratification and support for individual ambitions such as education or vocational advancement are less specific tasks which create bonds. While many tasks are discrete and random, the process of task bonding is ongoing and cumulative. In other words, task bonding is less a response to one event than the result of many major and minor events which confer continuity on family interactional patterns.

Both membership gratification bonds and task bonds tend to be formed pragmatically for utilitarian purposes. Where, then, are the emotional needs of persons involved in the bonding process? Part of the answer can be found in the development of appropriately named *person* bonds. The typology of person bonds is dichotomous and consists of *identity* bonds and *response* bonds. Identity bonds are formed when one individual sees in another traits which appear highly desirable or valuable. These perceived traits become the precursers of identity bonds, which may be reciprocal or unilateral. In the latter situation the valued individual does not respond to the appreciation of the other. One individual may identify with another because of appearance, social status, financial assets, or character traits. Classically the identity bond which is not reciprocated by the admired person is known in song and legend as unrequited love.

A person seen as desirable by another may respond in kind. If the response is made in a manner acceptable to the self-concept of the admirer, a response bond will be formed. It can readily be seen that when an identification bond is followed by a response bond, each will strengthen the other. A functional family dyad generally exhibits healthy identification and response bonding. Strong but unhealthy bonds may exist if a partner with little self-esteem forms identity bonds with an individual whose response bonds are expressed in physical or psychological abuse; this response reinforces the low self-image of the first individual.

Crescive bonds are the last category to be reviewed; more than any other type, these are continuity bonds. Other types of bonds may weaken according to circumstances, but crescive bonds become stronger with time. Five types of crescive bonds are discussed here. The first type stems from the amount of time the participants invest in one another or the extent of their shared history. This would include memories and feelings of cohesiveness experienced by members of the family unit. The second type involves the number of planned but uncompleted events in which the family is engaged. When the family system endures, and pervades the life of its members, opportunities for this type of bonding increase. Saving for a car or a vacation home, or planning for the education of children are examples of not yet realized events which contribute to this order of crescive bonding. Uncompleted activities and objectives which are meaningful to more than one family member allow for renewal of crescive bonding in established family systems.

The third type of crescive bonding is the interlocking of roles or interdependence between members. Roles are often described in terms of enactment or performance of overt behaviors, but families often engage in covert role taking which is supportive of the system. Covert roles would include ascribed roles such as the "supportive" member, the "rebellious" member, or the "competent" member. Within the system, members become increasingly dependent on the continuation of these roles. While rigid role enactment promotes homeostasis, it may cause disequilibrium when family members or family circumstances are in need of change.

The responsibility felt toward other members of the family creates the fourth type of crescive bonding. What this entails is concern for the well-being of others arising from the consequences of one's own actions. The fifth and last type of crescive bonding involves communication. This area encompasses subjects which may be discussed within the family system, and the freedom or restrictions surrounding the discussions.

Bonding is a mechanism through which a family is established and maintained. Bonding can occur on many levels and with many people simultaneously. If the bonds between two persons are multiple and strong, a vigorous interactional potential will be present. The individuals involved in the bonding come to depend upon one another in diverse ways, and the resultant system is an interdependent social unit which enables members to meet their needs.

A family system can assume a variety of complex forms. Establishing a family may be a conscious joining with another individual either through the ritual of marriage or through a more loosely structured living arrangement. A single adult may make a conscious or unconscious decision to remain closely connected with the family of origin. Or a conscious or unconscious choice may be made to invest in a relationship other than marriage with another person or group, thus creating a meaningful support system. Occasionally these indefinite relationships are identified as family systems, but more often they are not. Identification problems may result from deliberate efforts by the participants to avoid social censure, as in the family system of a homosexual couple. At times, the conventional stereotype of the family may not readily be applied to the support system an individual has selected. An astute and knowledgeable professional will be able to identify alternative family systems and thus alleviate the distress of clients whose life-style includes unusual models of family organization.

ASSESSMENT OF FAMILY SYSTEM

The comprehensive nature of family assessment means that the professional must utilize effective and sensitive interviewing techniques. Data gathering must be rapid, yet must not be accomplished at the expense of rapport. A nonjudgmental attitude and careful timing are facilitative when sexual, ethnic, or provocative personal problems are being discussed. During the exploratory phase of assessment, a careful application of bonding and systems theory concepts will help the interviewer make an accurate and complete family assessment.

In determining intervention strategy, a health professional may find it relevant to review the major theorists in family work, most of whom conceptualize the family as an interactional unit. From this general premise it follows that intervention should be aimed at changing dysfunctional interactional patterns. Changes in interaction are reflected in the system, whether the structure follows or deviates from conventional forms. The methods selected to alter interactions will vary with the professional and with the exigencies of the system undergoing change. However, the overall goal of intervention is to encourage family members to adopt new modes of interaction and communication. Family patterns are the result of the interplay of structure and function, which in turn represent accommodations between individual needs and system requirements. Because of the influence of structure upon family functioning, several alternative forms of family organization must be considered as new families are established.

THE CHILDLESS MARRIED COUPLE SYSTEM

The married couple without children offers a natural starting point for discussing family systems. The family structure of the legally married dyad consists of husband and wife; their family system is acknowledged by the two participants, the community, and the state. Legal and social recognition of the married couple may have either a positive or negative effect on the system. If, for example, a high cultural value is placed on procreation, the married couple that chooses to be childless may be regarded in some quarters as socially deviant. Childlessness may cause the spouses to spend most of their time together, or conversely, to become involved individually or together with various groups. The career of one or both partners may become an essential feature of the marriage. Other aspects of dyadic function which are affected by childlessness are resources (financial, collateral support networks, coping mechanisms), environment (social, physical, cultural), and communication (quality, quantity, exclusiveness, or inclusiveness).

The rules under which the married couple operates are worthy of attention because rules have the power to sustain or destroy a marriage. The question of procreation is momentous in most marriages. A marital dyad may have been formed in which only one partner is truly committed to the expectation of procreation. The wish to remain childless may be entertained by one of other of the partners. In other situations the partners may be in agreement to remain childless, but have not communicated this decision to their families of origin.

The childlessness of a married couple is rarely without serious ramifications for the partners and their extended families. At times it may be expedient for the practitioner to deal with several factors that impinge on the childless family structure. If the couple desires children but is physically incapable of producing them, one may ask in what ways the roles of husband and wife have changed in order to cope with the unfulfilled hopes of being parents. Has the dyad bonded so as to be all-consuming and protected from peripheral involvement, or have the childless partners diffused their relationship so as to include extended familial or extrafamilial systems? With procreation in dispute, does one partner sabotage the goals of the other in reprisal? If being childless has been a mutual decision and constitutes a dyadic boundary, does the decision not to have children cause intergenerational dissension? In the latter case a voluntarily childless couple may avoid interaction with disapproving parents or engage in intergenerational transactions which are fraught with difficulty.

Tensions within a childless dyadic system often fluctuate, and it is not unusual for one partner to experience crisis around the issue of procreation. When tension mounts in a childless family, the precipitating cause may lie within the system or originate in an external locus. As is common in crisis, the usual coping mechanisms fail and professional intervention may be required. If the bonding mechanism or system functions were marginal before the crisis, it may be necessary to address these deficiencies in the course of crisis intervention. The extent to which dysfunctional patterns can be altered depends on the nature of the procreation crisis and the capacity of the partners for insight. The construction of a hypothetical childless marital system may elucidate the concepts being discussed.

CLINICAL EXAMPLE: THE CHILDLESS DYADIC MARRIAGE

Jim and Lisa were married 4 years ago and are childless. They married during their senior year in college; after graduation Jim entered graduate school and Lisa worked as a teacher to support them. She enjoyed her job and was therefore willing to tolerate the fact that Jim's studies left them little time together. When he finished graduate school and obtained a promising position, Jim believed that he and Lisa were ready to become parents since they now had economic resources to provide for a child. Lisa, on the other hand, was ambivalent about motherhood. She was reluctant to give up her satisfying work and wanted more time before becoming pregnant. In the early years of the marriage Jim had been the dominant decision maker, and Lisa became very anxious over the tension between them because of her hesitation. Believing that their parents would actively support him, Jim announced to his own and to Lisa's parents his eagerness to have a child. As a result both sets of parents offered frequent hints and suggestions to Lisa that she should become pregnant. Their interference infuriated her. She especially resented Jim's actions because the couple had always handled their own problems in the past. Jim also talked to a number of their friends who were parents, in the hope of obtaining information which would overcome Lisa's reluctance. This, too, was considered objectionable by Lisa.

Bonding Analysis

Membership Gratification Bonds   Jim and Lisa both derived considerable gratification from their respective career activities. Jim was delighted to give up his student status. He looked forward to being a wage earner and to joining the ranks of young parents.

Task Bonds   Jim was the overt decision maker in the family, although there had been endeavors to engage in cooperative decision making.

Person Bonds   Lisa was offended by Jim's apparent indifference to her feelings. In addition, she interpreted the intrusion of their parents as a violation of a basic rule of the marriage.

Crescive Bonds   Lack of crescive bonding was reflected in the inadequate amount of time Jim and Lisa spent together as a couple. Each partner fulfilled individual needs through independent career activities. Neither partner had much sense of responsibility for the other, nor much willingness to accommodate personal needs to system needs.

System Analysis

Structure   The marriage was dyadic in structure with substantial input from significant others such as the parents of the couple, and from friends who already had children.

Function   Jim was accustomed to asserting dominance in decision making. Lisa's wage-earning activities had been crucial during the first 4 years of marriage, but Jim discounted this in his eagerness to assume the role of primary provider. Teaching had not been a burden for Lisa; on the contrary, it was a rewarding occupation psychologically as well as financially. It seemed to Lisa that she was being asked suddenly to renounce her meaningful career in order to begin the unfamiliar childbearing function. Moreover, an established boundary pattern was disrupted when Jim solicited the support of their parents on this very intimate issue.

Intervention

Within the marriage there was excessive tension, anger, and anxiety. The strong feelings of the partners were not dissipated through rational discussion of their divergent viewpoints, and each partner believed the other to be selfish and inconsiderate. Communication was fragmented and nonspecific. Since each partner was aware of one viewpoint only, objective feedback was necessary to restore equilibrium. The intrusion of the couple's parents was injurious because their bias contributed to Lisa's feelings of being misunderstood.

As a couple, Jim and Lisa were undergoing rapid change in two respects. The first change resulted from Jim's new role as family provider, the second from his expressed desire to have a child. Although the couple had accepted Jim as the major decision maker, they had also agreed that Lisa would share in the decision process. The problematic issues resided in the areas of person and crescive bonding. The objectives of intervention were to balance the wishes of the two partners. Lisa was encouraged to share her negative feelings about Jim's use of parental pressure against her and to reveal her fears of giving up the job she enjoyed so much. Jim was helped to realize that Lisa's aversion to motherhood was not irrevocable but merely a form of temporizing. In essence this was a married couple who had led separate lives during their first 4 years together. Shared activities and a period of adjustment to Jim's new role of provider were suggested as precursers to the important step which Jim wanted immediately and which Lisa resisted for the moment.

THE UNMARRIED HETEROSEXUAL SYSTEM

Alternative family systems, besides being plagued by the same stresses as conventional families, are subject to special problems. The married and unmarried heterosexual couple have much in common, but the absence of a legal commitment imposes special strains on the unmarried heterosexual pair who have decided to live together. It may prove difficult for a health professional who is working with one or both partners in such an arrangement to ascertain the structure of the system because of the couple's fear of social or cultural stigma. However, this problem may arise less frequently at present than in former years. Indeed, some groups in our society now attach prestige to living together without marriage, and it is helpful for the practitioner to note how participants in these liaisons relate to their original families, and to peer and reference groups. A practitioner might ask whether the participants are comfortable with their dyadic arrangement. Is it considered a temporary or permanent commitment by one, both, or neither of the partners? Much of the initial assessment may center on two issues: (1) the relationship of the partners to their families of origin and to society in general, and (2) the permanency or impermanency of the relationship in the minds of the participants.

The functioning aspects of the "living-together" family system are similar to those of other couples of comparable age and station. Couples, married or unmarried, will generally have preferred ways of spending time together and some individualistic involvement in career or school. Occasionally financial concerns markedly affect the structure and function of the living-together system. College students who fear losing parental aid by making an unapproved marriage may choose to live together. The same considerations may influence a welfare mother who would forego support payments if she were to marry, or an elderly couple who would lose social security benefits in the event of a remarriage.

When a couple must hide the true nature of its relationship, there are inevitable repercussions. For the purposes of concealment, the amount of interaction between the dyad and other systems must be reduced, sometimes causing the couple to become overly involved with each other and to restrict their responsiveness to others. The issue of permanence may cause additional threats to adequate system functioning. Because crescive bonds depend in part on the promise of continued interaction, a prolonged threat of fragility in the system is often dysfunctional. Crescive bonds are continuity bonds which become stronger with time, as shared memories and ambitions accumulate. In the absence of legal commitment, one or both partners may suffer feelings of insecurity which may threaten the relationship. The result may be enmeshment within the dyad or outward movement toward subsystems that appear to offer guarantees of continuity. Role or task bonding may be hindered in the unmarried heterosexual system because the traditional roles of husband and wife cannot be strictly followed. New bonds must then be formed around these traditional roles so that the system can remain functional.

CLINICAL EXAMPLE: AN UNMARRIED HETEROSEXUAL COUPLE

Ann and Bob were an unmarried heterosexual couple who attended a college in their home town. Both were from middle-class families and both lived on campus during their first year at college. In their second year they leased an apartment together, and after graduation they continued this arrangement for 3 years. Both were employed and their combined incomes permitted a comfortable existence. Bob had not spoken to his parents for several years because of their strong objections to his living arrangements with Ann. She had maintained some communication with her family, although living with Bob was never mentioned. The couple shared many interests and household responsibilities; each placed a premium on open communication. They had relatively few friends and spent almost all their free time together. Both indicated that they were content and happy living together without marriage, but added that they might want to have children some day and would probably marry then.

Bonding Analysis

Membership Gratification Bonds   There was apparent satisfaction in the dyadic relationship with little involvement of the participants in subsystems or in their extended families.

Task Bonds   No apparent threat to task bonding was discernible, and an equitable balance had been established between individual and dyadic orientation in tasks.

Person Bonds   Information in this area was somewhat limited, but no obvious problems emerged.

Crescive Bonds   The continuity bonds seemed to be quite strong, as shown by the value the couple placed on honest communication, the large amount of time the two spent together, and their recognition of mutual dependence.

System Analysis

Structure   The dyadic structure was stable because of the strong commitment of the partners to each other. There was limited interaction with others outside the dyad.

Function   Ann and Bob had developed a cooperative sharing of responsibilities which allowed some independence of action. Each was involved in a separate career. Communication was highly valued and considered essential to preserving the relationship. A tentative rule was in effect that they would marry when they decided to have a child. The system was in a state of homeostasis under present conditions.

Intervention

Ann and Bob had established a harmonious family system with potential for growth and self-actualization. They agreed that structural and functional changes in their system would take place when they decided to have a child. The bonding between Ann and Bob was strong and multifaceted. One weakness of their family system was the relative isolation from their parents and from other subsystems. The possibility that Ann and Bob would experience guilt or regret for disappointing their parents could not be totally discounted. Intervention objectives would include fostering interaction with others, particularly with the two families of origin who represent a potential problem area for the couple.

THE SINGLE SYSTEM

Single persons offer an extensive range of alternate family system models. The ranks of single persons include the never married, the widowed, and the divorced, and most of these persons have support systems identifiable as families. Admittedly, it is easier for the health professional to recognize formal family systems, but single persons who relate primarily to their original families have support systems which are readily identifiable.

In some situations a single person may never have broken ties with the original family. However, many single persons whose marriages were dissolved by death or divorce return to their extended families for primary support. Included in this group are single persons who are psychologically close to their families, engage in social activities with them, and seek their assistance or counsel in time of trouble. Some individuals may be tied to the family of origin because, as unmarried persons, they cannot turn to others without breaking cultural or ethnic rules. In some families, the single person may be mature in years but fettered by lack of marital status. The single person who is young but has not yet found a mate may also be relegated by the parental system to the same ambiguous status. This transitional period may be trying for the young single person, particularly if there is family pressure to marry and the single person is not actively looking for a mate.

A single person who lives some distance from the family of origin usually finds a support system of sorts, but a discriminating practitioner may be required to identify it. Sometimes the support systems of single persons are unexpectedly casual, as exemplified by one elderly man who had no communication with his grown children but relied on his neighborhood barber for friendship and support. The barber was unaware of the significance of their interactions to his elderly customer, but he was listed as next of kin and was the only visitor when the elderly man was hospitalized. Generally, however, the support system of an individual is less one-sided and more recognizable to the practitioner.

A friend or a reference group may be the most available support system for the single person. These relationships may be deep or superficial, permanent or transitory, and they may be more meaningful to the single person than to the others involved. A single individual may have difficulty explaining the import or meaning of the supportive relationship. Couples clearly identify with one another and have shared expectations of the partnership. Single persons may not openly identify the significant others in their lives because of vague expectations, especially in regard to person and crescive bonds. Because the support systems of single persons are often implicit rather than explicit, assessment may be a difficult and tedious procedure.

CLINICAL EXAMPLE: A SINGLE-FAMILY SYSTEM

Jean attended an urban college several hundred miles from her home town. After graduating, she found a job and an apartment in the same city and remained there. Her closest friend was Chris, a divorced woman whom Jean had known for about 15 years. Jean was active and popular in several circles, but Chris was her special confidant. The two women had dinner together every week or so just to talk things over, and they frequently took short vacations together. Chris, who was more restless than Jean, began to talk of moving to another city. When asked to comment, Jean responded that a move might be advantageous for Chris but she avoided discussing what the move might mean to their relationship.

Bonding Analysis

Membership Gratification Bonds A great deal of mutual gratification resulted from the bond between Chris and Jean. Other subsystems were active in the lives of both women through social and professional relationships.

Task Bonds The friendship between the two women was warm and supportive. Each evidenced respect for the other. There were many mutual indications of concern and solicitude.

Crescive Bonds Jean and Chris had known each other for 15 years. During this period each pursued individual interests but managed to organize her life to include the friendship. The women shared many memories and experiences. Chris's discussion of moving to another city introduced a threat to the relationship.

Systems Analysis

Structure Jean and Chris were single women who lived some distance from their families of origin. Both interacted with various subsystems and reference groups, but each provided enormous support for the other.

Function The two women consistently organized their schedules to make time for each other. Although receptive to other relationships, they adhered to rules about allocating time to one another. As capable working women, they exhibited high energy levels with little dysfunctional tension. A threat of disequilibrium was introduced by the proposed relocation of Chris. This eventuality was not discussed openly by either woman. It is possible that expressing regret would have been regarded by both women as a violation of system boundaries.

Intervention

The loss of her best friend did not become a severe crisis for Jean, who had access to other resources to offset the loss when Chris finally did leave. For some time Jean used the mechanism of denial to ignore the consequences of the projected move. When Chris did relocate, Jean became restless and irritable. With brief counseling she worked through the depressive reaction which followed the departure of her friend, and was able to renew other friendships. She realized that her early failure to admit or discuss losing Chris ultimately intensified the pain of her loss. When Chris returned for a short visit, Jean was able to express her feelings of anger and abandonment. Finding that Chris had undergone similar mourning, Jean was able to complete the grieving process and accept her separate existence.

THE HOMOSEXUAL SYSTEM

The problems a homosexual couple must face, like those of certain other alternate family systems, include issues of permanency and of being at variance with cultural mores. The exploration of sexual relationships between partners in any family system requires sensitivity and discretion on the part of the health professional, and perhaps should not be undertaken unless sexuality is an issue disturbing the system. A practitioner who intimidates a client by probing before trust has been won endangers therapeutic effectiveness. Questions which are worded in nonthreatening ways help allay the anxiety of the client. Referring to the homosexual partner by nonspecific names such as "housemate" may elicit information about the structure and function of the system without denoting sexual prejudice. As always, a practitioner will wish to learn how the individual relates to the community, and find out about the satisfactions and dissatisfactions derived from the system. The homosexual client may reveal freely that the significant other is a sexual partner. If this is acknowledged, the practitioner may begin to explore some dimensions of the relationship. Is the liaison a permanent or a temporary one? Do the families of origin know of the relationship, and if so what is their reaction? Are the partners candid about their relationship or have they decided to remain "closet" homosexuals? If disclosures regarding the sexual aspects of the relationship are not freely offered, the practitioner may be content to obtain other information about the system and later return to the sexual relationship if it is germane.

CLINICAL EXAMPLE: A HOMOSEXUAL FAMILY SYSTEM

Jane was a professional woman in her mid-thirties, divorced and the mother of two children, aged 7 and 5. A year previously, Jane had purchased a home jointly with her friend Lynn, a single career woman whom Jane met after her divorce. The children and the two women lived in the house and were apparently well adjusted. Although Jane and Lynn were involved in community and social activities, priority was placed on spending family time together. Jane regarded her life as untroubled until the children's father threatened her with custody proceedings, charging that she and Lynn were lesbians. Jane admitted during counseling that she and Lynn were lovers as well as friends, but she insisted that she was a good mother to the children and that they were not being harmed by her relationship with Lynn. She was very worried about the effect of scandal on her children and also feared its effect on her professional future. Lynn was reported as solicitous but insistent that the decision must be Jane's, saying that she would understand if Jane separated to protect her children.

Bonding Analysis

Membership Gratification Bonds The relationship between the two women was rewarding but involved risk to them both, especially to Jane.

Task Bonds   Tasks and responsibilities in the home were shared harmoniously. In the past decisions had been made jointly by Jane and Lynn. However, Lynn was reluctant to influence Jane in the crucial decision related to the custody suit.

Person Bonds   Jane had strong, positive feelings for Lynn, which were reciprocated. Both evidenced deep concern for the other and complementarity was obvious in their interactions.

Crescive Bonds   The relationship between the two women was not entered into lightly. Great importance was placed on shared time and activities, and Lynn was almost as devoted to the children as Jane. There was great affection and respect between the women, and they regarded their lives as idyllic until the threat of custody proceedings.

Systems Analysis

Structure   Jane was a divorced woman who had functioned in the capacity of a single parent. Lynn's entrance into the family system improved Jane's financial position, helped provide a comfortable home for the children, and fulfilled many of Jane's needs. Lynn and Jane became a couple in every sense of the word.

Function   The two women worked out an equitable sharing of financial and family responsibilities. Each pursued an independent career and socialized with other friends. Rules were established about family time and family obligations and these rules were respected even though input from other systems was allowable. Jane and Lynn were discreet about their sexual relationship, and did not flaunt it in the community. A high energy level characterized the family system, but this was vitiated by the custody threats of Jane's former husband. In general systems terminology, feedback from other systems was disrupting the equilibrium of this family.

Intervention

Jane and Lynn formed a system which seemed stable and functional. Responsibilities were discharged capably, and open boundaries were maintained with other systems. Disequilibrium loomed because of the action of Jane's former husband. Bonding between Jane and Lynn was present except in the realm of membership gratification; this was denied them due to the social stigma attached to homosexuality. Intervention objectives with this dyad consisted of helping Jane make her decision. Lynn did not wish to coerce or influence Jane, but her failure to participate in the decision was not helpful. Jane needed to know Lynn's feelings about being involved in the custody case, since this was inevitable unless the women separated. The importance of the dyadic relationship had to be measured against its potential cost to Jane, Lynn, and the children. It was important that Lynn be involved in the decision, and that she not withhold support from Jane. Legal counsel was mandatory to guarantee Jane and the children their rights, and to protect both women to the fullest extent. Whether she decided to stay with Lynn or to separate, Jane needed help in coping with the consequences of her choice.

COMMUNAL FAMILIES

Communal families are usually a form of countercultural movement which exists apart from the mainstream of life. The term *counterculture* was used by Roszak (1969) to refer to a heterogeneous and changeable set of conditions which nevertheless possessed an insistent reality. In a study of marriages in the counterculture, Kafka and Ryder (1973) included couples who were legally married but adopted a deviant life-style by emphasizing the intimate aspects of their relationship and deemphasizing the utilitarian aspects such as jobs, money, living space, and possessions. Thus the couples who adopt the life-style of the counterculture may be legally married but deviant in various other aspects of their lives. For example, their attitudes toward material resources may be communistic rather than capitalistic. Whether wed or unwed, couples of the counterculture may not be restricted to serial monogamy but may engage in open sexual adventures in which one or both partners participate.

The activism of the 1960s was accompanied by an observable trend among young people toward communal living arrangements. It is widely assumed that communal families of the counterculture were and are characterized by sexual permissiveness and promiscuity. A more reassuring observation was made by Kafka and Ryder (1973) who wrote that participants in counterculture marriages were likely to be more sexually active than conventional persons, but that sexual activity was not the focal point of their existence. Unlike so-called swingers, the lives of communal couples were not necessarily centered on sexuality. Indeed, for many counterculture couples sexuality was considered as somewhat inconsequential in that it was the object of neither reverence nor fear.

Although the impetus toward communal living has somewhat abated, the movement is far from exhausted. Perhaps the desire for communal living springs from the universal human wish to belong and to relate in a more than ordinary way. Many communal groups begin vigorously but are short-lived. Those which do survive involve idealism and commitment, and do not thrive merely on the exploitation of weaker members. The kibbutzim of Israel are examples of communal living which respects traditional family values while preserving group idealism and commitment. Unfortunately in many communal societies a charismatic leader becomes the substitute for an ideal. Identification with the leader induces rank and file members to renounce property rights and personal freedom in return for acceptance from the leader who may or may not be sincere.

American society has often been described by critics as materialistic and lacking in relatedness (Melville, 1972). Communal living offers disenchanted individuals reduced material rewards in exchange for expanded social relationships. Members of communal families seem able to make this adjustment by reducing their expressed need for material resources and by deriving greater satisfaction from affectional or idealistic bonds with the group. This was expressed in somewhat psychoanalytic language by Kafka and Ryder (1972) who explained that counterculture allegiance replaced anal-genital possessiveness with more generous oral-genital attachments. From this phraseology it may be inferred that commune members express counterculture attitudes toward persons and possessions by sharing rather than by proprietorship.

The mainstream culture tends to be distrustful of communal family arrangements. This fear may be based on ignorance, on envy, or on the belief that communes release the repressive forces which society uses to control our instinctual drives. Certainly the history of communal movements includes some inglorious episodes such as the conquest of the weak members by the strong. It would, however, be unfair to consign all communal living arrangements to the same ash heap. There are many cooperative communes which effectively harness group capabilities and distribute group responsibilities, thereby achieving a degree of economic and social success. Although some communal families achieve the longed-for transcendental experience mainly through hallucinogenic drugs and self-serving sexual exploits, other groups are mutually supportive, and serve as clearinghouses for shared ideas and problems. Most communes are too short-lived or impenetrable to allow objective investigation of their long-term effects on members, whether adult or child. Disaffected members are probably no more reliable as reporters than are the happy participants of a communal movement. As representatives of the counterculture, communes have not been very receptive to objective researchers from outside.

Detractors of communal living see the arrangement as an infringement of personal liberty and a threat to society's stability. Such criticism is not likely to terminate communal living as individuals continue to attempt to regain paradise by building a new community with its own folkways. All that can be said with any accuracy is that within the dominant society there can be found a number of individuals who wish to eliminate the struggle and isolation of modern life by adopting an alternative life-style in which the family is neither nuclear nor extended, but is established through common ideology or commitment rather than legality or consanguinity.

CLINICAL EXAMPLE: MARITAL SHARING
IN A COMMUNAL FAMILY

Susan and Jim lived with six other couples on a ramshackle farm. Two of the men in the group had jobs in town while the rest of the group worked on the farm. Susan was exempt from farm work because of her skilled weaving which could be sold to tourists in the summer. Most of the sexual relationships in the group were monogamous even though no couple was legally married. Occasionally there was some mate swapping but Susan and Jim expected fidelity from each other. Both of them complied with this expectation until Judy's partner, tired of the group life, packed up his van and headed west. Susan was worried and upset by this. Judy and Jim got along well together and Susan was afraid that an unattached woman might be tempting and seductive to the men, especially to Jim. Her fears were well founded, for in a few weeks Jim told Susan that he was helping Judy adjust to her unattached state and that his help included having sexual intercourse. Susan was furious and for a time rejected Jim's overtures to her. Eventually, however, she capitulated and confessed later that she was excited by the idea of sharing Jim with Judy. The arrangement continued without change until an unattached male joined the commune and entered a sexual relationship with Judy. This development reduced but did not altogether terminate Judy's sexual encounters with Jim, to which Susan no longer objected.

Bonding Analysis

Cohesion among commune members was based on alienation from mainstream society rather than bonds between partners. Members had tasks which also helped to hold them together.

System Analysis

Structure   The dyad composed of Susan and Jim was triangulated by the sexual liaison between Judy and Jim. This relationship was attenuated but not altogether destroyed by the arrival in the commune of a regular sexual partner for Judy.

Function   The expectation of the group was that couples who were members of the communal family would be monogamous, even though not legally married to each other. This implied commitment to fidelity was broken by Jim. Thus the relationship of Jim with two female group members violated an established norm. Although she was angry at first with Jim, Susan recovered and then became erotically stimulated by sharing her partner with another woman. The arrival of a male partner allowed Judy to form a new sexual relationship, and clearly made Jim's sexual connection with Judy secondary to his relationship with Susan. This reassured Susan that she was first in Jim's affection, and allowed the sexual encounters between Jim and Judy to continue in a manner acceptable to all four principals. An unknown variable was the attitude of other members of the communal family toward the involvement of Jim and Judy. Judy's acquisition of a partner permitted the group to pretend that the norm of monogamous commitment was upheld. In actuality it had not been preserved.

Intervention

No intervention was sought but the stability of the communal family was threatened. There was a brief period of disequilibrium for Susan until she resolved her feelings, and an important group norm was violated by Jim. When a partner appeared for Judy, a precarious triangle was transformed into a structural arrangement which diffused the tensions of the triad. There seemed to be a return to earlier group norms, but the potential for disequilibrium remained. Since Jim was enjoying the sexual favors of both women, it was possible that the new man might seek the same privilege. This would necessitate a decision from Susan to agree or refuse.

As the group deviant, Jim could be subject to pressure from Susan or the communal family to give up Judy as a sexual partner. Failing this, Jim might be expelled from the group. On the other hand the actions of Jim might persuade the communal family to renounce monogamy as a norm and to adopt freer sexual habits. The sexual practices of Jim, which were welcomed by Judy and condoned by Susan, introduced change and possible fragmentation into the communal family.

SUMMARY

Concepts drawn from bonding and from general systems theory were utilized in this chapter to help professionals understand the establishment and maintenance of some alternative styles of family organization. Alternative styles considered included the childless married couples, unmarried heterosexual couples, single persons, homosexual couples, and communal families. The point was made that these alternative models constitute family systems which are viable and meaningful to the participants. The need for open-mindedness and sensitivity on the part of professionals was stressed. The application of bonding and general systems theory to alternative family models was presented as a method of increasing cognitive and objective awareness during the assessment process.

REFERENCES

Kafka, J. S., & Ryder, R. G. Notes on marriages in the counter culture. *Journal of Applied Behavioral Science,* 1973, **9**(1), 321–330.

Marcuse, H. *An essay on liberation.* Boston: Beacon Press, 1969.

Melville, K. *Communes in the counter culture.* New York: Morrow, 1972.

Roszak, T. *The making of a counter culture.* New York: Doubleday, 1969.

Turner, R. H. *Family interaction.* New York: Wiley, 1970.

Chapter 9

Entry of Children into the Family System

Judith Ann Moore
Phyllis Noerager Stern

This chapter concerns the effect on the family social system of the addition of a new member. It is also concerned with the effects on the new member as he or she is socialized to fit into the system. In other words, it deals with the process of integrating a new member into a group.

The integration of a new member changes both member and group. This can be illustrated by an example from another kind of social situation. Two teachers engage in conversation; a student joins them and attempts to participate. Although all three persons are part of the school system, they belong to separate subsystems. The faculty members can either include or exclude the student. They may turn away, leave the scene, or include the student in the group. Regardless of the decision to include or exclude, the original pair alters its behavior. They may talk more guardedly or change the topic which was being discussed when they were alone. Meanwhile, the student may act in a way that will ensure a welcome. For example, the student may attempt to please by imitating the manners of the faculty group, but with a respectful stance. In any case, all the members of the new three-person system begin to act in a new way. The system has been altered by the entry of the newcomer.

If on the other hand, the joining person is another teacher, less altera-tion of interaction is required, since all three members have been socialized into the teacher role. They speak the same language. However, if the third faculty member is from another department, or is not a peer, this person will represent a different subsystem. In this case, the action of all three per-sons changes to accommodate to the addition of the outsider.

A child entering a family system causes change which is both qualitative and quantitative (Blood, 1972). The helplessness of the newborn and the de-mands produced by its dependency cause changes in priorities of work, finances, and time. Moreover, these changes are not a matter of choice, since a newborn will not survive without care. Adding a new member often throws the family into disequilibrium. The family regains a semblance of balance only when members become comfortable with the new system. This occurs when the family can accommodate to the demands of the new mem-ber, and when the new member is integrated into the system.

Families acquire children in a variety of ways: through birth, *biological children;* through adoption, *adopted children;* or through the marriage of single parents. The new spouse then becomes parent to *stepchildren.* Although there are differences in these three types of parental relationships, the transcending variable is socialization. All parents interact with children on a social level, regardless of whether they are biological, adoptive or step-parents.

The concept of the social parent is what makes the biological, adoptive, and stepfamily work. It is through parent-child interactions that family members become joined to each other and are held together by social ties. In the following section, some social changes which affect the character of these three kinds of families are considered.

BACKGROUND AND CURRENT TRENDS

Family Patterns

Social trends influence patterns of birth, divorce, and adoption. More births are planned today than ever in the past, and an increasing number of couples postpones childbearing until they are well established in their respective careers. A class of older parents has evolved from the zero population movement of the late sixties. Many a woman who announced in 1970 that she would refuse to add to an overburdened earth may find herself 30 and childless in 1980, and say, "I didn't mean I was *never* going to have a child!"

Older first-time parents require different kinds of services from health professionals. Older couples tend to be better informed, and to know what assistance they need. The chances are good that they have learned how to make the social system work for them, and that they are more adept at getting their demands met than younger couples. Older, more sophisticated couples shop around until they find the kinds of services they require. When they demand alternative, homelike birth centers, hospitals tend to respond. When they balk at limited hospital visiting, old restrictions may be lifted.

In this time of consumerism many couples approach the birthing experience with expressed preferences. Younger couples, too, are enrolling in childbirth education classes, and requesting natural births with less ritualized medical intervention.

Other social movements of the sixties which have influenced patterns of childbirth and child care are the equal rights movement and the women's movement. These have had an effect on the continuing involvement of the father in birth and child rearing. Typically, women suggest that their mates attend preparation for childbirth classes, but frequently it is the fathers themselves who get caught up in participating in the birth process and in the rearing of their children. With the new emphasis on role flexibility, fathers have come to consider involvement their right.

Adoption

Contemporary social movements have had a profound effect on adoption, decreasing the number of babies available. As a result, the adopted child of today tends to be older, of different race, and sometimes handicapped. Social workers are warning parents of adopted children of another likely change: the Adoptees Liberty Movement Association (ALMA), founded by Florence Fisher, may soon force the opening of adoption records. If this happens, there will no longer be a choice about telling children they are adopted.

The availability of abortion and effective birth control also helps account for the small number of adoptable babies. Of the 80 children placed through the San Francisco Department of Social Services in 1976, only 9 were under 1 year of age. This contrasts with the 280 children under 1 year of age who were placed through the same agency in 1969.

Changing mores are making it easier for the single woman who decides to continue her pregnancy to keep her baby. Unfortunately, the single parent is most often a teenager for whom the multiple pressures of parenthood, interrupted schooling, and earning a livelihood may prove overwhelming. Mothers who are scarcely past their own childhood sometimes have no realization of the needs of a baby. From this immature, unprepared age group the largest number of battering parents emerge. The result is that a child from such an environment who is finally offered for adoption is not only older, but may also be psychologically or physically traumatized.

In the early seventies, Caucasian couples began to adopt children of other races, particularly black children, because of the myth that black children were seldom adopted by black couples, and that therefore they would be available to whites. For years, however, black families have taken "outside" children into their homes without the formality of legal adoption proceedings. In fact, blacks adopt proportionately more children than do whites in terms of their percentage of the total population. In 1972, black social workers responded to the growing number of transracial, black-white adoptions with a position paper decrying the damaging effects of these adoptions on the racial identity of the child (Berman, 1974).

Transcountry adoptions have provided a partial answer to the lack of available young children in this country. In California, for instance, there were 250 transcountry adoptions in 1976 according to the California Department of Health. Most of these children were from the Orient, but a new source of adoptable children has recently been found in South America. At one time the number of adoptable Korean children was almost limitless. Recently, however, Korea has reacted with regulations restricting the number of children allowed out of that country. No children are arriving from Vietnam at this writing because diplomatic relations between Vietnam and the United States have been severed. Children from the Orient are generally adopted by Americans of European, Japanese, and Chinese ancestry. Filipinos tend to adopt only Filipinos, usually relatives from the home islands.

Stepfamilies

Stepfamilies are increasingly commonplace in the United States, where over a million marriages end in divorce each year, and four out of five divorced persons remarry. National records are not available on the number of these marriages which involve children. Studies in San Diego (Bohannan, 1975; Bohannan & Erickson, 1978) showed that 9 percent of all the families in that city were headed by a stepfather. The father in divorce is granted physical custody of his children about 10 percent of the time; most divorced fathers see their children on weekends. When men who do not have custody remarry, their spouse typically becomes a weekend stepmother or a vacation parent. Of the three types of families—biological, adopted, and step- the latter has the least external assistance. Preparation classes are available for pregnant couples and for adopting parents, but classes or groups for remarrying parents are almost nonexistent and the problems faced by such families are manifold.

SYSTEMS MODIFICATION IN THE GROWING FAMILY

In any growing family, constant readjustment is the order of each day. One is forced to think in terms of dynamic rather than static conditions. The processes which determine the family's rules, its communication patterns, and its contact with the outside world are derived from the sentimental order of the family of origin of the spouses.

Sentimental order

Sentimental order is a term used to describe behaviors based on the interactant's conception of the proper way of doing things (Glaser & Strauss, 1965). Sentimental order is what feels right, what seems to the family member to be normal. It is a sentimental attachment to the way things have always been done. Sentimental order is akin to a value system, but it goes beyond that concept to include cultural and ethical viewpoints, and a feeling of familiarity; only obliquely does it include moral outlooks. What was "right" at home, is the yardstick by which normalcy in the new home is measured. Normalcy for family members covers a vast range of possibilities. One family may consider the evening meal a meeting at which stimulating conversation takes place, while another uses the mealtime to discuss family members' transgressions. A third family may have a rule which forbids talk by children while at dinner. Sentimental order determines the family's social-structural processes or the way structure is negotiated. Sentimental order determines social-psychological processes, that is, the way persons involved feel about the social interactions. If one spouse comes from a father-dominant family, and the other from a democratic family, their sentimental orders may differ. A spouse who believes shouting is allowed when making a point has difficulty understanding the silent withdrawal employed by the other spouse. These dissonant communication patterns make social structuring difficult. From a social-psychological point of view, divergent ways of interacting may make each mate think that the other is impossible to deal with. It may also make each wonder if there is something vaguely amiss in his or her own behavior.

No couple comes together with identical sentimental orders, because the original families are different. And couples who have succeeded in negotiating a working social order often find that conflict starts again when children appear. One parent's ideas about how a child should be socialized may differ from the beliefs of the other parent. A period of conflict and disequilibrium may ensue until the couple negotiates a compromise.

PATTERNS OF STRUCTURE AND FUNCTION

Function

The goal of a healthy family is the optimal growth of its individual members. Therefore, family groups are less efficient at getting work done than other institutions which are more concerned with productivity than growth. In healthy families, rules about family functions such as chore assignments tend to be flexible rather than static. Jobs can be shifted to suit changing times. If, for instance, Mother is a wage earner or a student, someone else may be assigned to prepare dinner, or the family can eat take-home food. If Father is sick, Junior can do the lawn work, and if Jane is practicing for the school play, Mother and Dad will probably do the dinner dishes.

Structure

Social-structure processes determine who is in power, and what positions the other members of the family hold. These processes determine, and are determined by, the communication patterns in the family. When the father holds the charge position, he passes his orders to the second in command, generally the mother, whose job it is to communicate the orders to the children. Families fall more or less into patterns of father dominance, mother dominance, or a democratic arrangement in which both parents share power.

Complementary and Symmetrical Relationships Another way of talking about power relationships is to refer to them as symmetrical or complementary. In a *symmetrical* relationship, the partners enjoy equal status. "Weakness or strength, goodness or badness, are not relevant here, for equality can be maintained in any of these areas" (Watzlawick, Beavin, & Jackson, 1967, p. 68). In a complementary relationship, one partner assumes a "one-up" position, the other a "one-down" status. Both interactants agree to play out their particular parts in a complementary relationship, that is, one-up does not force the other to submit to a one-down position; rather, one-down volunteers for the role. "It is important to emphasize the interlocking nature of the relationship, in which dissimilar but fitted behaviors evoke each other" (Watzlawick et al., 1967). Spouses in a marriage, then, can assume symmetrical positions, or they can take on complementary male-dominant or female-dominant roles.

Male Dominance Traditionally, the man of the house held the most power because of superior physical, economic, and political strength. Some families still retain this traditional power structure. Problems with male-dominant structure stem from the counterbalancing of this power by the woman of the house who is in the one-down or inferior position. To counter the man's power, the woman resorts to meeting her needs through subterfuge and manipulation. In this complementary relationship, often she does not state her demands directly. For her children, she frequently plays go-between, interceding for them with their father. The result is that in many families the mother is the switchboard through which all messages are transmitted. This communication pattern creates social distance and distortion between father and child. An additional problem ensues when the picture of a manipulative mother and a distant father becomes part of the child's sentimental order.

Female Dominance   At the other extreme is the home in which the woman assumes the charge role. The message emitted from this structural style is that men are weak while women are strong. It has been suggested in psychoanalytic literature that the male who grows up in a mother-dominant home tends to identify sexually with his mother, and to seek out males as love objects. This suggestion has been disputed, however, and certainly, it is impossible to demonstrate a single cause and effect in these structural conditions. However, it is safe to say that weak men and strong women are not acceptable norms for the larger society; therefore, a child from a female-dominant home gains a concept of family life that is at variance with the norm.

Symmetry   In democratic homes, parents share power. It is probably closer to the truth to say that each wields power some of the time. A symmetrical relationship occasionally deteriorates, with each partner taking opposing positions. Generally, when a power struggle threatens to erupt over an issue, the relationship converts to a complementary one for a time. The temporary one-down partner may retreat in order to plan a strategy for the next discussion of the problem.

A great deal of communication is needed to make a democratic family system function. Since every decision must be talked out, children tend to participate more in family negotiations. The message given to children in these homes is that everyone's opinion is important: the mother's, the father's, and the children's. This is not to say that the children have an equal vote, but rather that they are allowed to express their point of view in some of the decision making. Some families permit children to gain power and influence as they age. It is rare for very small children to be involved in family matters, but the contributions of the older child are increasingly respected. The child is allowed to assume a status position which increases with age.

Single-Parent Dynamics   The single-parent home generally represents a variation of the mother-dominant home. In the United States 90 percent of single parents living with their children are female. In this power structure, the mother-child dyad becomes the working social system. Children in single-parent homes miss the opportunity to observe the give and take of married life. They are unable to learn the political strategy men and women use in interactions (Adams, 1973). The child fails to experience the important skill of playing one parent against the other, which is the first step in learning to manipulate the social world. When a single parent marries, the child brings along a sentimental order learned in a home of single rule. This child may have worked out a symmetrical relationship with the parent which included a pseudoadult role for the child. Such a young person rarely welcomes the new rule maker, who brings his own sentimental order into the family.

Adoptive Homes   Structural patterns in adoptive homes do not differ from patterns in the home into which a child is born. However, older children who are adopted bring with them a sentimental order from a past life. Such children may perceive the new way of doing things as foreign, and therefore not normal. The same can be said for stepchildren, who have developed an idea of fitness and propriety from their family of origin.

Stepfamilies   In a study of stepfather families, Stern (1977) found five social structural patterns. Stepfather families generally start their life together with the mother in charge of the child, because she and the child have shared a life apart from the stepfather. The mother usually plays go-between for stepfather and child. Because she knows both of them best, she explains the behavior of one to the other. If this communication pattern persists, however, family integration will be impaired.

When the family first moves in together, the stepfather usually asks the mother what role he should play regarding the child. "After all," he says, "it's not my kid." Ideally the mother will suggest that they make no radical changes, that they respect each other and resort at times to trial and error. If the stepparent moves slowly, and makes a friend rather than a rival of the child, the family can move toward an integrated pattern resembling the democratic pattern of biological homes. In this pattern, no one is left out, and even the child shares in rule making.

If the stepfather is harsh or the child rejecting, the mother may be torn between her husband and her child. A period of disequilibrium may ensue and, if balance is not restored, a chaos pattern will emerge. In this pattern, the mother plays go-between, and everyone makes rules, but no one observes anyone else's rules. Family members either communicate by shouting, or get their message across by retiring behind closed doors. Estrangement replaces reconciliation and an escalated symmetrical relationship involving all family members appears.

Some mothers ask the stepfather to assume the role of disciplinarian of the home. This may mean an imitation of the traditional pattern in which the man of the house is the announced boss. The mother then plays go-between and carries out only the rules made by the stepfather of which she approves. The role of stepfather-in-charge is a titular one only. Other women, who have difficulty managing a small child on their own, ask the stepfather to take charge. This may be called the child-left-out pattern, because a child who has lost his biological father now is turned over by his mother to a disciplinarian who is a stranger. The message passed to the child by the mother is that she does not feel able or willing to manage her youngster, and she has called in a disciplinarian to help her. The child is left with the impression that only a very bad person would receive such treatment.

Boundaries and Tensions

Boundaries   Ideally, before becoming parents, mates form an identity as a couple. They establish bonds through love, shared experience, sexual pleasure, and private jokes. This is called a couple coalition. The arrival of children strains the primary couple relationship, because the demands of children erode the time and privacy available to the couple. In the healthy family, the spouses' coalition allows them to support one another in their parental efforts. Although the demands of children must be met, healthy parents are able to sustain their adult love relationship. Children are nurtured, but are not allowed to intrude on the parent coalition. Strong parental boundaries preclude intrusion by children into their parents' special relationship.

When parental boundaries are weak, parents can be pulled into bonds with children which become stronger than the primary coupling. According to Satir (1967) the marital union is dysfunctional when a person of low self-esteem marries to complete a sense of self, hoping to find an enhancement of self in the other. If both partners look to their mates to provide what is lacking, both will be disillusioned. When one partner turns to the child for fulfillment, a new dyad is formed which excludes the other spouse. When both partners turns to the child, the child is caught in a triangle which transcends generations. An example of a parent-child dyad can be found in the case of a woman who solicits unqualified love from her child to the extent that the needs of her husband become her secondary concern. As the child is pulled into a close relationship with its mother, the husband moves away from his spouse, becoming involved in business or perhaps another sexual liaison. If the husband also focuses his attention on the child as a primary love object, the child becomes the ploy between two parents. This condition is not uncommon among divorced parents who fight one another through the child. Tremendous pressure is placed on the child to meet parental needs and children are ill equipped for the weight of this responsibility. Something has to be sacrificed, and often it is the child's sense of reality. The child is ensnared in the overwhelming love of one or both parents. When the time comes for the child to leave home and form relationships of its own, it cannot escape easily. The danger of being a parent's primary love object is especially great for a child living with a single parent. Often the child assumes the position of surrogate adult, sharing the responsibility by helping the parent, and feeling that the parent would perish without the child's presence. Because of this feeling, some exploited children never dare to leave home.

Boundaries in stepfamilies are established over time and follow the lines drawn in the structural patterns described in the previous section. Such families report that structural patterns and boundaries are established over a period of 1½ to 2 years. In stepfamilies, the couple forms its relationship in the presence of the child. Parent and child have already formed dyadic bonds, which may have become stronger by divorce. The child who has lost one parent may cling to the remaining parent desperately for fear of total abandonment (Kransler, 1973). Parent and child share a history in which the stepparent has no part. Thus, in stepfamilies, the husband-wife and parent-child subsystems are usually kept separate until the family becomes integrated. Some stepfamilies never become integrated, but maintain separate subsystems with the parent taking care of "my" children, and then separately fulfilling the role of spouse.

Go-between communication is not limited to stepfamilies; it also occurs in adoptive homes and in biological families. This communication pattern inspires a kind of cold war between the walled-off parent and child. Since they communicate through a switchboard in the person of a go-between, neither parent nor child knows the other fully. Go-between communications indicate an effort to sidestep tensions, as one parent attempts to keep a feuding parent and child apart. At times, these communication patterns represent a power tactic by the mediating parent.

Tensions   Tensions within families fluctuate and change as the family grows. The numerical growth of the family increases the potential for sibling rivalry. No matter how well parents handle the situation, the fact remains that a single child gets more parental attention and material goods than a child with siblings. Most parents strive to favor children by turn. Some parents have full-time favorites, and children know this only too well. Children can cope with sibling conflict if each child in turn is allowed to feel special, and equal to the other children, in parental love.

Special tensions for adoptive and stepfamilies stem from problems of boundaries and origins. Both kinds of families resist certain intrusions from the outside world, and both have to deal with the fact that the child has experienced at least one parent outside the home.

Adopting parents feel the weight of social control from the very beginning. Hammons (1976), citing the theory of Kornitzer, writes that the adopting couple operates with certain disadvantages. Adoptive couples initially are placed in a dependent role in which they must be approved as good parents. This scrutinization may undermine parental confidence at the outset and inject dependence into a role otherwise considered to be independent.

Once a couple adopts a child, they often worry about what to tell the child about its origins. A source of tension for the adoptive family lies in the fear that a neighbor or relative may tell the child it is adopted before the parents are ready to reveal this vital information to the child. Couples must decide for themselves when to tell their child about its origin.

Most adopted children today fall into the older or other-racial categories. There is no question about telling these children they are adopted; they know. In several states, laws have been changed to allow children of 14 or older to open their adoption files. This may encourage parents to tell their children in a matter-of-fact manner, an approach which is considered preferable (Braff, 1977).

Adoptive parents fear that children who know their true origins will transfer affection from adoptive to biological parents, but this fear is usually groundless. The social parent-child relationship which has existed over the years is not easily shaken.

The associates of adoptive families often create problems for them. It is sometimes suggested that the adoptive family is viewed as socially inferior (Klibanoff & Klibanoff, 1973; Hammons, 1976; Anderson, 1971). For this reason, adoptive parents often tend to err on the side of overdisciplining. Blood (1972) stated that children in their biological families are allowed to speak their minds and behave freely, whereas adopted children are overdisciplined.

Misgivings arise over the matter of genetic health, particularly since adoptive files are often scanty in the matter of medical information. Even though agencies do not attempt to conceal problems, it is possible that the biological mother may not have been aware of genetic diseases. Inherited talents also remain a mystery. There is no question that the adoptive parents suffer from uncertainties that are unknown to biological parents.

Reproduction is an issue in adoption. Adopting parents may grow tense as the child nears adolescence and becomes sexually mature. According to Schechter (1970) the parents are reminded again of their own barrenness, and may even resent the child's ability to reproduce. Another fear which grips adoptive parents as their child nears adolescence, according to Schechter, is that the child will marry and the couple will be childless again. As a consequence, adoptive parents tend to be more restrictive regarding dating practices of their teenagers.

Couples in stepfamily homes are faced with working through the problems of any new marriage, but they have the additional encumbrance of a child and a past unshared with each other. The children, for their part, must accept the company of a stranger with whom the parent must be shared.

Children seek support from peers and often show no compunction in telling a friend that a new stepfather is a "dirty rat." The remarrying parents are more reticent and are reluctant to share any marriage problems with their social group. To fail in a second marriage suggests to remarrying couples (and to their friends) that they may have contributed to the downfall of the first marriage. The wish to keep marital problems secret deprives these couples of peer support which might be valuable.

Stepsiblings in working-class homes are usually more compatible than those in middle- or upper-class families. A reason that has been suggested for this is that children in these families are more accustomed to visitors (Duberman, 1973). Problems between stepsiblings are similar to, but more pronounced than those between biological siblings. Real or imagined favoritism is frequently an issue. These children not only battle over property, but over prior ownership of the parents. "He's not your dad," says the biological child of the father, "he's mine!" Issues over favoritism extend to the parental pair when children living with the divorced mate visit on weekends and seem to receive preferential treatment.

Equilibrium Sources of disequilibrium can arise from within or from outside the system, but the family has to learn to cope, to make do, to get back to normal, or the system cannot survive as a family. Satir (1972) likened the family group to a mobile in which the members, although attached, are freely moving. By shortening or lengthening the strings, the family can be kept in balance or equilibrium (p. 119). Satir recommended that a family have more than one way to maintain balance. Flexibility in chore assignment to allow for individual needs is one example of this. A family which has dysfunctional ways of restoring balance may add too much weight to one member, or pull the string too short on another. In such cases, equilibrium is reestablished at the expense of one member. Jackson (1957) contended that homeostasis in a sick family is maintained by assigning a "sick" status to one member. If that member starts to become well, the balance is upset. Therefore, the family struggles to keep that member in the "sick" role.

When an older adopted child or stepchild comes into a family, a honeymoon period occurs as problems are tabled and everyone makes allowances for others for a short while. The honeymoon is over when the stepparent demands a change in the stepchild's behavior, when the adopted child refuses to eat unfamiliar food, or when the mother complains of the attitude of the stepfather toward her child (Stern, 1968). After the honeymoon period, the family must learn to resolve their differences during the period of disequilibrium. No matter what the cause of disequilibrium, if a family is to survive, it must find a way to return to normal, or to accept new standards for what is normal.

THE GROWING CHILD AND THE FAMILY

Infancy

In this section, the effects of the arriving infant on the family system are discussed, together with ways in which the family accommodates to restore equilibrium.

Preparation The amount of disruption caused by the entry of a child into the family is determined by financial circumstances, preparation, and the personality of the individuals involved. Whether the child is born to a couple, adopted, or a stepchild, preparation begins before its arrival. Whether the pregnancy is planned or unplanned, the gestation period is one of waiting and preparation. More and more pregnant couples attend classes designed to help them through labor and delivery of their infant. However, the most important preparation for parenthood is the parenting the couple themselves have received. The couple's socialization of their children provides intergenerational continuity.

Tensions at Arrival The first 4 to 6 weeks after the arrival of an infant is a stressful period, as the couple strives to "get organized." The infant's inability to speak English leads to what Blood (1972) calls diagnostic problems: "What is he crying about?" "What does she need (if anything)?" "Should we call the doctor?"

Whether the arrival of the child constitutes a crisis depends on a variety of factors. Reserves of energy, material well-being, and the health of the participants vary from family to family. Parenthood may be viewed as an "extensive" or "severe" crisis (Blood, 1972). Dyer (1963), however, views the crisis as moderate for most couples. A more recent study by Russell (1974) showed that most couples do not consider the first year of parenthood a crisis. Thomas and Chess (1977) contend that the temperament of the infant largely determines how the couple copes with parenthood. Parents and children mutually influence one another from the beginning in a constantly evolving process of interaction.

Increasingly, fathers assist in baby care and household tasks; nevertheless, for the mother who quits her job and assumes full-time child care, the loneliness, in addition to the burden of always having to be available, constitutes a stress. The amount of help a mother receives varies from culture to culture and from age to age. Filipinos, for instance, provide help for one another, and in the first 30 days after birth the mother's only task is nursing her infant while relatives or maids assume responsibility for housework. In our society, the older first-time mother, who is less likely to have an older relative for child care, may have special problems. Young women may also find it difficult to obtain the help of their middle-aged mothers, since so many women are now employed.

Development of Nurturing Patterns   Infancy provides the occasion for an awakening of sensual pleasure, as parent and child respond to skin touch, caressing, closeness, and the sight of the loved one. Sensual pleasure learned in the arms of a parent is the source of all loves which follow. Failure to learn this predisposes one to a life of shallow emotional and physical responsiveness. Parents and children begin to respond to one another at birth. Within a few weeks, the principal care giver, who is usually the mother, is able to distinguish between various vocalizations and expressions of the infant, and to respond appropriately.

During the first 3 months of life the mother must understand the needs of her infant to ensure its survival. Bowlby (1951/1966) claimed that the infant and mother had to form an "attachment" in order for the child to develop normally. Although recent studies (Lynn, 1974) have demonstrated the vital role of the father, a symbiotic relationship between the mother and child exists for a time. Even when she is separated from her infant for a short while, the mother is preoccupied with thoughts of the child.

Around the third month of infancy, the father expects the mother to renew her interest in him and in the larger world. He may suggest that she involve herself with a class or a job, spend more time on meals, or pay more attention to her person. The mother's first response is that her mate is unreasonable, that she has too much to do, and the baby needs her. In the healthy family, the mother soon realizes that an afternoon off to shop while the father or baby-sitter takes over child care is a boon to her spirits. She returns feeling revitalized. In the troubled family, the mother is unable to make this separation, and clings unnaturally to her infant, refusing to believe that the child can manage without her.

The Maturing Infant   The mind and body of an infant grow at an amazing rate. Every day the baby acquires new accomplishments. The child learns to smile, laugh, turn over, creep, crawl, sit, stand, and walk. A family system designed to promote the growth of its individual members can strike a balance between safety and freedom. The growing infant learns what "no" means, how to make parents laugh, and what parental limits are. By the end of the infancy period, the child has learned a number of social graces, which allows some control over the world, and ingratiates the child in the social system of the family.

Variations in Adoptive and Stepfamilies   A principal difference between adoptive and stepfamilies is that the mother of an adopted child is not worn out physically from the birth experience. Because adoption is a prolonged process, the waiting period for a suitable child represents a gestation period for the parents. The adopted child, like the stepchild, is a youngster whose socialization has already begun. Therefore, both child and parents must unlearn as well as learn from each other.

The Preschool Child

The childbearing years of the family begin with the birth of the first child and end when the last child enters school. Many families have one or more preschoolers, aged 3 through 5, to care for and nurture. Regardless of the form of the family unit, the family is central in the life of a preschooler, who exerts influence on all the family members. At this stage of family life, parents are still developing their skills and roles. Because preschoolers have considerable verbal facility, the frustration many parents feel in the infancy stage may decrease considerably. Preschoolers ask both simple and complex questions, and mispronounce unfamiliar words, activities that delight parents and grandparents. Such behaviors endear preschoolers to their family and provide source material for stories in years to come.

For certain parents, frustration may increase because of the preschooler's mobility and use of language. If parents have not done so before, they will begin to come to grips with what they feel toward the child. A struggle for control, lasting from 1 to 3 years, develops between parent and child. Parents continue to use their authority and power with young children; a contest of will related to discipline and family rules may arise between parent and child, or between parents for the control of the child.

Preschoolers are usually emotionally and physically close to their parents and it is at this stage that the family enters what Freud called the "oedipal" romance or the stage of the family triangle (Murray & Zenter, 1975). During this period of pregenital sexuality the child directs strong loving feelings toward the parent of the opposite sex, and the parent of the same sex is the recipient of competitive feelings from the child. The child imitates the adult roles and tries to become "daddy's girl," or "mommy's boy." For a preschooler with a single parent, this may be an especially difficult period. In this regard, Dresen (1976) wrote that it is common for the single parent to make either or both of two maladaptive responses. One is overcompensation to the children; the second is denial of one's own personal identity.

The single parent may focus on the parenting role, withdraw from outside social activities, and temporarily shelve many personal needs. Sexual needs may be negated or become "an issue surrounded with logistical problems" (Dresen, 1976). Most preschoolers resent live-in arrangements that their parent makes with another person.

If a potential or actual stepfather can survive the honeymoon period in which the couple ignores child-rearing conflicts in order to show the idyllic quality of their stepfamily relationships, he will be tested further by his spouse and the preschooler. The stepfather may try to make what Stern

(1976) called "friending overtures," which are defined as making a friend of the child while attempting to enforce rules. The wife still has the power regarding discipline; she may deny, grant, or withdraw permission for the stepfather to discipline her child. As soon as she trusts his discipline and rule making, the mother will be less watchful of his behavior, even though she continues to regard the child as her responsibility. In the reconstituted family, the members will negotiate and renegotiate for 1½ to 2 years. Through these interactions family members work out a master plan for structure and discipline. Fewer crises may occur if the stepfather and spouse are knowledgeable about the normal development of preschoolers. Stern (1976) found that abrupt, intense efforts by the stepfather to change child behavior were disintegrative. Accepting children's faults as well as their virtues is necessary if the family is to remain integrated and viable.

Before a new baby or an adopted child enters the family of a preschooler, the child should be prepared for the changes that will shortly occur.

During the preschool period, parents may not be totally involved in home life. Most fathers of preschoolers are settling into their work during this phase of family life. One third of the mothers of 3- to 5-year-olds are employed (Gorman, 1978). Mothers with preschoolers often decide to return to work, and investigate day care programs, baby-sitters, or nursery schools. In some instances, members of the extended family may assist with child care. If thoughtful arrangements have been made, contacts such as these which extend outside the home expand the preschooler's world and aid his or her socialization.

The School-Aged Child

During the child-rearing years of the family, when the child is between 6 and 12 years of age, a major task is the development of a nurturing pattern for all family members. Adults as well as children need to be nurtured in an emotional sense. Being available to young children means listening, answering questions, supervising activities, and protecting their health. Responsible, mature adults with inner resources can manage to fulfill these obligations. A vital role of each spouse is to provide a caring environment for the other so as to create opportunities for refueling. If their emotional and physical reserves are not replenished, parents become self-absorbed and neglectful of both their children and their mates (Rhodes, 1977). An essential function of the family is to share nurturing among all members and to foster mutual support between the partners. The single-parent family is at risk during this phase, because the solitary parent is especially dependent on sources outside the family to replenish psychological resources.

As children become more self-sufficient and competent, they seek greater freedom and independence. This causes the family to extend its boundaries so as to include churches, schools, and neighborhoods. Children who have established their role identity within the family structure need to progress to an identity which is not defined only by roles and responsibilities within the family (Rhodes, 1977).

The progressive independence of the last school-aged child may create new disequilibrium in the family. Some women experience a crisis if they view themselves as losing their highly invested care-giver role. If they have been engrossed in family life, they see the wife role as their only other identity. To complicate matters, the father may be so involved in his work or professional role that he provides little support for his wife during this crisis. In turn, the wife may be so stressed over her own role losses that she fails to provide support and encouragement to her spouse regarding his career or his approaching mid-life crisis.

When a couple decides to adopt a school-aged child and succeeds in doing so, there are reverberations throughout the newly formed family system. The pattern of relationships (*Structure*), communication (*Function*), and the use of resources will be altered, thus creating tension and disequilibrium. It is normal for a child who has been separated from his or her biological mother to feel mistrustful and to grieve this separation and loss. Parents need to acknowledge the grief, accept the child's feelings, and realize that the child is concerned with identity and acceptance. Furthermore, the child may think that the separation and loss which have occurred already may be repeated.

New adoptive parents will wonder whether they have the capacity to meet the child's needs and whether the child will respond to their love and attention (Moss & Moss, 1975). They may be painfully aware of being substitutes, and this may lead to overindulging the child. Time is needed to develop confidence in parenting and to adjusting the marital relationship to include a new talking-feeling member. If the marital coalition is strong enough for the parents to accept their inability to produce a child, or to forego having their own child in order to provide for a homeless child, and if the parents can accept the adopted child's social and genetic endowment, they will be well on the way to establishing a new triad in equilibrium.

In cases where transracial adoption occurs, the system will probably feel strong reverberations. Many critics consider a white home to be an inappropriate place for a black child because white parents are considered incapable of fostering ethnic awareness in the child, or teaching survival strategies in racially hostile environments (Chimezie, 1977). The child may be the object of social cruelty in school, church, or neighborhood activities because of differences in ethnic origin. When this occurs, the parents may close the family boundaries against outsiders until equilibrium is reestablished following the anger and pain. If the family boundaries are not subsequently reopened, further complications may ensue.

Divorces are frequent in families with school-aged children. Although some friends and members of the extended family may rally in support, divorce tends to disrupt friendships since individuals find it difficult to be loyal to both parties involved (Walker, Rogers, & Messinger, 1977). During the period of separation and divorce, family members must renegotiate relationships and goals. The periods of tension and disequilibrium fluctuate in unpredictable ways based on the level of emotional and functional upheaval experienced by individual family members.

Simon (1965) has written that most parents remarry 2 to 5 years after the end of the previous marriage. Some parents may regard the presence of their child as an impediment to remarriage, but others seem to take the position of "Love me, love my kid! Or no marriage." Stern (1976) wrote that a stepfather needs to accept the complete mother-child "package." In Stern's study, one potential stepfather advised another that the most important consideration in a stepfamily is whether the stepfather likes the child before he takes the plunge. Few romances seem to be broken up due to children's disapproval; rather, when potential spouses doubt the relationship, the protests of children serve as reinforcement.

It is interesting that school-aged children are more accepting of a new parent than are preschoolers or adolescents. Why is that? First, most school-aged children have developed some social graces which inhibit direct rudeness. Secondly, they are mature enough to give the stepparent a chance and to see what the prospective parent may be like as a person. Thirdly, they are interested in things outside the home; the home scene is less central and they are less demanding of total parental attention. Prior to marriage, the child and the potential stepparent need time to know one another. The parent needs to share information with the child about loving the new partner and hoping that the child will accept the stepparent-to-be (Simon, 1965).

The stepparent family must expect adjustments of many kinds. For example, the stepmother may resent having to cope with the consequences of what she considers poor child rearing; the stepfather may be concerned about seeing his new wife hug a smaller edition of her first husband. Favoritism or neglect of children may occur; children may test the parents to discover where they fit into the system (Simon, 1965), and some children may fear the new stepparent. Stern (1976) found that children used their friends and siblings for advice and support until the crisis of readjustment had passed. On the other hand, parents who had serious problems of adjustment rarely used their friends or other stepparents for advice. They "never thought of it" (Stern, 1976, p. 194). Many subjects in the study supported the idea of having *classes* not *groups* for remarrieds because "groups" suggested problems (Stern, 1976, pp. 194–195). Nurses and others involved in family prevention and intervention work might well follow this lead regarding classes.

If a child's parent has "married up or down in the social, cultural or economic scale or across religious or geographical lines" (Simon, 1965, p. 220) the family structure, function, and boundary changes become very complex. The reconstituted combination family consisting of the father and his biological children, the mother and her biological children, and possibly the couple's biological children has been referred to as the "forest primeval" (Simon, 1965).

Adolescence

Two processes occur during the adolescence of a child which cause drastic alterations in the family system: the physical upheaval of sexual maturation, and the growing independence of the budding adult. To add to the stress, the time at which the child of the family passes through adolescence coincides with transitional developmental periods in the lives of the family adults. The man of the house may have reached the peak period in his career involvement, or he may be moving into mid-life transition as described by Levinson, Darrow, Klein, Levinson, and Braxton (1974). Women examine new careers, return to school, or move to more fulfilling jobs during the child's teen years. The life crisis of adolescence holds possibilities for abundant but hazardous growth for the entire family.

Sexual Maturation   The effect of chemical messages sent by the gonadotrophic hormones to the testes of the male and the ovaries of the female becomes increasingly apparent around the twelfth or thirteenth year of life. No longer children, young people begin to look different, sound different, and smell different. The changing body of the young adult affects every family member. The rising breasts of the female and the falling voice of the male alter the interaction between parent and child, brother and sister.

Having one's body change in this dramatic fashion has a disquieting effect. One teenage boy may accept whiskers or pubic hair with equanimity, while another may despair over a croaking voice. Custom in the United States expects a sexually maturing body to conform to a different set of behaviors. In the absence of prescribed rituals for the transition to adulthood, the young person must try on one role after another in a ceaseless quest for a suitable adult identity.

Search for Identity and Independence   In the expanding family, the system accommodates to the arrival of new members; in the launching family the system prepares for members' departure. In achieving their developmental tasks, teenagers prepare for their identity as persons independent of the family.

A Gallup study (1977) showed that parents of teenagers worry most about discipline, motivation, work and study habits, and drug and alcohol abuse. Adolescents consider the use and abuse of drugs the most important problem, but they also consider the inability of parents and children to communicate or to get along with each other a close second. The whole family is affected as the young person experiences the pain and the pleasures of growing up. Ravenscroft (1974) found in a study of adolescents and their families that there is a normal family regression at adolescence. The various members recall their own struggles during teen years and, given the example of the child, find it necessary to work through their own teen problems once again.

The child struggles for an identity and is faced with the teenage question, "Who am I?" Erikson (1968) describes the process as a selection of ever-narrowing choices from a range of possible identities. The search for identity continues into the second or third decade according to Erikson. Coles (1970), writing about Erikson's work on identity, stated that the young person had to gain a sense of confidence that somehow, in the middle of change, he or she would find an "inner sameness and continuity," and become certain that it could be recognized by others and taken for granted.

Identity has many components. It is derived from one's family, with its genetic variety and patterns of behavior and structure. It is influenced by the social flavor of community and one's place in it. A sense of self, especially during adolescence, is gained in the reflected appraisal of peers. The constant question of the adolescent is "What do they think of me?"

Sexual Identity   Sexual identity comes from training which begins at birth. It includes the family romance of the preschool years and, during adolescence, an awareness of oneself as a sexual being is gained through association with peers. Psychoanalytic theory posits that adolescents and their parents finally resolve oedipal conflicts begun during the toddler years. Teenagers discard the family romance and search for mates of an age nearer to their own. The young person's preoccupation with sexual matters adds to the disquiet in the family. Some parents adjust to the tensions of adolescence with outward calm, but the new sexuality in the family makes all members a little tense. Mothers may compete with daughters for masculine attention; fathers may find fault with a son's appearance and obvious virility.

By traditional standards, indulgence in sexual intercourse has been permissible for teenage males, while female sexuality has been restricted. However, adequate birth control methods have brought changing patterns of sexual activity. Welches (1977) in a study of teenage women, found that over a third of 18-year-old women had experimented with intercourse. Experimentation with intercourse may be one way of separating from the family and taking on a more adult role.

Regaining Equilibrium   The conscientious family attempts to temper demands for freedom with rules that create a balance between safety and the freedom to grow. Threats posed by drugs and sex pose a dilemma to a family that knows it must avoid overprotection. The confusion and ambivalence of parents give rise to rules which err on the side of strictness or else on the side of excessive permissiveness. Often a decision is tabled with a parent's exasperated cry, "Oh, I don't know, I don't want to talk about it right now!" Young people learn to adust rules to avoid confrontation, while parents gradually learn to deal with the separating adolescent, and the transition to adulthood proceeds.

Variations in Step- and Adoptive Families   Stern (1976) found that discipline proved to be especially troublesome in dealing with teenage stepchildren. The teenager feels imposed upon by paternalism from a stepparent, while the stepparent feels at a disadvantage in setting limits for the behavior of an adolescent. A stepfather who is welcomed by a schoolaged child may find that the child's teenage sibling reacts rebelliously to disciplinary attempts, or else ignores them.

In step-, adoptive, or biological families, the prospect of losing teenage members is a disturbing influence on the system. It is only after the adolescents have moved out of the home that the couple system can resume patterns which existed before the arrival of children. Once again the parents are able to give each other the attention which the demands of children had denied them for years. In a healthy family, the couple will have matured over the years and will be able to enrich their relationship at this stage. In an unhealthy system, the growth of the couple may have been in directions which moved them away from each other.

CLINICAL IMPLICATIONS OF THE ADDITION OF A CHILD

Functional Reactions

Occasionally more time is spent educating health professionals about pathology and dysfunction than about the health and functions of individuals and families. Authors, researchers, and clinicians are still struggling to define and understand family health, function, dysfunction, and pathology. Researchers studying "normal" families or "nonlabeled" families have usually defined these families as having several of the following characteristics: (1) no arrests or police contact in recent years; (2) no family member currently or previously in psychotherapy or psychiatric treatment; (3) no apparent pathological symptoms as determined by an interviewer; (4) all family members in good physical health; (5) no family member identified by the community as having problems; and (6) all members performing the roles expected of them by the community (Riskin, 1976). Boszormenyi-Nagy and Spark (1973) concluded that health and pathology are jointly determined by (1) the nature of the multiperson relational laws, (2) the psychological characteristics ("psychic structure") of individual members, and (3) the interlocking between these two realms of system organization. A degree of flexibility and balance contributes to health, while inflexible system patterns may predispose individuals to pathology.

Stachowiak (1975) believed that health care workers need not know the "perfect" way to be a family, but should be aware that there are myriad ways of being a family. The essential criterion is that family members work out problems in their own interacting system.

With the thought in mind that there are countless variations in healthy families, some typical functional reactions of the family system, and some dysfunctional reactions related to the entry of children will be discussed. Examples of assessment and intervention will be provided.

Infant   The couple which decides to have a baby in order to have the pleasure and responsibility of rearing and relating to a child is starting the parenting experience with admirable reasons and attitudes. Parenting has been defined as "sharing the emotional and physical aspects of the total experience of bearing and rearing children" (Nichols, 1977, p. 30). Since parenthood involved redefining and readjusting roles, parents who cope effectively with the arrival of an infant will have given some thought to the effects of parenthood on their life-style. Decisions must be made on questions such as the following:

1   Can the father remain at home during the postpartum period to assist with early family adjustment, or can a relative of choice help the family in the first few weeks after birth?

2   Will the mother work outside the home during the first year of the infant's life?

3   What restrictions will the presence of the child place on the couple's freedom?

4   Will others be involved in the caretaking process? If so, will they share infant care and household chores?

   5 Is there space for the baby in the household?
   6 Is money available to pay for extra expenses incurred? Have plans been made to help the couple adjust to decreased income if a previously working parent does not continue?

   Even with careful planning, the birth of a child or the adoption of an infant will disrupt the homeostatic equilibrium of the family. However, a couple which has considered the foregoing questions will have an easier time coping with the event.

   Maternal attachment—the process by which the mother forms an affectional relationship with her infant—usually takes place during the first 3 months of the infant's life. Following delivery of the baby, the mother touches and looks at the infant and this is the maternal sensitive period (Kennell, 1975). When the infant is about 3 months old, the mother is emotionally committed to it, accepts her maternal obligations, experiences love and warmth toward the infant, and feels protective toward it. Proximal attachment behaviors (touching and holding) and distal attachment behaviors (looking, talking, smiling, and laughing) are the major pathways by which the attachment is made (Curry, 1974, 1976; Leiderman, 1975). It is normal for the mother to have some ambivalent feelings as well as some hostile impulses and thoughts about the infant. One young woman whose 2-week-old infant son had kept her and her husband up most of the night had just settled down and was almost asleep when the baby began to wail once again. The mother screamed, "Oh, that kid! I could murder him!" Whereupon, the husband leaped out of bed and flew to the side of the infant and began to comfort him. Both parents realized that the mother would not murder the child, but that she had reached the limits of her tolerance. Gradually, by means of the normal attachment process, ambivalence is suppressed and warm, nurturant behaviors predominate (Sideleau, 1978).

   Clinicians and researchers are beginning to look at both paternal and parental attachment. Fathers who are heavily involved in the care of the infant profess to be attached to their son or daughter in ways similar to those of their wives. Parental attachment, the process by which enduring bonds between parent and child are developed, is a concept which has been observed (Jordan, 1976). It should be noted that parents who have adopted an infant will experience an attachment similar to that felt by natural parents, but the process may take longer because of feelings of ambivalence about the adoption (Bello & Obrig, 1978).

   During the period in which the biological mother is becoming attached to the infant, mother and infant go through a phase of normal symbiosis. The infant experiences a state of undifferentiated fusion with the mother from about the third to the fifth month of life. Between the fifth and ninth months the child will be more alert when awake and there will be more locomotor action. In the following 8 months, the child is most highly involved in separating from the mother. Patience and understanding will be needed in this toddler period to allow the child to develop autonomous functions. The negativism of the toddler is considered by some to be a behavioral reaction that marks disengagement from symbiosis with the mother (Mahler, 1968). One result of adequate mothering is that the infant will develop the ability to distinguish between self and others (Nichols, 1977).

During the expanding phase of family life, the functional family develops cohesiveness and continuity, successfully incorporating extended family members and adjusting to parents of the spouses moving into grandparent roles. The parents establish a mutually satisfying sexual relationship, and show pride in the offspring, whom they nurture through beginning separation and individuation. The couple moves from an adult-centered peer organization into a child-centered organization and develops a satisfactory division of labor.

Preschool The preschooler's environment must be a place where the child is safe physically and emotionally. The child needs to be allowed autonomy and individuality, for out of this will evolve self-responsibility, initiative, and a sense of identity. Parents will need to accept the fact that their children may be quite different from earlier parental fantasies. Parental responsibility includes allowing the child to express a variety of feelings, while helping him or her gain some control over negative aggressive feelings. The latter becomes especially necessary if the impact of sibling rivalry needs to be moderated, a problem which is most intense when children are of the same sex.

Since even the most well-adjusted parents become exasperated by the continuous demands of a young child, it is important that they seek activities which will provide some relief. To prevent total preoccupation with the family, its boundaries should be expanded to include and serve the needs of others. Usually the couple will discuss whether to have more children, and evaluate this in terms of their goals and resources. The parents may also start to prepare themselves for the child's entry into school. Maintenance of effective communication becomes a matter of special importance. Tasks in the household can be shared with the child as a way of helping the child learn responsibility. In spite of occasional exasperation, parents will have many happy times as they enjoy their preschooler's eternal curiosity and amazement at each new experience.

School-Aged Child The functional family that has children in school is organized so that the children are provided with parental support and opportunities to develop both within and outside of the family. The child needs to be secure and free enough to become a member of a peer network at school, since the identity of student will give impetus to the individuation process (Rhodes, 1977). As children become progressively more independent, self-sufficient, and socially competent, they venture beyond the family boundaries into neighborhood and community. This requires that parents allow the boundaries between home and community to be bridged. The child will introduce new thoughts and behaviors into the family, which may produce temporary tension. For example, one child returned home to tell about witnessing the birth of kittens in a neighborhood home. Her description was both thorough and replete with correct medical terms. A neighboring parent in the health field had been teaching the children about the event as it occurred. Though the girl's parents thought their daughter still too young to watch the birthing, they kept this to themselves and were able to understand their daughter's excitement. These parents were allowing a "morphogenic process," which is explained as a change made in form, structure, or values in order to permit viability (Speer, 1970). They did not let their own values and sentimental order about when it was proper for their daughter to learn about the birth process mar the occasion for their child.

Even after resolution of the oedipal struggle, it is not unusual for a family romance to develop during the child's latency period. A common form the family romance takes is that the biological child wishes he or she were an adoptee in order to overcome disappointments in the relationship with parents (Wieder, 1977). The child's fantasy includes elements such as: "These aren't my parents, I've been stolen or separated from them. Or maybe I'm adopted. Someday my real parents will come and get me and I'll see them. Why, they may be a king and queen in some other place!" Wise biological parents realize that this phase will pass. They do not rob the child of the comforting fantasy nor react emotionally or neglect him during this tense period. The emotionally attached adopted child has an opposite fantasy. This child usually establishes a fantasied blood relationship to the adoptive parents, thus erasing the humiliation of being adopted (Wieder, 1977). In most instances, adopted children will be upset when told they are adopted. Tolerating this distress and answering questions as thoughtfully and truthfully as possible will reassure the child and help reestablish family equilibrium.

When parents adopt an older child, they and other family members need to know that tension and disequilibrium may be present for a while, because the child is likely to attack the new family system where it is vulnerable by changing the pattern of family alliances or by acting-out behaviors (Katz, 1977). Here again a firm balance between tolerance, limit setting, and loving support are needed until the adoptee learns his or her place and functions in the family organization.

The stepparent family whose members become friends has an excellent chance of becoming an integrated and adjusted family. During the "friending" process, the stepparent wins over the cooperation of the stepchild and the stepchild learns that the stepparent can be a source of family strength. Usually the addition of a stepfather means that the stepfamily has its living standard raised; nevertheless, it is helpful to the development of new family relationship patterns (*Structure*) if the child has special toys, trinkets, or gifts which come directly from the new parent (Stern, 1976).

Adolescence   Each member of the family has important developmental tasks to accomplish during the launching period, particularly since the emotional crisis of adolescents often coincides with the parents' crisis of middle age (Moore, 1974). Turmoil occurs as adolescents fluctuate between dependence and independence. They usually resent parental authority and guidance, turning to the peer network for approval and direction. Their boundaries expand to include peers, but at times they exclude their parents. One way in which adolescents establish identity is through opposition to others. Parents with a strong marital coalition can support one another as they encounter the turmoil of adolescent crises. The fluctuating tensions in families with maturing adolescents create accentuated periods of disequilibrium. If communication between parents and adolescents remains good, many of the problems can be alleviated.

Parents whose youth is over may be envious of the adolescent's opportunities and experiences. While adolescents are sorting out feelings about both parents, they may identify with or reject parental standards and values. In finding their own identity, adolescents may question parental standards, develop new ones of their own, or adopt those of peers or of some admired adult.

Adopted adolescents are sensitive to their special status. Being both adopted and an adolescent may cause excessive emotional pain, which is shown at times through fighting with parents or through running away. Family members may react with angry impulses, and punish the adolescent (Katz, 1977). Patience, tolerance, and maintenance of communication on the part of parents are essential to restore equilibrium and allay the fears of a troubled youngster.

An adolescent who becomes a stepchild has special difficulty adapting to the stepparent. It is generally agreed that the role of stepmother is especially difficult, for the stepmother usually has more contact with the children than does her husband. In order to decrease potential problems, the mother should not move quickly into the role of substitute parent. Evidence has been offered that a new stepfather is less of a problem for an adolescent, and that adjustment is easier if the stepparent replaces a divorced parent rather than a deceased one (Walker, Rogers, & Messinger, 1977).

Whether the young person is adopted, a stepchild, or a biological child, the parents will have to set limits. The adolescent complains about limits in order to establish independence. At the same time parents must not insist upon established rules merely to maintain the status quo (Murray & Zentner, 1975). Parents who do so create a morphostatic family system which is unresponsive to change (Speer, 1970).

Dysfunctional Reactions

When parents and family members fail to adjust to the addition of new members, the resulting dysfunction has negative consequences for all, and especially for the children. Hirschowitz (1974–1975) has identified some unhealthy patterns that families create to deal with change. They include the following:

1 Data received about needed change are distorted and obscured.
2 Data are ignored or tuned out by members who withdraw.
3 Energy is dissipated as family members try to retain the past or fantasize about the future.
4 When the need for change cannot be denied, the family searches for a scapegoat.
5 The father may abdicate his parental role and invest most of his time at work.
6 Members may anesthetize pain with drugs, alcohol, or food.
7 Ultimately the family may request that someone else take over, and may become dependent on an individual or agency.

It is safe to say that one or more of these patterns will be evident in the specific dysfunctional reactions which will be discussed next.

Among these dysfunctional reactions are disorders of maternal attachment such as maternal deprivation, failure-to-thrive (FTT) children, and parental child abuse. Other dysfunctional reactions are parent-child symbiosis, the replacement child phenomenon, and the consequences of prematurely informing a child about being adopted.

Disorders of Maternal Attachment   During the first few years of a child's life, as the family structure shifts, parents and child enact a drama which may have tragic consequences. These consequences include maternal deprivation, failure-to-thrive infants, parent-child symbiosis, and parental or sibling abuse. All these are related to the failure of the mother and infant to attach.

A primary responsibility of health professionals is to assess the progress of maternal-infant attachment. To do so, certain observations must be made.

1   Does the mother inspect the baby to see if it is whole, to identify the baby as a reality and not as a fantasy? Does the mother identify characteristics in the baby that were found in the families of origin?

2   Does the mother seek and maintain some eye-to-eye contact with the baby?

3   Does inspection include fingertip touching, then whole hand touching, and finally embracement of the child to her body?

4   Is the baby usually held so that the mother's and baby's eyes are on the same vertical plane?

5   Does the mother proceed with caring for the baby by feeding the child and changing diapers? (Bello & Obrig, 1978)

Some mothers may be so dismayed by the child's needs that they wonder about their ability to mother. Young mothers have seldom resolved their own identity problems and may wish to be dependent and free of responsibility. Teenage mothers, whose husbands may not give needed support, require consistent support and continuity of care from the nurse and other professionals. Gentle encouragement of early contact with the infant facilitates assumption of the mothering role (Iorio, 1975). The young mother deserves attention and praise for each task done well. One experienced maternity nurse has suggested that if nurses were to admit being less than perfect in their handling of newborns, young mothers might feel more comfortable. Nurses who do not seem all-knowing may contribute less to the anxiety of a mother who fears she can never manage her baby as well as the nurse (Curry, 1978).

Parents who are mentally ill, who use alcohol or drugs excessively, or who are mentally retarded may have children whose survival is at risk (Gorman, 1978). In premature infants, the attachment process is often delayed. The need for care in the premature nursery and concern about the fragile infant may lead to the mother's withdrawal from the infant. Mothers of premature infants are more hesitant and clumsy in learning mothering tasks and may feel that the baby belongs to the doctors and nurses (Kennell, 1975).

The infant labeled as difficult and temperamental may be rejected and deprived of mothering because attachment does not occur. Characteristics of such an infant include:

1   Unpredictable sleeping and feeding patterns
2   High intensity of reactions or responses
3   Tendency to withdraw in the face of new stimuli
4   Negative mood
5   Slow adaptability to changes or environment (Thomas, Chess, & Birch, 1970).

Mothers experience strain in relating to infants with unbalanced rhythms who are not soothed by "mothering" measures (Light, 1978). Once the nurse has assessed the presence of these characteristics, appropriate steps to be taken are as follows:

1 Determine if the mother fails to respond to the infant because of her own needs.
2 Determine the level of anxiety that the mother may be communicating to the infant during mothering activities.
3 Investigate the level of the mother's frustration and the methods of coping used to deal with the problem.

After the initial assessment, the health professional can explore with the client what seems to be needed to improve the situation. Does the mother need to develop consistency in her attention to the child? Is additional support required from husband, relatives, neighbors, or a health professional? Does the mother need to visit the pediatrician to discuss the infant? What methods of soothing the baby are effective? Does the mother need help in accepting the uniqueness of her infant? Does she need reassurance regarding the infant's behavioral repertoire?

The infant who fails to thrive "suffers from generalized retarded growth and malnutrition despite the availability of adequate food" (Greenberg, 1970, p. 101). The following clinical criteria are used to identify failure-to-thrive children:

1 Weight below the third percentile, with subsequent weight gain in the presence of appropriate nurturing
2 No evidence of systemic disease or abnormality on physical examination to explain growth failure
3 Developmental retardation with subsequent acceleration following appropriate stimulation and feeding
4 Clinical signs of deprivation which decrease in a more nurturing environment
5 Presence of significant environmental psychosocial disruption (Barbero, 1975, p. 9).

Infants who fail to thrive display numerous bizarre eye behaviors such as continuous scanning of the environment and avoidance of eye-to-eye contact. These babies tend to be either rigid, flaccid, or immobile. Hospitalization of the infant is in order. Intervention usually includes investigation by a pediatrician for a possible systemic disorder as well as exploration of psychosocial factors. Nursing intervention includes education of the parents and supportive counseling during hospitalization as well as planned follow-up care. In extreme situations, the mother may need to be referred for individual therapy or the family for family therapy.

In the case of the adopted child, rejection sometimes results when the child has been adopted by relatives who were impelled by duty or impulse. Younger adopted children may show signs of deprivation in these circumstances. They may engage in attention-seeking behavior, aggressive outbursts, food fadism, compulsive disorders, and petty pilfering. An adolescent adoptee who feels deprived may become moody, delinquent, or despondent. These signs represent the child's rejection of the adoptive parents following their rejection of the child (Lewis, 1965). When such behavior becomes apparent to the professional, investigation to determine causation is in order. Gathering a history from the parents, and then from the child or adolescent, is essential. Parents respond differently to their adopted child's behavior when the behavior is relabeled by a professional. For example, "Johnny is bad because he steals money from the cookie jar" can be relabeled as follows by the health professional working with a concerned mother and her 7-year-old: "Johnny doesn't think you care about him or love him, and he may be taking money to get your attention. It is his way of saying, 'Mom and Dad, notice me!' " The child's actions have been relabeled as attention-seeking and love-starved behavior.

The neglected child is often encountered by professionals. Negligence and deprivation frequently are rooted in the background and personality of the parents, especially in the degree to which the mother can be warm and nurturing. When nutritional, sensory, or dependency needs of the child are not met, physical growth slows, motor development is delayed, and social and emotional withdrawal follow. Other forms of child neglect result from poor hygiene, inadequate immunization, inappropriate clothing, and poor communication with the child, all of which decrease self-esteem and acceptance. These conditions can be noted by school nurses, community health nurses, pediatric nurse-practitioners, and family health nurse-practitioners. Health providers may react angrily to negligence and deprivation, but their anger should be reduced through objective discussion with other professionals. Unless strong feelings are controlled, the professional will be impeded in attempts to assess and intervene effectively.

Another blatant attachment disorder is parental or sibling abuse of an infant or child. There is no dearth of documented stories about child abuse. Infants have been thrown out of second-story apartment houses; children have been burned with irons, suffocated with pillows, burned with cigarettes, and beaten. Battering may start as early as the postpartum period. Lynn (1974) described child abuse as nonaccidental physical injury to minor children by persons responsible for caring for them.

Statistics on child abuse are unreliable; abuse may occur six times in every 1000 children (Sideleau, 1978). A substantial number of abused children are eventually killed. Brain damage is a frequent occurrence. The height and weight of abused children are on the average lower than those of 97 percent of children the same age (Ackley, 1977).

Some salient characteristics associated with parents who are child abusers can be of help in identifying the abusers.

1   The abusing parent was an abused child (Ackley, 1977; Sideleau, 1978; Lynn, 1974; Helfer, 1975).

2   The abusive parent is a solitary or isolated individual (Ackley, 1977; Lynn, 1974; Helfer, 1975.)

3   Potential abusers bear a child in an attempt to fulfill their own emotional needs (Ackley, 1977; Helfer, 1975).

4   Families of lower socioeconomic and educational status are more often abusive (Sideleau, 1977; Lynn, 1974).

5   The ethnic distribution of the child-abusing parents is approximately that of the general population (Lynn, 1974).

6   Abusive parents tend to have several children (Lynn, 1974).

7   In an intact home, the father or substitute father is the perpetrator of nearly two-thirds of the child abuse incidents, and fathers inflicted the most severe injuries (Lynn, 1974).

8   A parent is more likely to abuse a child of the same sex (Lynn, 1974).

9   Beating with a belt or paddle is a frequent method of abuse (Lynn, 1974).

10   Parents expect behavior from their children which is more mature than the child's age warrants (Lynn, 1974).

11   Abusive parents have low self-esteem and poor marital relationships (Helfer, 1975).

12   The mother who allows her husband to abuse the child is frequently abused by him (Sideleau, 1978).

13   Abusive parents may exhibit characteristics as follows: immaturity, impulsivity, dependency, hostility, aggressiveness, and rigidity (Sideleau, 1978).

14   Alcohol abuse decreases inhibitions of the child abuser; more impulsive, assaultive sexual behaviors may then occur (Sideleau, 1978).

Any parent with a number of the characteristics mentioned above runs the risk of becoming an abuser.

Families may not report the assault of siblings on a younger child. The family may deny such events. In order to maintain intrafamilial solidarity, parents may make a preconscious judgment that the assault was unintentional or merely "horseplay" (Tooley, 1977). The older sibling may be acting out the mother's unconscious resentment of the young child. The child in a violent family who kills a sibling has been described as the unwitting agent of an adult, usually a parent, who unconsciously encourages the child to kill so that the adult can vicariously benefit from the fatal act (Sideleau, 1978).

Certain characteristics and behaviors of children increase their likelihood of being abused. Among these are the following:

1 An infant or child who cries inconsolably
2 An infant who has colic or is cranky
3 A child whose sex is opposite to the one the parents desired
4 A child who reminds a parent of a hated parent or sibling
5 A child who fails to recognize the parent's warning signs of being upset (Ackley, 1977)
6 An infant who is born prematurely (Kennell, 1975; Blumberg, 1977)
7 A toddler who is untidy and difficult (Sideleau, 1978)
8 An infant who is the product of an unwanted pregnancy, or the child of a partner by a previous marriage (Blumberg, 1977)

A child with one or more of the above characteristics may well end up in an emergency room before the age of 3. In the emergency room, the abused child has injuries which do not fit the parent's description of the accident. Bruises or burns are often evident. X-ray reports demonstrate that old fractures have healed. Upon hospitalization, the child does not protest and cry when the parents leave, and adapts quickly to the hospital unit (Sideleau, 1978). On the other hand, the abused child may seem devoted to the parent, for the child has learned that failure to show affection may increase abuse.

Legislation has been enacted to protect children from abuse, and health care professionals are required to report suspected cases. Intervention with the child requires physical and emotional care in the hospital; the child needs protection from further abuse until the family can be evaluated. Based on the family assessment and evaluation, the health professional offers sustained intervention to the family. Intensive long-term care is usually indicated, and includes such goals as building parenting skills and helping the family understand growth and development so they may make reasonable and age-appropriate demands on the child. Abusing parents must be helped to turn to other adults rather than to the child in time of emotional need. With professional assistance, parents can become more effective problem solvers. Involving the parents in support groups in which they can share their experiences with professional group leaders and other child abusers has been shown to be helpful.

Ideally, to eliminate child abuse by attacking its causes, society must confront the problems of poverty, unemployment, and racism that aggravate the abuse-prone parent. Lack of nursery schools and day care centers means that overburdened mothers have little chance for temporal relief from their children. More crisis hot lines are needed to provide immediate help for potentially abusive parents. Care givers and health professionals must function as social and legislative advocates if these changes are to be effected.

Parent-Child Symbiosis When the infant and the mothering figure continue fusion and undifferentiation beyond the sixth month of the infant's life, the symbiosis is considered pathological. When boundaries between the mothering one and the older infant lack permeability, the child may demonstrate a symbiotic psychosis.

A conscientious but very dependent mother will have a hard time allowing her child to become separate and independent. Mothers who have had tubal ligations for which they are not emotionally prepared, and who lack support from husband and relatives, may handle their conflict by retarding the child's move toward independence (Bello & Obrig, 1978).

The clinical symptoms of symbiosis may not be apparent until after the first year of the child's life. Light (1978) suggested questions to be addressed in the assessment process.

1 Do incidents of separation elicit excessive anxiety and problematic behavior?
2 Does the child exhibit temper tantrums inappropriate to the developmental age?
3 Do the parents exhibit problems or express fears about normal separation from the child?
4 Is the child's speech appropriate to the developmental age? (p. 567).

After an initial family meeting to explain the purpose of the sessions, it is advisable to interview the parents separately, and to spend time alone with the child. This allows the interviewer to compare how the child behaves with and without the presence of parents. During the interview it is crucial to assess the marital relationship. It is always possible that the parents or the family system require a disturbed child to maintain its equilibrium.

Therapeutic goals should focus primarily on helping the child separate and individuate. This means that the mother will need help in managing her anxiety during the separation process. Such mothers should be encouraged to invest time and energies in activities outside the nurturer role. The child needs to experience and gradually to tolerate increased time away from the mother. The child should be helped to develop satisfying relationships with others such as relatives or playmates. Parents will need help with their own communication and with their ability to resolve conflict (Light, 1978). If the child is older than 9 or 10 and is still symbiotically attached to the mother, multifamily group therapy with a qualified professional may be the treatment of choice. Sibling support often can aid differentiation and individuation. Family therapy and multifamily group therapy can make very good use of such support to foster separation and individuation.

The Replacement Child   Mr. and Mrs. Jones have lost their firstborn, who died of pneumonia when he was 2 months old. A nurse says, "You are young and healthy. It won't be long before you can be pregnant again." Mr. and Mrs. Lopez have just been told that their daughter Angela died on the way to the nursery. Every attempt was made to save her but it was just one of those strange events. In an attempt to be consoling, the doctor advises the parents to have a new baby in order to get over the loss of Angela. The advice is well meant in both cases, but both the nurse and the doctor are using poor clinical judgment. It is not wise to encourage parents to have a new baby to replace their dead child immediately. Parents require a period of 6 months to a year or more to mourn a dead child before having or adopting another child.

Of their own volition, parents may decide to decrease the pain of loss by quickly conceiving a new infant or beginning adoption proceedings. However, introducing a new infant into the family may disrupt or delay the mourning process, without resolving it (Legg & Sherick 1976). The replacement child enters a hazardous situation, literally walking in the shadow of death. Life begins while the parents are still in mourning, and the child must establish his or her identity in the shadow of another identity which is projected on the child by the family. To make things more difficult, the parents, having just lost one child, may overprotect the replacement child (Pinkerton, 1965).

It is not too early to ascertain during the early mourning period whether the parents are thinking of having another child in the near future. If the parents say they are contemplating conception within the next 6 months, the health professional may elect to share some information. For example, the professional might comment that it is the parents who must decide about conception, but that they might consider the wisdom of having a child so soon. The parents might be advised to give themselves time to mourn the dead child and to resolve their loss. If the parents decide to have another baby as soon as possible, they should be assisted in avoiding potential difficulties and observed for possible complications.

On Hearing of Adoption   Children who are over 6 years of age are old enough to assimilate basic information about their adoption. When younger children are told of being adopted, they may react with severe separation anxiety and confusion, which produces regression and behavioral changes. Dependency and passivity may persist for quite some time; sleep disturbances may occur. There is danger of conflict of identification when a child realizes that he or she has two sets of parents (Wieder, 1977a).

Intervention should be focused on prevention. When a child is adopted, the parents may need to plan how information about the adoption will be shared. Is the child of an appropriate age? Are there intervening fears or worries? By anticipatory planning, consensually validating appropriate plans, and discussing the fears and worries of the parent, the professional may help to avert a dysfunctional reaction in the child.

CLINICAL EXAMPLE: A CHILD-LEFT-OUT FAMILY

Structure

Nola and Hoyt have been married for 6 years. It is the second marriage for both. Living in the home are Nola's 9-year-old son Eric, Hoyt's 11-year-old daughter Heather, and 5-year-old Iva, a child of the present union. Hoyt, 35, holds a middle-management position with thirteen employees under him, whom he says he "fathers." Nola, in her late twenties, keeps herself occupied with her children and her church work; she became a born-again Christian 2 years ago (*Suprasystem*). Nola prides herself on her immaculate house. She is a talkative woman who describes herself as "absentminded" and "a nut."

Function

Hoyt moved in with Nola when Eric was 3½ years old. Nola was unable to handle Eric, and when Hoyt observed the screaming matches between the two, he asked Nola if she wanted him to help her control the child. Nola accepted Hoyt's offer because, she said, "Eric was real hyper, and he needed discipline." The enforcement technique Hoyt used on Eric consisted of beating the child with a belt. This method made sense to Hoyt since he had been similarly beaten by his mother, his father, his stepmother, and the nuns at the Catholic schools he attended (*Sentimental order*). Eric protested for a time, but eventually he became subdued, and obeyed the rules except when he "forgot." In his presence, Eric's parents described him as "very absentminded" (*Feedback*). Eric has not seen his departed father, a long-haired, marijuana-smoking musician, in 4 years. The father lives

500 miles away, and Eric is not allowed to visit, because of the father's life-style. Eric said he misses his father "very much."

When Eric was 6, Heather joined the family, because her step-father had made sexual advances to her. Heather has not seen her mother since the move, because the mother lives some distance away and cannot afford the trip. In addition, Heather is not allowed by her stepfather to visit her mother even though Heather says she misses her. Heather is never beaten for infractions of the rules, because Heather "always knows when to quit" (*Feedback*). Nola was angry that only her child received corporal punishment (*Scapegoating*), but she could not bring herself to inflict this means of control upon Heather. She and Heather once faked a beating for Hoyt's benefit, using sound effects from a bedroom. Both Heather and Nola describe their relationship as "close" (*Alliance*).

Nola carries out Hoyt's household rules when he is at work, and formulates a number of her own rules. Nola allows Iva to disobey many of these rules because "she's just a little girl, and she means to do the right thing." Privately, she confessed that she thought Hoyt had been too strict with Eric, but, she added, "There's nothing I can do about that now, I can see that it doesn't happen to Iva" (*Go-between function*).

Eric is handsome and eager to please. He presents a shy demeanor, and moves his hands nervously. Although Hoyt speaks directly to Eric, his stepson answers in a muffled voice (*Feedback*). Nola often answers questions directed to Eric (*Go-between function*). A recent IQ test showed Eric to be exceptionally bright, but his school performance is poor. He is unable to tie his shoes. Friends do not visit Eric at home, because his mother demands the phone number of all visiting children in advance, and Eric is too shy to obtain this information (*Boundaries*). The other two children are outgoing and speak directly to Hoyt. When therapy for the family was suggested to Nola, she said she might consider it, but she was sure Hoyt would not agree. She has attended a group for stepparents, however (revised from Stern, 1976, pp. 129–131).

Assessment

Structure The husband-in-charge in this household was instrumental in creating alliances between the wife and the two female children. Eric is the child-left-out who receives most of the punishment. He has no champion or healer, which is typical of the scapegoated position. The family boundaries indicate limited accessibility to outside assistance.

Function The mother is a go-between in communication between the father and children. Feedback is short-circuited through the mother and feedback to the stepson is consistently derogatory. The energy level is the family is within normal limits. The sentimental order indicates a pattern of beating the male child.

Planned Intervention

Structure Family structure should be adjusted to allow for shared leadership of the marital pair. The stepson should be allowed a higher status position to promote his integration into the family. Boundaries should be opened to the outside, so that Eric can have the privilege of his friends' visits. Arrangements should be made for the children to see their absent parents.

Function Direct communication should be increased between all family members. The family should be helped to develop a sentimental order which forbids child beating and substitutes other disciplinary measures.

SUMMARY

The family system undergoes many changes as new members are added and as individual members change over time. Modifications that occur in structure and functioning as the family grows were discussed. Similarities and differences in biological and stepfamilies were described, with emphasis on the variations in boundaries and developmental tensions. Professionals should be alert and sensitive to potential problems over the family life cycle. Nurses, in particular, because of their opportunities for close contact with children and their families, are in a position to use sound clinical judgement, to implement the therapeutic process, and to evaluate the outcome. Individual, family, and group counseling (in stepparent groups, for example) were suggested as a means to ease the tension associated with stressful transitional periods.

REFERENCES

Ackley, D. C. A brief overview of child abuse. *Social Casework,* 1977, **58**(1), 21–28.

Adams, P. L. Functions of the lower class partial family. *American Journal of Psychiatry,* 1973, **130**(2), 200–203.

Anderson, D. C. *Children of special value. Interracial adoption in America.* New York: St. Martin's Press, 1971.

Barbero, G. Failure to thrive. In M. H. Klaus, T. Leger, & M. A. Trause (Eds.), *Maternal attachment and mothering disorders: A round table.* New Brunswick, N.J.: Johnson & Johnson Baby Products, 1975.

Bello, A., & Obrig, A. M. Promotion of mental health in families. In J. Haber, A. Leach, S. M. Schurdy, & B. F. Sideleau (Eds.), *Comprehensive Psychiatric Nursing.* New York: McGraw-Hill, 1978.

Berman, C. *We take this child. A candid look at modern adoption.* Garden City, N.Y.: Doubleday, 1974.

Blood, R. O. *The family.* New York: Free Press, 1972.

Blumberg, M. Treatment of the abused child and child abuser. *American Journal of Psychotherapy,* 1977, **31**, 204–215.

Bohannan, P. J. *Stepfathers and the mental health of their children.* (Summary of findings for NIMH Grant No. RO1M H 21146, 1975). Western Behavioral Sciences Institute, 1150 Silverado St., La Jolla, Calif. 92037.

Bohannan, P. J., & Erickson, R. Stepping in. *Psychology Today,* January 1978, pp. 53–59.

Boszormenyi-Nagy, I., & Spark, G. *Invisible loyalties: Reciprocity in intergenerational family therapy.* New York: Harper & Row, 1973.

Bowlby, J. *Maternal care and mental health.* New York: Schocken Books, 1966.

Braff, A. M. Telling children about their adoption: New alternatives for parents. *MCN The American Journal of Maternal Child Nursing,* 1977, **2**(4), 254–259.

Chimezie, A. Bold but irrelevant: Grow and Shapiro on transracial adoption. *Child Welfare,* 1977, **56**(2), 75–86.

Coles, R. Profiles. The measure of man—1. *The New Yorker,* November, 7, 1970, pp. 51–131.

Curry, M. A. Maternal attachment: An eclectic theory. Lectures at University of California, San Francisco, November 27, 1974, March 4, 1976, & February 7, 1978.

Dresen, S. Adjusting to single parenting. *American Journal of Nursing,* 1976, **8**, 1286–1289.

Duberman, L. Step-kin relationships. *Journal of Marriage and the Family,* 1973, **35**, 283–292.

Dyer, E. D. Parenthood as crisis: A re-study. *Marriage and Family Living,* 1963, **25**, 196–201.

Erikson, E. H. *Identity: Youth and crisis.* New York: Norton, 1968.

Foley, V. *An introduction to family therapy.* New York: Grune & Stratton, 1974.

Gallup, G. What worries today's parents most. *San Francisco Chronicle,* September 30, 1977, p. 27.

Glaser, B. G., & Strauss, A. L. *Awareness of dying.* Chicago: Aldine, 1965.

Gorman, J. Secondary prevention in families with infants and children. In J. Haber, A. Leach, S. M. Schurdy, & B. F. Sideleau (Eds.), *Comprehensive Psychiatric Nursing.* New York: McGraw-Hill, 1978.

Greenberg, N. H. Atypical behavior during infancy: Infant development in relation to the behavior and personality of the mother. In E. J. Anthony & C. Koupernik (Eds.), *The child in his family.* New York: Wiley, 1970.

Hammons, C. The adoptive family. *American Journal of Nursing,* 1976, **76** 251–257.

Helfer, R. The relationship between lack of bonding and child abuse and neglect. In M. H. Klaus, T. Leger, & M. A. Trause (Eds.), *Maternal attachment and mothering disorders: A round table.* New Brunswick, N.J.: Johnson & Johnson Baby Products, 1975.

Hirschowitz, R. G. Family coping patterns in times of change. *International Journal of Social Psychiatry,* 1974–1975, **21**(1), 37–43.

Iorio, J. *Childbirth: Family-centered nursing* (3rd ed.). St. Louis: C. V. Mosby, 1975.

Jackson, D. D. The question of family homeostasis. *The Psychiatric Quarterly Supplement,* 1957, **31**(Pt. 1), 79–90.

Jordan, C. The process of parental attachment, part 1. *Pediatric Nursing,* 1976, **2**(4), 8–15.

Katz, L. Older child adaptive placement: A time of family crisis. *Child Welfare,* 1977, **56**(3), 165–171.

Kennell, J. Evidence for a sensitive period in the human mother. In M. H. Klaus, T. Leger, & M. A. Trause (Eds.), *Maternal attachment and mothering disorders: A round table.* New Brunswick, N.J.: Johnson & Johnson Baby Products, 1975.

Klibanoff, S., & Klibanoff, E. *Let's talk about adoption.* Boston: Little, Brown, 1973.

Krantzler, M. *Creative divorce.* New York: Signet, 1973.

Lamb, M. E. *The role of the father in child development.* New York: Wiley, 1976.

Legg, C., & Sherick, I. The replacement child—a developmental tragedy: Some preliminary comments. *Child Psychiatry and Human Development,* 1976, **7**(2), 113–126.

Leiderman, H. Mother-infant separation: Delayed consequences. In M. H. Klaus, T. Leger, & M. A. Trause (Eds.), *Maternal attachment and mothering disorders: A round table.* Johnson & Johnson Baby Products, 1975.

Levinson, D. J., Darrow, C. M., Klein, E. B., Levinson, M. H., & Braxton, M. The psychosocial development of men in early adulthood and the mid-life transition. In D. F. Ricks, A. Thomas, & M. Roff (Eds.), *Life history research in psychopathology* (Vol. 3). Minneapolis: University of Minnesota Press, 1974.

Lewis, J. The psychiatric aspects of adoption. In J. G. Howells (Ed.), *Modern perspectives in child psychiatry.* Springfield, Ill.: Charles C Thomas, 1965.

Light, N. The family with a psychotic child. In J. Haer, A. Leach, S. M. Schurdy, & B. F. Sideleau (Eds.), *Comprehensive Psychiatric Nursing.* New York: McGraw-Hill, 1978.

Lynn, D. B. *The father: His role in child development.* Belmont, Calif.: Wadsworth, 1974.

Mahler, M. *On human symbiosis and the vicissitudes of individuation* (Vol. 1). New York: International University Press, 1968.

Moore, J. A. Developmental reactions in the middle years. In M. Kalkman & A. Davis (Eds.), *New dimensions of mental health-psychiatric nursing.* New York: McGraw-Hill, 1974.

Moss, S. Z., & Moss, M. S. Surrogate mother-child relationships. *American Journal of Orthopsychiatry,* 1975, **45**, 382.

Murray, R., & Zentner, J. *Nursing assessment and health promotion through the life span.* Englewood Cliffs, N.J.: Prentice-Hall, 1975.

Nichols, B. B. Motherhood, mothering and casework. *Social Casework,* 1977, **58**(1), 29–35.

Pinkerton, P. The psychosomatic approach in child psychiatry. In J. G. Howells (Ed.), *Modern perspectives in child psychiatry.* Springfield, Ill.: Charles C Thomas, 1965.

Pulitteri, A. *Nursing care of the growing family: A child health text.* Boston: Little, Brown, 1977.

Ravenscroft, K. Normal family regression at adolescence. *American Journal of Psychiatry,* 1974, **131**(1), 31–35.

Rhodes, S. L. A developmental approach to the life cycle of the family. *Social Casework,* 1977, **58**(5), 301–311.

Riskin, J. 'Nonlabeled' family interaction: Preliminary report on a prospective study. *Family Process,* 1976, **15**, 433–439.

Rossi, A. Transition to parenthood. In P. J. Stein, J. Richman, & N. Hannon (Eds.), *The family: Functions conflicts and symbols.* Reading, Mass.: Addison-Wesley, 1977.

Russell, C. S. Transition to parenthood: Problems and gratifications. *Journal of Marriage and the Family,* 1974, **36**, 294–301.

Satir, V. *Conjoint family therapy* (Rev. ed.). Palo Alto, Calif.: Science & Behavior Books, 1967.

Satir, V. *Peoplemaking.* Palo Alto, Calif.: Science & Behavior Books, 1972.

Schechter, M. D. About adoptive parents. In J. Anthony & T. Benedek (Eds.), *Parenthood: Its psychology & psychopathology.* Boston: Little, Brown, 1970.

Sideleau, B. F. The abusive family. In J. Haber, A. Leach, S. M. Schurdy, & B. F. Sideleau (Eds.), *Comprehensive Psychiatric Nursing.* New York: McGraw-Hill, 1978.

Simon, A. W. *Stepchild in the family.* New York: Pocket Books, 1965.

Speer, D. C. Family systems: Morphostasis and morphogenesis, or 'Is homeostasis enough?' *Family Process,* 1970, **9**, 259–278.

Stachowiak, J. Functional and dysfunctional families. In V. Satir, J. Stachowiak, & H. A. Taschman (Eds.), *Helping families to change.* New York: Jason Aronson, 1975.

Stern, P. N. Integrative discipline in stepfather families (Doctoral dissertation, University of California). San Francisco: University Microfilms, 1976. No. 77–5276 *Dissertation Abstracts International,* 1977, **37**.

Stern, P. N. Stepfather families: Integration around child discipline. *Issues in Mental Health Nursing,* 1978, **1**(2), 50–56.

Thomas, A., & Chess, S. *Temperament and development.* New York: Brunner/Mazel, 1977.

Thomas, A., Chess, S., & Birch, H. G. The origin of personality. *Scientific American,* 1970, **223**, 102–109.

Tooley, M. The young child as victim of sibling attack. *Social Casework,* 1977, **58**(1), 25–28.

Walker, K. N., Rogers, J., & Messinger, L. Remarriage after divorce: A review. *Social Casework,* 1977, **58**, 276–285.

Watzlawick, P., Beavin, J. H., & Jackson, D. D. *Pragmatics of human communication.* New York: Norton, 1967.

Welches, L. Teenage sexual behavior and the family. Paper presented to the First Regional Congress of Social Psychiatry, Santa Barbara, Calif., September 7, 1977.

Wieder, H. On being told of adoption. *The Psychoanalytic Quarterly,* 1977, **46**(1), 1-22. (a)

Wieder, H. The family romance fantasies of adopted children. *The Psychoanalytic Quarterly,* 1977, **46**(2), 185-200. (b)

Chapter 10

Stresses of
Postparental Couples

Sandra A. Chenelly
Ellen H. Janosik

In recent years interest in studying the developmental tasks of middle-aged adults has surged. Most practitioners have become familiar with the concept of a mid-life crisis, a term culled from the growing body of literature dealing with the transitional issues of middle age. At present the mean age of the American population is rising, reflecting both an increase in the numbers of persons surviving into the later years and a decrease in the birth rate. "The graying of America" (1977) has stimulated exploration of significant events in the later years of adulthood, as the importance of helping older adults deal with their special problems becomes more apparent.

POTENTIAL PROBLEMS

One difficult problem which middle-aged adults must face is the departure of the last child from the parental home. The cyclical nature of individual and family development is obvious when one considers the middle-aged couple who find themselves alone after 20 or 30 crowded years. Earlier periods of childbearing and child rearing give way to a contracting family system which eventually returns to its original dyadic structure. Unlike the newly married pair beginning life together, the postparental couple has a shared history which may either assist or impede adjustment during this period of reassessment, clarification, and change.

When the family again becomes a dyad, the postparental couple may have to deal with problems arising from renewed intimacy and divergent personal goals. Throughout family life, the biological and social differences between men and women necessitate crucial adjustments by the partners and by other members in order for the family system to survive. This remains true as couples move into the fourth and fifth decades of their lives. Frequently the wife who sublimated her own ambitions to family needs sees the postparental years as a last chance to express herself. Some husbands are heavily involved with their work at this period, while others may want their lives to be more family-centered, and therefore may be reluctant to accept the wife's personal goals. Neugarten (1968) aptly described the differences between middle-aged men and middle-aged women.

> Important differences exist between men and women as they age. Men seem to become more receptive to affiliative and nurturant promptings, women more responsive toward and less guilty about aggressive and egocentric impulses (p. 98).

Disparity between the value systems of couples in their middle years was also noted by Sheehy (1974) who wrote that it is essential for the second half of life to have its own significance. Menopause and separation from the last child find some women eager to pursue ambitions outside the context of family life. Other women, who gladly lived for and through their families, may feel superfluous and unwanted by husband and adult children, yet fear embarking on new ventures. In some cases the responses of the couple are congruent, with the husband encouraging the vocational aspirations of his wife. In others, the man may resent having his wife commit herself to a developing career. Lifelong patterns of adaptivity in certain men, as well as in certain women, have been described by Sheehy (1974). Individuals who are adaptive consistently find a way of enacting family roles adequately while pursuing their individual goals and interests. Because they balanced personal and family obligations well before the children left home, such persons are called *integrators,* and they are more likely to move into the postparental years without imposing undue strain on marital relationships and without compromising the integrity of the partner.

The postparental stage has been labeled in various ways. Labels such as the "deserted parents stage" or the "empty nest stage" imply a time of loss or abandonment. Less doleful are terms like the "middle-years family" or the "launching family" (Duvall, 1977). Whatever their implication, the terms are generally applied to the interval of family life when children no longer reside primarily in the family home, but parents have not yet entered the vaguely defined period called old age.

The diversity among the labels attached to this stage of family life reflects the conflicting views surrounding the impact of parenting and postparenting on the marital relationship. Most research in the area has attempted to study the effect of the departure of children on marital satisfaction and individual adjustment. However, no definitive data have emerged to determine whether this period in the family life cycle does indeed constitute a crisis of major proportions. What can be said with some assurance is that any drastic alteration of roles or role performance constitutes stress on the family system, and that adjustment depends on the ability of the couple to accommodate to each other.

In an early study, Axelson (1965) compared a "quasi-parental" group in which one or more children over 18 years remained at home with a "true postparental" group of individuals whose last child had left. The men and women in both postparental and quasi-parental groups reported a significant lowering of concern around children and finances, and a significant heightening of marital satisfaction and shared activities. Both groups reported a decrease in community participation and involvement, supporting the assumption that the presence of children deepens the family's roots in the community. The study supported the view that the empty nest stage is a time of ascendency for the marital relationshp. On the negative side, postparental women reported a significant increase in loneliness. This finding might be related to the fact that males in this study reported more interest in their daily work than they had felt previously.

Lowenthal and Chiriboga (1972) studied transition to the empty nest stage, concluding that for most couples few new frustrations accompanied the loss of active parenting. Males and females in their sample reported continued satisfaction with parenthood and in their relationships with their grown children. Again, males and females reported different problems, with men being more concerned about jobs and finances. Some of this might be attributed to an urgency to achieve in their careers in the face of approaching retirement. Regardless of whether they worked outside the home, women reported interpersonal or marital problems as most troublesome. Women were twice as likely as men to speak negatively of spouses and only three of fifty-two respondents mentioned current satisfaction with the marriage.

A later study (Thurnher, 1974) of empty nest couples found other differences in the adjustment of men and of women. Despite the fact that children were no longer present, both husband and wife focused first on *interpersonal-expressive* values centering on home and family. However, the men focused next on *instrumental-material* values related to job and finances, while women focused on *ease and contentment* values. Women in the study were more reluctant than men to foresee or admit any possibility of their decreased commitment to family in the future. Men, on the other hand, anticipated a gradual increase in their strong job orientation, accompanied by an increase in hedonistic pursuits. In contrast, women believed interpersonal-expressive values would remain paramount, with no increase in hedonistic activities. These findings are somewhat at variance with those of Neugarten presented earlier, but again they indicate disparity between the attitudes of husbands and wives.

The preceding discussion illustrates the lack of consensus on the question of whether the postparental stage of family life represents a crisis, a challenge, or a relief for the middle-aged couple. Spanier, Lewis, and Cole (1975) advanced a logical explanation for the frequent disclosure that postparental couples report increased marital satisfaction in the empty nest years, while disagreeing on priorities for the future and for personal adjustment. Since most studies of the postparental period are cross-sectional, not longitudinal, in design, there is a gradual elimination from the potential sample of marriages which terminate in divorce. As a result, the marriages included in the samples may consist of couples who have learned to work out differences and have been relatively well adjusted throughout the marriage.

In most studies, generational differences have not been adequately considered. Couples who are now in the later stages of life married and raised their children in a more traditional social climate. These older cohorts have been characterized by lower divorce rates regardless of dyadic or extramarital pressure to divorce. Spanier et al. (1975) proposed that older couples might be more likely to affirm their high marital satisfaction because of a "social desirablity response set." Discrepancies in the responses of men and women indicate that the transition to the empty nest years may require some degree of discomforting reappraisal by the partners. Systems theory concepts indicate that any family that experiences the permanent loss of a unit in the form of separation will undergo some disruption of homeostasis. As Stevenson (1977) has suggested, the prevalence of depression, psychoactive drug dependence, alcoholism, obesity, and divorce among the middle-aged demonstrates that life may not always be rewarding for the postparental couple.

Some couples seem able to move tranquilly from active parenting to a life that remains rich and fulfilling. Others find that the loss of children is traumatic in terms of self-esteem and marital compatibility. Who, then, are the couples most likely to require help in adapting to the departure of children from the home? In order to understand potential problem areas for postparental couples, it may be helpful to review the developmental tasks of the middle-aged family.

DEVELOPMENTAL TASKS

Duvall (1977) was the first theorist to organize and define the tasks of the family in middle age. Duvall categorized eight stages of family development which encompass the entire life cycle of individual members. During the early years of establishing and expanding the family system, the marital couple either moves toward resolution of divergent loyalties and goals, or remains conflicted by failure to accomplish resolution. This means that the marital couple enters the postparental years with an alliance which has been weakened or strengthened by past experience. If problem solving has been an endeavor in which both partners participated, this coping behavior is available to them. If the couple has not been able to acknowledge differences, or if the opinions of one partner have always prevailed, the postparental years may be quite difficult.

The developmental tasks (Duvall, 1977) of the middle-aged family may be summarized as follows: (1) rebuilding the marital dyad, (2) maintaining ties with older and younger generations, (3) providing security for later years, and (4) reaffirming the values of life which are meaningful. Another framework was offered by Stevenson (1977) who formulated a model of developmental tasks as seen from the perspective of the adult family members. This framework emphasizes the importance of developing and maintaining interdependent relationships between the members of the marital partnership. Also regarded as essential were relationships between the postparental couple and their children, as well as between the postparental couple and their aged parents. An additional task was identified for the middle-aged adult, namely that of adapting self and behavior to the signals of an accelerated aging process. A couple having difficulty with any of the foregoing developmental tasks is likely to be at risk. Troubled couples may need professional intervention of a supportive nature so that the potential for renewal in the marital relationship becomes an opportunity rather than a threat.

PRACTITIONER GUIDELINES

Evaluating the performance of the developmental tasks of the individual and the family during the launching and postparental years is one way of assessing the marital relationship. A practitioner using developmental concepts might employ structural interventions to enable the couple to move toward interdependence. Distances could be closed by encouraging joint activities and by establishing clear communication habits. Without children in the home to function as intermediaries or help preserve the isolation of the partners, the couple must begin to deal more openly with their concerns. Avoidance tactics are more difficult to employ when the children are gone from the home. The postparental couple in difficulty must be helped to learn or relearn the art of effective communication. Recognition of the rights of both partners should be included in the therapeutic approach, since interdependence is not attained by one dominant and one submissive spouse.

Stevenson (1977) thought that the problems encountered by middle-aged couples might arise from lack of available role models to help in the transition from parenthood to postparenthood. As longevity increases in our society, this assumption may be questioned. Since most couples have ample opportunity to watch others move into the postparental stage of family life, other variables besides the scarcity of role models may be operating. Sussman (1965) stated that middle-class families tend to have less family continuity than lower-class families. This is probably because lower-class couples have more opportunity to observe their own parents as role models, since lower-class families seem to spend more time together because of lack of money for baby-sitters, separate vacations, or non-family-related activities.

Nevertheless, observing their own parents does not provide lower-class couples with opportunities to plan for alternative roles. Many lower-class couples are caught up in the responsibilities of child rearing to such an extent that there is no opportunity for extrafamilial roles. Middle-class families, on the other hand, have resources which permit couples to spend more time in pursuits outside the family. This advantage encourages planning for the empty nest period by giving couples a chance to develop outside interests of their own while building an interdependent dyadic relationship which will be satisfying in their later years. Adjustment to postparenthood may be somewhat easier for middle-class couples not only because they are able to give more attention to the dyadic relationship but also because alternative roles are possible for the couple.

Any assessment of the marital couple in the empty nest stage must include the exploration of viable alternative roles for each spouse. It is likely that women who have never been active outside the home will be vulnerable to stress when the mothering role has to be discarded. This is especially true for women who equate selfhood with motherhood. Some marriages become stronger as the interdependence of the couple grows over the years. Other marriages are sustained mainly by the presence of the children to whose welfare both parents are devoted. When the children leave, the parents are left only with their own relationship. In the absence of the children tensions may mount, and it may become more difficult for the partners to deny that the marriage is friable.

The role transition of the postparental couple is not limited to discarding active parenthood. Just when a couple has achieved a satisfactory interdependence, the wife has begun a new career with her husband's support, or the husband has found a balance between work and home, the problem of senescent parents may intrude. Most middle-aged couples are able to adjust to the additional role transition which follows the deterioration of aged parents. If relationships between the two generations are good, and the interdependence of the middle-aged couple is sound, this period of role reversal will be less trying. Realization of the cyclical nature of life is a factor which alleviates the turmoil of caring for aged parents. Middle-aged couples tend to treat their own parents as they would wish to be treated in turn. One well-adjusted middle-aged woman described her awareness of her place in the parade of generations as follows:

> It is as if there are two mirrors before me, each held at a partial angle. I see part of myself in the mother who is growing old, and part of her in me. In the other mirror I see part of myself in my daughter. . . . It is a set of revelations that I suppose can only come when you are in the middle of three generations (Neugarten, 1968, p. 98).

Neugarten listed the executive processes of the successful middle-aged. These included selectivity, control of one's environment, and competence. Experience brings to middle-aged people a realistic awareness of what is possible and, for many of them, a mastery of immature impulses. As Neugarten explained, "The successful middle-aged person often describes himself as no longer 'driven' but as now the 'driver'—in short, 'in command'" (1968, p. 98).

The practitioner who intervenes in a dysfunctional postparental relationship is advised to adopt an eclectic approach based upon developmental frameworks, role theory, and general systems theory. Because the postparental couple shares a common history, it is important to discover what the marriage was like over time. Marriages characterized by relatively low levels of satisfaction throughout each family stage are most sensitive to the strains of the postparental period. Attention should be paid to coping mechanisms that were successfully utilized in former years, and to individual dissatisfactions that may not have been expressed earlier.

CLINICAL EXAMPLE: OVERREACTION IN A POSTPARENTAL FAMILY

Bill Johnson, the last child in the family, finished college the same month that his mother received a master's degree in business administration. Soon after, Bill moved out of the comfortable family home and into a place of his own. Trudy, his mother, continued to supervise the care of the home, but most of her time was taken up by her new job as a financial analyst. Fred Johnson, Trudy's husband of 27 years, was a fairly successful academician, a tenured professor who spent about half his time on campus and the other half at home turning out books on erudite subjects. Fred's books never made much money, but that was not important to the family. The family was able to go to Europe every few years and to afford good schools and colleges for the three children. There was enough money for annuities and insurance to make the world safe, and for books and music to make it interesting. Trudy's belated entry into the business world was accepted by Fred and cheered by the children, who wanted their mother to have a chance to prove herself.

Trudy's father had been a successful businessman, and at 45 Trudy was discovering her own talents. She found the business world exciting; there weren't enough hours in the day for all she wanted to do. From the first week Trudy felt at home in the supercharged corporate world but, looking around her, she felt self-conscious about her appearance. An exercise salon and a rigid diet promptly became part of her daily schedule. Because she left earlier in the morning than Fred, they were not able to have breakfast together. Lunch for Trudy was a diet drink taken at her desk, and during the week many of her dinners were part of a business evening with a client.

Trudy was so happy in her job and so self-engrossed that she failed to notice the changes in Fred. As she became more involved in her work, Fred became quieter and more remote. He lost interest in his appearance and when Trudy was not home for dinner, he usually did not bother to eat. Fred felt his life was closing in on him just as Trudy's began to open up. The three children were gone, and called infrequently. Every day, Fred's students seemed younger to him, and less interested in the obscure historical data which had always fascinated him. A generous man, he was unable to restrict Trudy, even though he was accustomed to a warm family life. Only now the pleasant home was always empty. Trudy was a well-groomed stranger talking animatedly about accounts and customers. Fred hid his feelings even from himself but sometimes he felt that his life was over. Alcohol eased his loneliness but also made him more morose. Things might have continued like this for much longer except that Bill came home to do his laundry one night and found his self-contained father sobbing uncontrollably in the family library, an empty bottle of Scotch not far away.

Structure

With the last child gone, Trudy and Fred Johnson were a couple again in the literal sense. In reality they became two separate people living in the same house. As a result of Trudy's new career the marital relationship was attenuated, in her case almost to the point of disengagement. Fred was at the end of a long, productive career, but he no longer felt the commitment and enthusiasm which his work had aroused in him 30 years earlier. After Trudy started her job, she functioned as a free and separate individual. Freed from the rigors of parenthood, she was like a 20-year-old setting out to conquer the world. The demands of Trudy's job and her enthusiasm blinded her to Fred's loneliness. In effect, the dyadic structure was disrupted so as to make each partner an isolate. The family structure before intervention is diagrammed in Figure 10-1.

Function

The family life of the Johnsons had been happy and successful for many years. Fred was able to combine an academic career with a strong involvement in the lives of his wife and children. In the early years the family system was characterized by complementarity and responsiveness to the needs of every member. Trudy was pivotal in the operation of the family system. When Fred wrote books or articles, it was Trudy who typed and edited them. Her name appeared on every dedicatory page, and Trudy knew, as did the children, that Fred meant every word. An active clubwoman and community worker, Trudy appeared to have established a perfect equilibrium. Until her last child left the family home, Trudy did not reveal her deep-seated dissatisfaction with her own accomplishments.

The departure of Bill removed from Trudy any feelings of responsibility. Fred had always been supportive of Trudy's independent activities and, in her zeal for a successful career, she forgot that her responsibility to her marriage was not over. Freedom from parenthood was interpreted by Trudy as freedom from wifehood as well.

Fred could be called an integrator rather than a totally committed careerist. This meant that his wife and family were essential to his well-being. Fred had shared his life with his wife and family to an extent which few men attempt. His hard work and unselfishness had

Figure 10-1   Overreaction in a postparental family before intervention.

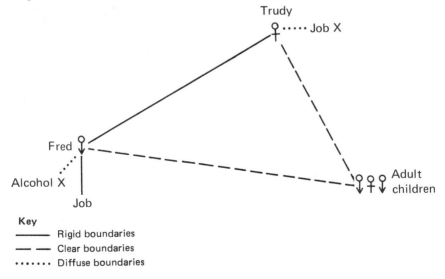

Key
—————— Rigid boundaries
— —   Clear boundaries
••••••• Diffuse boundaries

helped his wife and children become independent and successful. The reward for Fred was a nest with no one in it except himself. Fred found himself looking into a bleak future full of lonely evenings. Unwilling to ask more from Trudy than she volunteered to give, Fred slipped deeper into a state of mid-life depression. As marital and social interaction declined, Fred's intake of alcohol increased proportionately.

Intervention

1 The first step in dealing with the problems of this marriage was to arrange for a medical work-up for Fred. Depression in mid- and late life may be a precursor or an indicator of organic disorder.
2 After the initial step, the following objectives were pursued:
   a Help Trudy limit her excessive involvement with her job by learning to say no to some of the demands made on her. Because her experience with paid employment was limited, Trudy was sometimes reluctant to refuse evening meetings for fear that her superiors would be angry.
   b Encourage Fred to verbalize his feelings of loneliness and his need for companionship. Because he had never told Trudy how much he disliked having dinner alone, she did not realize how deprived Fred felt.
   c Increase effective communication and interaction between the couple. Fred's academic world and Trudy's business world were miles apart. Trudy and Fred had once spoken the same language—his. Now it was Fred's turn to learn the vocabulary

Figure 10-2 Clear boundaries after intervention.

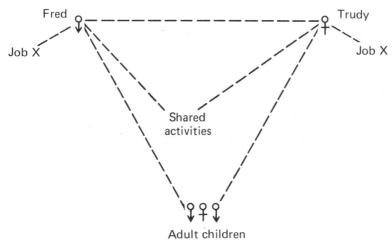

Key

—— Clear boundaries

which was meaningful to Trudy. Instead of ignoring Trudy's efforts to share her experiences, he learned to be an avid listener. Because of his scholarly habits, Fred was occasionally able to analyze issues in ways which were helpful to Trudy.

d   Assist Trudy in moderating her total involvement with work. There was never any question of forcing Trudy to choose between Fred and her job. What was necessary was for Trudy to set some priorities so that she was able to regulate her life at home and at work.

e   Interpret Fred's depression and Trudy's egocentricity as mutually maladaptive. Each partner overreacted to change. Trudy behaved as if her life were just beginning, while Fred reacted as if his were over. Each was helped to understand the maladaptive nature of their behaviors, and the reciprocal nature of their responses.

Figure 10-2 shows family boundaries after intervention.

SUMMARY

Guided by Duvall's and Stevenson's formulations of developmental tasks appropriate for middle-aged couples, the practitioner will be equipped to deal with tasks with which a couple is experiencing difficulty. For example, a wife who is beginning a new job or career might be helped to keep some perspective about her other commitments. Referring a husband to a preretirement planning group might help him deal with financial matters as well as expand his overall range of interest. Intervention could include reassurance about the normal changes which accompany middle age, particularly if a husband is concerned about a diminished sex drive. Because the incidence of illness and disability rises markedly in the middle years, attention to physical complaints may be required before the couple can address other matters.

The postparental couple should be allowed to discuss individual as well as relationship problems. Attention to projected wishes for the future helps the partners to communicate and to arrive at mutually acceptable compromises. The postparental phase of family life can be a time of diminished satisfaction or of a revitalized relationship. In *The Joys and Sorrows of Parenthood* (Group for the Advancement of Psychiatry, 1973) there is a compelling description of the hazards and rewards of postparental life.

> The active phase of parenthood . . . fades slowly, like the dimming of house-lights in a theater. Whether that dimming proceeds to total darkness or the curtain lifts on a new and brighter scene depends on how husband and wife have weathered the storms of parenthood, how they have matured, and how they will take up their new roles (p. 117).

REFERENCES

Axelson, L. Personal adjustment in the postparental period. In C. Vedder (Ed.), *Problems of the middle aged.* Springfield, Ill.: Charles C Thomas, 1965.

Duvall, E. M. *Marriage and family development* (5th ed.). Philadelphia: Lippincott, 1977.

The graying of America. *Newsweek,* February 28, 1977, pp. 50–65.

Group for the Advancement of Psychiatry. *The joys and sorrows of parenthood.* New York: Scribner, 1973.

Lowenthal, M., & Chiriboga, D. Transition to the empty next: Crisis, challenge or relief? *Archives of General Psychiatry,* January 1972, **26,** 8–14.

Neugarten, B. L. The awareness of middle age. In B. L. Neugarten (Ed.), *Middle age and aging.* Chicago: University of Chicago Press, 1968.

Sheehy, G. *Passages.* New York: Dutton, 1974.

Spanier, G., Lewis, R., & Cole, C. Marital adjustment over the family life cycle: The issue of curvilinearity. *Journal of Marriage and the Family,* May 1975, **37,** 263–275.

Stevenson, J. *Issues and crises during middlescence.* New York: Appleton-Century-Crofts, 1977.

Sussman, M. Intergenerational family relationships and social role changes in middle age. In C. Vedder (Ed.), *Problems of the middle aged.* Springfield, Ill.: Charles C Thomas, 1965.

Thurnher, M. Goals, values and life evaluations at the preretirement stage. *Journal of Gerontology,* January 1974, **29,** 85–96.

Chapter 11

Losses in the Family System

Elta Green

Every one of us sooner or later experiences a form of physical or psychological separation from our family or from a beloved family member. The separation may result from normative situations such as attending school, leaving home to find employment, or marrying and establishing a new nuclear family, or from idiosyncratic losses occurring under unusual or adverse circumstances. Alienation, desertion, divorce, war, chronic mental or physical illness, and death from natural or accidental causes are less normative developments which constitute losses in a family system. Separation and loss, with their ramifications for the total family system, are discussed in this chapter. Clinical examples of the social, psychological, and economic effects of loss on the family system are presented, together with concepts pertaining to assessment and intervention. The suggested interventions are not intended as a list of quick remedies; instead, the purpose is to delineate some problems and pitfalls that may beset the practitioner who is dealing with family losses. The interventions are also intended to be used as guidelines for the development of a therapeutic attitude on the part of the clinician.

SEPARATION OF CHILDREN

Aside from birth itself, the most important step in the differentiation of infant from mother occurs when the infant becomes aware of being separate from the mother; this realization comes at approximately 4 to 6 months of age. At this point of differentiation, the concept of *boundary* becomes significant. Thus begins a gradual process in parent-child separation which eventually culminates in the physical and psychological emancipation of offspring from parents.

Separation is a process which involves a number of developmental stages over the years. Both child and parent must go through these stages in order for the child to achieve genuine personhood. If the parents had trouble separating from their own families of origin, they may bring their unresolved problems into the relationship with their children. A primary goal of family life is to help children differentiate and individuate from parents, so that they can eventually separate from their original families in order to establish families of their own. Some families of origin help their children accomplish various developmental tasks, until the time comes for the child to make the major break, leaving home for good, whether for college, a job, or marriage. At this time a family which previously functioned well may become dysfunctional as parents and the young adult reinforce in each other the fear of separation. The separation may occur, but it may be complicated by ambivalence and contradiction.

The child entering first grade takes a major step away from home and family. The 6-year old brings part of the new world of school home to parents and, in so doing, shares experiences with the parents in order to obtain their recognition and approval. For their part, parents must learn to share their authority with teachers, who are important and essential to the child's development.

The process of separation is a progressive one; at later stages, the child's entrances into high school and college become important milestones in family life. An individual's educational achievement has particular social and emotional significance for the family. When a child's education exceeds that of the parents, parental pride may be insufficient to overcome the disparity of interests between parents and child. The child who is unwilling or unable to attain the academic standards of the parents may also experience alienation from parents because of disparate interests.

A certain amount of alienation or rebellion in adolescents is normative because young people must repudiate some of their parents' values in order to achieve a separate identity. Teenagers go through a stage in which they experiment with how far they can challenge parental ideas and values. They may test family rules and values by arguing, defying, staying out late, or even dropping out of school. However, this last behavior may have more complicated motivations than the mere testing of parental values. Very often the onset of the period of adolescence is difficult for both the developing child and the parent. It is unfortunate that the crisis of adolescence often coincides with the parental crisis of middle life. As the children leave the nest, the mother experiences menopause, and the father reaches the plateau of his career. Parents must watch their children's vigor and sexuality increase as their own physical powers and sexual attractiveness decline.

Parents do not always behave constructively with children who are alienated from the family. In fact, the alienation process is usually shaped by both parents and child. The estranged child's behavior is determined by many inner forces, conscious and unconscious, personal and interpersonal, which affect and are affected by family patterns.

Parents sometimes hold on to children to meet their own emotional needs, and have marked difficulty in letting a child or an adolescent separate. In overt and covert ways a parent may see the child as a replacement for his or her own lost parent. This process, called "parentifying" the child, makes heavy demands on the child for dependency gratification. A parent may invest an inappropriate amount of erotic feeling in a child of the opposite sex and become very attached to the child. Such a relationship may have heavy sexual overtones which perplex and trouble the child. In more seriously disordered families, actual incestuous behavior takes place. The generational boundaries are broken and cultural norms are transgressed.

Disturbed behavior in children may represent an acting out of a parent's unconscious wishes or emotional conflicts. A mother may not have successfully separated from her family of origin and may be left with unresolved emotional conflicts. For example, a mother may not have dealt adequately with anger at her parents for their suppression of her normal sexual development as an adolescent. As a result, she may unconsciously encourage her daughter's sexually promiscuous behavior as substitute rebellion against her own parents. Family interviews may reveal the subtle exploitation of a delinquent girl, or a father's encouragement of a delinquent son's behavior. Through nonverbal cues and messages from his father, the son is encouraged to relate and repeat his exploits. Family interviews may also show how children divide the parents, destroying the dyadic coalition needed for effective parenting.

Alienation may go beyond the normative boundary by being extreme and prolonged. In such cases the emotional pain of family members is severe enough to require professional intervention. Examples of alienated behavior are running away from home, engaging in delinquent acts, or sexual promiscuity. Antisocial and delinquent behavior in preteenage children that merits the attention of outside agencies such as the school, the police or the courts is usually indicative of serious emotional conflict in the family. Some family systems are so disruptive that delinquent and destructive behavior are consciously or unconsciously fostered and condoned. One child may become the family surrogate who acts out a parent's unconscious wish or fantasy. In these difficult situations the child may be removed from the family by a court, and placed in a group home or correctional institution, which hopefully can offer a more neutral environment.

The adolescent's or young adult's movement from school or a small part-time job to full-scale employment has implications for increasing independence and separation from family. In poorer families the young adult who leaves home to work may be called upon to send money home. The family's economic need may prolong the psychological ties between family and young adults, making it more difficult for the young adults to separate and to establish family units of their own. At the same time the role reversal experienced as parents become economically dependent on children is a potential source of stress.

The selection of a mate is a complex process in which conscious and unconscious forces operate. Some persons marry primarily to escape from a family of origin in which the burdens and demands are too heavy. In getting married, some immature persons merely change from being children in the family of origin to being children in another family. Moreover, the timing of a marriage may result from factors which are as complex as the reasons for choosing a particular partner.

The marriage or departure of a young person often leaves loneliness behind in the home, a condition which has been described as the *empty nest syndrome.* As a consequence of the emptying of the nest, the nuclear family becomes once again the original parental dyad. This is a gradual phenomenon, with children leaving home one by one until the last child has departed. At times parents may hold on more tightly to the last child, since this departure symbolizes the end of the parental role. How parents assume their new roles depends largely on how they dealt with the vicissitudes of parenthood through the years, and how they have matured as individuals and as a couple.

When an adult child marries, the separation continues to be a mutual process. The clear task for the newly married couple is to establish themselves apart from both families of origin. For the families of origin it is to facilitate this process by encouraging the couple in their independent efforts. The couple needs to establish its own boundary lines, be intimate, really get to know each other, and learn how to both love and fight fairly. They need space in which to grow, without interference from in-laws.

Parents need to learn different behaviors with regard to their married children; the parental role diminishes as the adult child separates to start a new family unit. Married children usually turn to their spouses, not to their parents, as primary love objects. As a result of this change, many intergenerational conflicts erupt. At times emotional ties to the family of origin are strong, and parents may insist on continued loyalty to the family of origin, despite the marriage of their child.

CLINICAL EXAMPLE: SEPARATING OF AN ADOLESCENT DAUGHTER

Mrs. A., aged 50, entered the hospital for the third time in 6 months for exacerbation of bronchial asthma. Among the facts learned by the admitting nurse was that 18-year-old Laurie, the last of the family's four children, was to leave home in 3 weeks to enter college. The other three children had all graduated from college and were out of the house. Both Mr. and Mrs. A. had worked hard to send the children to school; Mrs. A. was especially proud of this accomplishment since she had not attended college herself. The nurse also learned that Mrs. A. had suffered an asthma attack just prior to other separations and losses. Severe asthmatic symptoms had developed when a son married, and again after her mother's death the previous year. Losses had special intensity for Mrs. A., who had lived with several sets of foster parents until she was 9 years old, at which time she was adopted by a family with whom she lived until adulthood.

Mr. A. was a shy, intellectual man who was a chemist for a small firm. He came to see his wife at visiting hours but spent most of his time there reading the evening paper. He gave monosyllabic replies to the staff, but responded in a friendly fashion to a young nurse who was about Laurie's age. Mr. A. commented that the student nurse reminded him of Laurie, "who is going away to college soon." The husband then added, "She is our last chick to leave the nest." This statement caused Mrs. A. to burst into tears. The nurse comforted the couple by asking more about their children. Mrs. A. talked about missing Laurie, adding that they were entering a new phase in their life. The nurse listened for a time, then asked about plans they might have for themselves after their family responsibilities decreased. This gradually led to a discussion of places they might like to visit in the future. What the nurse was encouraging was planning ahead for the empty nest days soon to come. The next day Mrs. A. told the staff that she felt generally much better and noted that her chest did not feel quite as tight. She indicated that she was looking forward to seeing some travel folders her husband was bringing that evening. "Even if we don't go away this year," Mrs. A. explained, "we can begin to make some plans for the future. There are some good things about being free."

General Therapeutic Guidelines for Child and Adolescent Separation Problems

Assessment A comprehensive evaluation has to do with defining the nature of the separation problem in terms of family relationships. One needs to ask the following questions:

What is the relationship between the parents? Is there coalition or conflict? Coalition in what areas? Conflict in what areas?

What does the child's or the adolescent's behavior mean in terms of his or her attachment to the parents? What are the dimensions of distance from the parents now and what were they in the past? What messages are hidden in the behavior, and what messages are revealed?

Are the parents' behavioral responses contradictory? For example, parents may express a wish for a child to be independent, but insist that the child is not old enough for an allowace and therefore must ask them for whatever money is needed.

What do the child's attempts to be independent mean to the parents? How does the child's growing independence intensify distress and conflicts within the family?

How attached are parents to their own family of origin? Is their failure to separate related to their opposition to the growing independence of their own offspring?

Intervention Allow and understand the parents' resistance to letting children go. This is a very complex task and hard to accomplish. Parents may be conflicted and ambivalent, but they rarely entertain conscious desires to impede the growth of a child.

Remember that adolescents may want to be dependent, and yet yearn for independence and autonomy at the same time. Their confusion exacerbates the confusion of the parents.

Adolescence is an emotionally painful growth period, but parenting can be painful, too. Change is not only painful but also frightening for the participants.

Do not expect separation of children or adolescents from parents and home ever to be quick, painless, and clean-cut.

Do not think that all rules for adolescents are necessarily bad even though the adolescent believes this to be so. Most adolescents need to rebel against the rules whatever they may be; yet the adolescent would flounder more if no rules or standards were available.

Do not side with an adolescent or become the advocate of the parents. There are always two sides to an issue, and this demands objectivity on the part of the health professional.

ALTERATIONS IN THE MARITAL SUBSYSTEM

When one considers what marriage is and what it is not, one sees that the myths are plentiful. These myths serve to obscure the reality of the marriage relationship and prevent the marital partners from viewing each other in proper perspective as human beings with needs, strengths, and vulnerabilities. The perpetuation of marriage myths blocks growth and change, and often breeds distance and resentment between the partners.

What are some of the prevailing myths about marriage? Several are popular enough to warrant definition and elaboration. Some people believe that problems will be resolved automatically when love is present in the relationship (Lederer & Jackson, 1968). This belief implies that no conscious effort or action is required to resolve differences or to establish and maintain a stable, working marital relationship. Some marital partners assert that there is a way of acting which guarantees satisfaction and bliss. Others believe that if only the right spouse is located the mysteries of life and love will be solved (Jourard, 1975). Another false notion often expressed is that one partner will always know intuitively how the other feels. Without discussion, one should know what reassurance or advice is needed by the spouse in every situation. In other marriages "negative" beliefs are held, such as the expectation that one partner will not be able to understand or meet the other's emotional needs, because no one can be trusted to give without extracting a heavy price in return. Therefore, one should be as self-sufficient and independent as possible, asking little or nothing of the partner. Along with this belief, which is usually learned in the family of origin, there will often be smoldering resentment, held over from the past, in the spouse who expects nothing, asks nothing, and hopes for nothing. The partner who does not trust is unable to give much emotionally, and may despise and reject the spouse who does make demands. As might be expected, spouses who perpetuate this negative system have considerable difficulty not only in becoming a couple, but also in enacting parenting roles. The entry of a child into such a system adds to the difficulties, which burgeon as the child grows and makes new emotional demands at each developmental stage.

Failure of the Marital Subsystem

Marriages fail for many reasons. According to Lederer and Jackson (1968), alienation between the married pair is usually precipitated not by deliberate, malevolent behavior, but by what the partners omit to say and do. In this paradigm, failure in marriage is attributed to two destructive omissions: (1) the failure of spouses to identify, determine, and mutually assign areas of competence and responsibility; and (2) the failure of spouses to evaluate their differences realistically.

Persons seeking divorce are sometimes forced to lie to satisfy legal requirements. At the same time they may be facing certain psychological realities about the decline of their commitment to each other which must be denied in order to fulfill the letter of the law. In some respects divorce laws in our society reflect a need to punish the principals in a failed marriage. Perhaps society sees these laws as a way of repairing marriages or of preserving an illusory view of a successful marriage. No-fault divorce is a more realistic approach since it clearly implies that two persons are required to destroy a marriage, just as two are needed to maintain a happy union.

Fersch and Vering (1976) state that no-fault divorce only legalizes the actual situation, and endeavors to move legal requirements closer to psychological realities.

Sooner or later, most couples become involved in power struggles over decision making, indicating that they have not established the allocation of tasks involved in living together. Incompatibility between partners is often a matter of unresolved differences. A marital relationship will generally become unsatisfactory when one partner cannot allow the other to think, act, or respond independently. The ability to be in touch with one's feelings, to express them, and to enjoy a degree of autonomy is necessary for the maintenance of individuality. Individual feelings and thoughts form the essence of what makes a person separate and distinct from others. For an individual to be denied this right by a partner predisposes to marital dissatisfaction. The behaviors of both partners require continuous accommodation, but feelings and thoughts are not synonymous with behavior.

There are other reasons why marriages fail. Couples may not know each other well when they are married. Those who marry very young, and have not completely separated from their family of origin, often enter the marriage relationship with romantic, unrealistic illusions about married life. These persons usually hope to achieve a sense of personal identity through marriage. Among the immature attitudes surrounding marriage is the need of spouses to project on each other images from past relationships. These images may represent the kind of person one partner wishes the other to be, or the way in which one partner wants the other one to change. Some partners gradually relinquish these illusions and accept each other as persons in their own right. When partners cannot give up their illusions, disappointment and anger will follow. The anger can accumulate to enormous proportions over the years. Fortresses are erected which isolate the partners; ammunition is stored for repeated battles. The marital relationship becomes a war game characterized by vindictiveness and suffering. Such a system may become entrenched and endure for years. Physical violence may erupt as a partner becomes a wife or husband abuser, and the marriage assumes the characteristics of a sado-masochistic relationship, in which vicarious and erotic pleasure is derived from inflicting and/or receiving pain. Some of these marriages last until a partner dies. Others end, usually when one partner no longer experiences pleasure of any kind and terminates the relationship. Marital partners mature and grow at different rates; one may change rapidly, while the other remains transfixed in an early developmental stage. In times of stress or crisis, one spouse may regress emotionally and be unable or unwilling, for complicated reasons, to grow or advance. The chasm between the partners then widens; they drift apart, realizing they no longer have much in common, and end the relationship.

Adultery is frequently the reason for the dissolution of a marriage. When one spouse finds out that the other is having an affair, the discovery may precipitate a crisis which can be used in marital counseling to look at what is wrong in the marital relationship. Occasionally both partners can learn and grow from the experience. At other times, the discovery of an adulterous liaison is taken as the final act of treason which severs the relationship beyond repair.

Types of Alterations

Alienation Lederer and Jackson (1968) emphasized that the crumbling of a marriage relationship takes place so gradually over the years that most couples do not perceive what is happening until their problems have reached enormous proportions. It is important to analyze what takes place in the alienation of spouses from each other. Misunderstanding, misinterpretation of actions and motives, a gradual decrease in verbal communication between spouses, or an increase in the frequency of verbal battles all become causes for and effects of alienation. Feelings of hurt and resentment accumulate. Avoidance of any constructive verbal communication causes isolation and emotional distance in the marital dyad. Physical distance often follows also, with the husband staying away from home or the wife seeking relationships or attachments elsewhere.

Separation The final separation of the couple may come only after prolonged periods of distress, many painful encounters, and mutual recrimination and vindictiveness. Often, episodes of separation are followed by attempts at reconciliation which may be spasmodic and temporary. Not all separations are planned; some spouses desert impulsively and never return. Regardless of the forms which alienation assumes, each partner involved in a failed marriage suffers loneliness, humiliation, loss of self-confidence, guilt, and depression.

In some marriages alienation persists for years before the separation takes place. Why does it take some couples so long to separate permanently even after years of a stormy and painful relationship? And why do couples renew acrimonious communication even after the divorce? Weiss (1975) wrote that these behaviors have to do with the nature and persistence of the attachment. Once the marital attachment is formed, no matter how stormy or destructive the relationship becomes some residue of the attachment survives, and it is extremely difficult to discount.

The breaking up of a marriage and a family takes heavy toll of the children, regardless of how well separation is handled by the parents. There are, however, ways of dealing with the trauma which are relatively constructive. There are also unhelpful ways of discussing the problems with a child which only serve to increase the child's fears, guilt, and confusion. Atkin and Rubin (1976) state that young children understand and interpret what happens with parents in relation to themselves. Children can be full of self-blame when parents quarrel and they often feel that they are the cause of problematic situations. Parents, for their part, often are certain that they have hidden marital discord from the children, but family interviews almost inevitably reveal the opposite. Small children are not easily deceived. They quickly notice and are affected by tensions in the atmosphere at home. Reddened eyes, hostile glances, or false politeness between the parents are indications of friction which children seldom fail to observe.

Children can be helped to face the painful reality of the parental separation. Most professional persons who counsel separated and divorced families say that children should be told when the definitive decision to separate has been made by the parents. Ideally, the separation should be discussed with the children by both parents together, who should then allow the children to express their feelings and to ask questions. The children's inquiries and the expression of their feelings can be very hard for their parents to endure. Atkin and Rubin (1976) conclude that it is better for children to be told the truth, no matter how distressful, than to have parents dissemble by concealing the situation or to avoid discussing it at all. When the latter happens, children can become very fearful and have fantasies which only increase anxiety and distrust.

Divorce   Divorce comes when the marriage fails. It is an open acknowledgement of failure. Divorce represents a change in the family system which is extremely difficult for every member. Parents and children alike may feel trapped, defeated, and frightened. Even under the best conditions divorce generally involves an expensive legal process and a court procedure. Although the grounds for divorce vary from state to state, an agreement must be reached, and a settlement made, about property, alimony, child support, and custody. The community and the courts generally assume one partner to be the guilty party and the other the innocent one.

The process of divorce and the concept of custody are undergoing major changes in this country. No-fault divorce and custody of children shared jointly by both partners are common in several states. These are fair and admirable changes, but nevertheless making divorce and custody agreements remains a complex process which requires careful attention. Fersch and Vering (1976) state that legal requirements regarding divorce, custody, and support are often in opposition to emotional realities.

Adjustments after Divorce   The period immediately following divorce is very difficult for the partners even when they have been separated for an extended period. This is a time when the divorced partners must begin to mend their broken lives, and to cope with the loneliness, regret, and depression that may accompany their feelings of relief. New social contacts must be inaugurated. For the spouse who has custody of the children, the role of single parent must begin. The newly divorced person is vulnerable and, when loneliness becomes intense, may too quickly become attached to another person of the opposite sex. A sexual relationship may develop rapidly, and sometimes a decision to marry is made before the divorced person has sufficient opportunity to work through the feelings of loss, or to develop an understanding of what went wrong in the first marriage.

The divorced person may choose a second partner who resembles the first spouse and repeat the mistakes of the failed marriage. However, some divorced persons learn from their failure, and their second marriage does not replicate previous errors, but develops into a mature and enduring relationship. Some individuals mature, and later choose partners with whom they can develop a mutually satisfying and lasting marriage. Even after remarriage, divorced spouses may continue to maintain some kind of relationship, however distant or destructive, for years.

Following separation through divorce, the family structure changes markedly. The divorced husband and wife must change their relationship, and relinquish a conscious commitment to one another. They also must assume different life roles, as each becomes a single parent, and often they find themselves in opposition to each other.

Functionally, in separated families, one parent, usually the mother, struggles to raise children alone, while the other, usually the father, attempts to be a part-time, weekend parent. Children no longer have united parents, but divided and alienated parents who differ over rules, privileges, and affection. Often children are used as pawns in the discontinued marital relationship. After separation and divorce, children are asked overtly or covertly to take sides. The mother may be secretly delighted when the children see her as the "good" parent and the father as the "bad" one, since in her view the father was the culprit. Her attitude encourages the children to blame their father, a practice which fosters doubt and guilt in the children.

Psychologically the afflictions of a failed marriage take a heavy toll from both partners. There is lessened morale, lowered self-esteem, and heightened guilt and depression.

A wounded or angry spouse is not inclined to make new friendships immediately after divorce, despite feelings of loneliness. When acutely distressed, separated spouses may at times exhibit "crazy" behaviors as they struggle with their feelings. Accepting the fact of single parenting is burdensome for both spouses, and exhausting at a time when they are already emotionally drained.

The change in the marital status of the parents has a major impact upon the children; guilt feelings and taking sides are inevitable. Children must be allowed to grieve the loss of the divorced parent who is no longer in the home. Children have a tendency to idealize and blame simultaneously, as they express confused feelings. Often the situation is incomprehensible to them and they search endlessly for answers and explanations.

Another problem for separated and divorced families is that they usually have less available money. A divorced mother may need to supplement support payments but be inadequately prepared to enter the job market. She must either accept a reduced living standard or find a way to obtain a marketable skill. Should she take courses or find a job, she will incur the additional expense of child care. A divorced father who pays child support or alimony has less money for his own needs. He too may be forced to accept a less comfortable standard of living. Divorced homeowners may have to give up the family residence and move to less expensive quarters. The deserted mother without access to support payments may have to apply for public assistance. Economic privation adds to the adjustment problems confronted by separated or divorced couples.

CLINICAL EXAMPLE: THE EFFECTS OF MARITAL SEPARATION ON ALL FAMILY MEMBERS

Mrs. B., age 37, separated for 2 months, phoned the family clinic to say she was having trouble with her son Bobby, age 10. Bobby was antagonistic toward her, fought with the other children at school, and had prolonged crying spells upon the slightest provocation. In the home were two older siblings: George, age 16, and Linda, age 14. Initially Mrs. B. stated that her husband left her; later in the conversation she explained that their decision to part had been made mutually after years of a stormy and unsatisfactory marital relationship. Both Mr. and Mrs. B. had seen their lawyers; papers for legal separation were being drawn up. Mrs. B., a teacher, said that she planned to return to work "as soon as things settled down."

Mrs. B. said both parents had "discussed" everything with the children, who "didn't seem to show any feelings." Therefore, she couldn't understand why Bobby was so upset and antagonistic. George had told her he "didn't care," since he would be going away to college in a couple of years anyway. Linda, whom the mother described as a quiet child, "seemed to accept the situation but spent a lot of time outside the home." She was often out of the house baby-sitting after school and on weekends. Mr. B. lived in the same city, but Mrs. B. did not think he would come for a family interview. When the family therapist explained that the purpose was not to reconcile the couple nor to place blame, Mrs. B. reluctantly agreed to phone her husband and invite him to the first meeting.

Several exploratory family interviews with the parents and the three children revealed both strengths and vulnerabilities in the system. Both parents were intelligent, and devoted to the children. The couple had married quite young and the children were born before the parents had time to adjust to each other very well or to strengthen their own relationship. Over the years the couple drifted apart. They had separated twice before but had been unable to make a final break. The crisis of the final separation had been very disruptive for all three children, but the children had not revealed their real feelings. Bobby, in fact, was now expressing the feelings of the whole family. The parents had "told" the children of the separation but had left no opportunity for them to express their feelings because "we were too upset ourselves." During the interviews the parents were encouraged to describe to the children the reasons for the separation, stressing the fact that they could no longer relate together as a couple, but that they cared deeply for the children. The mother at first tended to blame the father for the separation, but was later able to admit that she, too, wanted the separation. *Both* parents finally accepted responsibility for the decision to separate. This mean that neither could blame the other and appear as "good" in the eyes of the children, while making the other partner seem "bad." In particular, the mother expressed fear that the children would blame her, adding, "after all, I have to live with them." She also feared being the only parent at home.

In the supportive climate of the meetings, George for the first time shed tears, and spoke of anger at his father for "picking on" his mother. Linda said she always expected her parents would separate because "they had stopped fighting and did not sleep in the same bedroom any more." She surprised her parents by her extensive knowledge of what had been going on between them. Bobby was especially angry at his father and said bitterly that if his father really loved him, he would stay. The father was obviously moved; he also wept and openly expressed guilt that he could not be at home.

Weekly meetings took place with the family over a period of 4 months. The original goal had been to help the parents talk about the separation more openly with the children, to acknowledge their distress, and to learn how to respond less defensively. As the interviews progressed, family members were able to express their anger and sadness over the disintegration of the family unit. The father assured the children of his love and of his financial support, and told them he planned to see them often and regularly. He conveyed clearly that their relationship would remain meaningful. The mother became less angry with the father, reassuring him and the children there would be no interference with his visiting rights. She was subsequently referred to a group for separated and divorced women, so she could have some extra help for her own needs. In time the father eventually found some new friends, and his depression lessened. The older children adjusted fairly well, although George dropped out of high school and did not graduate. Linda's grades in school slipped somewhat. She had trouble making new friends, but her problems did not overwhelm her. Bobby stopped acting out his anger. He was depressed for a while, but this was felt to be normative and evidence of the grieving which he needed to do. After 4 months, mother and children met with the family therapist at monthly intervals only for the next 5 months. Not all problems were solved, but mother and children became a functioning unit and were able to cope satisfactorily with their changed lives.

General Therapeutic Guidelines for Families Separated by Divorce

Assessment   When determining how to be helpful, it is just as important to evaluate the *strengths* as it is to become knowledgeable about the *conflicts* and *weaknesses* in a family system. The following questions can be used as guidelines in the assessment of a family system with losses.

What is the nature of the current *relationship* between the separated spouses? The spouse and second partner?

What are the areas of difficulty (e.g., loss, grief, loneliness, loss of self-confidence, change in standard of living, shortage of money, problems in managing children)?

How has the separated or surviving spouse dealt with these areas? How are the children adjusting?

What are the support systems for the separated or widowed spouse with children, the children, the spouse who is living alone?

Intervention   The following suggestions are guidelines for intervention.

Encourage spouses to talk with a practitioner.

Encourage children to talk.

Allow for feelings of loss, grief, hostility, and disillusionment on the part of all family members.

Define the economic and social realities with the family.

Encourage social activities, other friendships, and time away from children for the single parent.

Encourage contact with extended family and help to establish it if there is conflict.

Do not be a judge.

Do not play the blame game.

Do not expect a single parent to be a miracle worker.

Do not shut the children out.

Do not shut the father out.

Do not make a plan in your own head and expect spouse or family to accept it. (Help them to make a plan of their own, at their own speed.)

LOSS FROM DEATH IN THE FAMILY

In the last decade, much attention has been paid to the subject of death and dying and to helping the dying person and the family. There is increased interest in how people die and concern about whether to prolong life for the terminally ill when death is imminent. We have advanced medical technology for saving life, but we are less advanced in our knowledge about how to deal humanely with the dying process. Bowen (1976) described three processes in operation around the terminally ill patient: (1) the intrapsychic process within the person in which there is always some denial of death, (2) the closed family relationship system, and (3) closed physician and medical staff communication system. Incurable disease is discussed with patients and families in greater depth now than previously, but much remains to be accomplished in teaching professional staff to deal with the difficult process of death and dying.

Death of a Child

One reads frequently in newspapers about the death of a child through an automobile accident, a drowning, the mistaken ingestion of poison, or cruel abuse from parents. Or one learns of a child stricken with a hopeless disease, an infant who was stillborn, or a child who suffered an unexplained "crib death." Such events arouse horror and disbelief. How untimely, how tragic such a loss appears and how unfair to those involved. One recognizes that old people die, but a child's death stirs the strongest indignation. The death of a child from accident or illness cannot fail to cause a major emotional upheaval in the family. The extent of its impact depends on several factors: age, the length of time the child has been part of the family's history, the child's role in the family and his or her relationship with the other family members, and the circumstances surrounding the death.

The loss of a child through death leaves an unfilled place in the structure of the family system, particularly when the child was an only child, or the oldest or youngest child. The death of an only child robs the marital couple of their parenting role, and they must revert to being a childless couple. The death of the oldest child has special significance for the parents since this was the firstborn, the child with whom parenthood was first experienced. A youngest child's death is significant also, since this child was the baby of the family, and often an especially favored child. Sibling positions shift with the death of a child. A usual consequence of the death is that the remaining offspring become more precious. The effect of these shifts depends upon the nature of the dyadic relationship, parent-child relationships, sibling relationships, and intrafamilial relationships of the entire system.

Following the death of a child there is an adjustment of functions of the surviving family members. A major question for the family is the way in which the dead child's role and functions will be distributed. For example, in a poor family, should the next sibling in line be delegated to replace the oldest sibling in working to contribute toward the economic support of the family? If the youngest and favored child has died, who now will be the favored one? If the scapegoated child has died, who must fill the role of being exploited, filling the gap between parents, or acting as a repository for hostile family feelings?

Professional persons are often in a quandary about how to deal with fatally ill children and their families. Significant advances have been made in the diagnosis and medical care of the terminally ill child, but our affective support has not kept up with our technical skills. It is difficult to know what to tell a dying child and family, and how to time certain disclosures. The inclusion of siblings in discussions poses problems for all health practitioners. Friedman (1974) states that the young child does not search for a diagnosis, but for assurance that he or she will not be abandoned. Older children can cope better with their disease if they know the diagnosis. Many older children seem aware of their diagnosis, even when not told. The inability of any dying person to discuss illness and pending death with parents, relatives, and friends may increase feelings of anxiety, confusion, and isolation. Children and adults who sense that they have an incurable disease may feel deceived by family members who deny, or give false hope. Siblings cannot help noticing a discrepancy between an inadequate explanation given to them and the treatment the dying brother or sister receives in the form of extensive medical attention and special privileges. It follows then, that the special status of the ill child may be resented by the confused siblings. This in turn will make the mourning process more complicated, since siblings will feel guilty about having resented the treatment accorded the dying child.

Extended family members may also experience painful loss when a child dies. For example, a grandmother may have a deep sense of deprivation at the death of a grandchild who represented a link to the future. The marital relationship of the parents is put to a serious test when a child faces terminal illness. Under such severe stress the strongest of marital relationships will be shaken. Parents can become closer under this strain and help each other, but the effects of the tragedy will clearly depend on the strength of the marriage. If the marriage is already unstable, the death of the child will probably not pull the parents together in a lasting way. Even a strong marriage will be tested, but it is more likely to weather the turmoil and pain. It is fortunate if there are other children in the family to assure the couple of their continuing parental role. Couples who are capable of having more children may also be able to deal more easily with their despair.

The loss of a child through death has a major social impact on a family system. Upon the death of an only child the parents become a childless couple among friends with children. Envy is added to feelings of sadness and loss. Sometimes the attention and affection given to bereaved parents by the children of friends or relatives can help. Where there are surviving siblings, particularly adolescents, the support of a peer group may be effective. A close girl friend may help console a grieving adolescent girl who has lost a sister. It should be remembered that siblings need to mourn, and that they need to do this within the family as well as with friends.

Death of Spouse

The death of a spouse brings a very different type of alteration to the marital subsystem. Whether death occurs after sudden or prolonged illness, or by accident, the loss of a spouse has tremendous impact upon the surviving partner and all the other family members. Death involves leaving and being left, and who is to say which causes greater suffering. Acute and profound grief can play havoc with the mourner's reason and sense of reality. In the case of a terminal illness, the task of the dying person is clear, whereas the tasks of the survivors are less so. As Elizabeth Kubler-Ross, a Chicago psychiatrist, observed, "The dying patient's problems come to an end, but the family's problems go on" (1970, p. 142).

A number of prominent persons have written about the experience of death and dying, and its implications for the dying person and the family. In 1917, Sigmund Freud presented the first original work about the psychology of the grieving process. Erich Lindemann (1944), a psychiatrist in Boston, discussed the management of acute grief. More recently, in her well-known book, *On Death and Dying,* Kubler-Ross (1970) related her experiences in working with dying patients and their families. Kubler-Ross encourages practitioners to interact deeply and extensively with the dying person and the family, pointing out that professionals often view death as an adversary whose arrival is met with denial and detachment.

After the death of a spouse, there are many psychological tasks to be performed by the rest of the family. The surviving parent may become overly preoccupied with his or her own distress, and be unable to give much to the children, whose grief around the loss may be equally intense. Frequently the persistent needs and demands of the children help the surviving parent to become less self-engrossed and to deal with pressing realities. People who suffer a loss eventually learn that the passage of time considerably diminishes the acute feelings of sorrow and loss.

The work of mourning the loss is the first order of psychological business for the family, and is a complex but necessary process. Immediately following the death of a spouse, there may be a period of disorganization in family life, but this is to be expected, and most families eventually settle back into familiar routines of daily life in the weeks following the funeral. "Normal" stages of the mourning process, as discussed by Engel (1962) include: (1) the stage of shock and disbelief, in which the reality cannot be accepted; (2) the stage of developing an awareness of the loss in which the bereaved person begins to face the emptiness, the painful void; and (3) the stage of restitution, in which the "work of mourning" takes place: mourning with family and friends, the funeral ceremony, and the preoccupation with the loss. Engel concludes that:

> The successful work of mourning takes anywhere from six to twelve months and the complete restitution of grief is indicated by the ability to remember comfortably and realistically both the pleasures and disappointments of the lost relationship. When successful, the survivor becomes capable of carrying on his life with new relationships, often having profited from the positive identification with the lost person (pp. 278–279).

The circumstances surrounding the death have much to do with the nature of the grieving process. The process is also affected by the relationships within the family before the death, which have the power to mitigate or exacerbate feelings of loss. A conflictual and highly ambivalent relationship with the deceased family member can complicate and prolong the mourning process for an individual or for the whole family. Family members who never had the chance to resolve a hostile and guilt-ridden relationship when the relative was alive are likely to experience a painfully prolonged mourning process which may last for years, unless the person seeks therapeutic intervention.

Both public and private mourning are necessary in the working-through process. Sharing the painful feelings of the grief and allowing friends to comfort relieves feelings of isolation. A person also needs to grieve privately; the pain of the loss needs to be experienced, and felt, since, when painful feelings are denied, or pushed aside, emotional complications may follow.

Death of Parents

Parents of a Family in the Formative Years At times, mothers and fathers die at an untimely age, either from accident or illness. Loss of a parent also follows when a parent commits suicide, is institutionalized for long periods, or deserts the family. The prolonged absence of one parent changes the structure and function of the family system. The family's task is then to cope with the loss in a way which allows for growth, individuation, and the acceptance of eventual separation. One-parent families do survive whether or not the remaining parent chooses to bring another person into the family unit as the spouse and stepparent. The death of both parents of a young family is a major catastrophe for the children and the family system.

The grieving process varies for each individual in the family because the relationship of each with the deceased person was different. Children need to mourn and to see their parents mourn. When a parent does not let children witness weeping as a reaction to death, children may feel they are not permitted to show feelings, and that crying is forbidden. In family system terms, the nature of the family's grieving indicates how well the family will heal when there has been a real working-through process. If pain and grief have been avoided, the grief will remain an unresolved problem.

In the family system, the original parental subsystem no longer exists when one parent dies. The remaining parent is left to raise the children alone. Roles need to be reorganized. Decisions have to be made about who will assume what responsibility for whom, and when. In the case of the death of both parents, surrogate parents need to fulfill the parental role—either extended family members or foster parents via an outside agency. Group homes and children's institutions are available sponsored by church, or federal, state, and county funds. Sometimes children who have lost both parents are legally adopted by relatives or foster parents.

A young, surviving parent may confront changed social status even when economic conditions are unchanged. The new status is not always clear to the surviving spouse who may continue to feel very much married. The widowed parent may try to find a niche in the former social group of couples and families. Single parents, whether widowed, separated, or divorced, have access to groups such as "Parents without Partners," which are formed to meet the social needs of single parents seeking relationships with persons like themselves.

Death of Older Parents   A person in the middle years (between 40 and 60 years of age) can expect parents' retirement, advancing infirmity, and finally death, although these events do not always take place within a short period of time. Old age is sometimes viewed as a completion of the life cycle which brings a sense of closure. Life review and reminiscences are often a part of the effort of the elderly to look back on their lives and accomplishments.

Parents grow old, and one of them eventually dies before the other. In some instances a widow or widower past 60 years of age remarries, and lives out the remaining years happily with a second spouse. More often, the surviving aging parent continues to live alone or with an adult child's family. In our culture, emphasis is placed upon independence from parents. Old people are not delegated to a position of honor, as in more traditional societies. Most couples' houses are not big enough to accommodate the older person's need for privacy. Three generations living together can be complex and adjustments are required from everyone when an older parent joins the household of a married son or daughter. The decision to provide a home and care for aging parents is a difficult and stressful one. Many factors—personal, social, and economic—must be carefully weighed in making the decision.

Some widows may continue to live alone for years, taking care of their own physical and social needs, and trying desperately to remain independent and "not become a burden" to the children. Widows who were extremely dependent upon their husbands may become even more dependent and helpless when they have to face life alone. Some widowed men continue to live in an apartment or house while others, not possessing housekeeping skills, move in with children, other relatives, or into a residence for the elderly. In actuarial terms, far more women than men outlive their spouses. Women are often somewhat younger than their mates and their life expectancy exceeds that of men.

The surviving older parent struggles with the loss of the spouse in addition to facing old age alone. If the relationship was of long duration, the loss is severe. Old persons have been known to say that part of them died with the spouse to whom they were devoted for 40 or 50 years. The social world of the old person gradually narrows as relatives and friends die or move away. Older persons tend to reduce their social activities and become less involved with people.

It is far harder for one person to live on a retirement income than for two. Subsidized housing for the elderly is a boon for those with limited incomes. The enormous cost of medical care and nursing homes for the elderly can cause catastrophic loss of life savings, which for some can mean their only recourse is to apply for public assistance.

The death of a parent is a milestone in life for a person of any age. With it comes a real break with the past, and the original family system enters another phase of its life. As long as their parents survive, middle-aged adults are not conscious of representing the older generation. But with the death of elderly parents, middle-aged adults feel their own mortality drawing closer. Occasionally they begin to see themselves as more vulnerable and their own children as ascendent.

CLINICAL EXAMPLE: LOSS OF A SON FROM DEATH

Mrs. D's 6-year-old son was dying of leukemia. She was a "problem" mother for whom few of the hospital staff could feel much compassion. The staff avoided her and cringed when she began her tirade against them. "The doctors are unavailable. No one will answer my questions. Why don't they try another medication? Why do I have to wait so long for results from the tests?"

Several other mothers (who also had leukemic children) sensed the reality in some of her complaints, agreed with her, and supported her attempts to complain to hospital officials. They also knew well the panic behind her hostile confrontations, and responded to this by comforting her at the bad times and telling her how scared they, too, were feeling.

This mother was angry to begin with about the fact that her child had the disease. She was angry about the defects in the medical system that cared for her son. The anger was also an easy mask to put on when she had to wait long hours in the hospital corridors with her crying son, and hear his screams when the bone marrow test was done. Her profound grief nearly drove her crazy and she wondered how much longer she could tolerate the anguish she felt so constantly. It weighed heavily upon her back and she could only shift it from one side to the other. When she was not enraged, she was filled with despair and cried for prolonged periods at home. She was divorced and her son was an only child.

CLINICAL EXAMPLE: A LOSS OF A DAUGHTER FROM DEATH

Lucy, age 18, was dying of sickle-cell anemia. She had many open lesions on her legs and arms and suffered a great deal from muscle and joint pains over most of her body. The disease had been diagnosed when she was 6 years old, and the family had made many trips to the hospital clinics since then. Lucy was the third of seven children born in an intact large black family. The family had been hopeful until recent weeks, but now they waited for the end to come. She was brought to the hospital in the last days because the pain was severe, although she had wanted to die at home. When she did die, her parents were with her. Both sobbed quietly at the bedside and allowed the staff to comfort them. The family had asked a lot of questions but had not understood much of the medical jargon with which their questions were answered. They were afraid to challenge any of the doctors. One of Lucy's older brothers did become angry at the hospital staff one day about some incident, and he never returned to visit her. Other family members were accepting and undemanding.

General Therapeutic Guidelines for Family Loss from Death

Assessment   Again, there is need to define the difficulties in the framework of relationships in the family.

What position in the family has the deceased person held?
What were his or her relationships with family members?
Where are family members in the grieving process?
Is their mourning normative or pathological?
Is the anger about the loss projected on to others—doctors, nurses, hospital personnel?

Intervention

Expect feelings of anger on the part of the survivors as part of the mourning process; do not try to "reason" the relatives out of these feelings.

Encourage all family members to talk about their grief, but remember that not all will be able to do so, even though they would feel better if they could.

Remember that some people are ready to die and do not fear death; they fear only life, particularly when all life holds for them is the agony of pain, discomfort, and further isolation.

Allow every human being the right to die in peace and with dignity.

The two clinical examples given in this chapter represent the "easy" and the "difficult" persons to help when a family member is critically ill or dies in the hospital. No case is easy, however. Knowing that nothing can be done to save a life, especially the life of a child, can be a very painful ordeal for even the strongest of professional persons. In both cases the health professional should accept the survivors' feelings of anger without trying to reason with them. Understanding the processes of grief can help the health professional console the mourning family.

SUMMARY

Losses are experienced in all families. The separation of children from the family through such normal experiences as school, employment, and marriage requires the family system to adjust structurally and functionally. Health professionals need to recognize normal resistances to separation as well as pathological behaviors of long duration. Parents can be helped to realize that adolescence is an emotionally painful growth period in which adolescents seek dependence, independence, and autonomy all at the same time.

Alterations in the marital subsystem occur when there is alienation between partners, separation, divorce, and death. Family members should be encouraged to express their feelings of loss, grief, hostility, and disillusionment during the transitional period. Other persons, such as extended family members and friends, also can be helpful at this time.

Changes in the family brought about by the death of a child or a parent can be very disruptive to the family system. Modifications must be made in roles, communication patterns, emotional relationships, and other behaviors. Health professionals can help the family make these adjustments through their understanding of the grief process and of the system modifications that must occur at this time.

REFERENCES

Atkin, E., & Rubin, E. *Part-time father.* New York: Vanguard, 1976.

Bowen, M. Family reaction to death. In P. J. Guerin, Jr. (Ed.), *Family therapy.* New York: Gardner, 1976.

Engel, G. L. Grief and grieving. *American Journal of Nursing,* September 1964, **64**(9), 93–98.

Engel, G. L. Psychological responses to major environmental stress. Grief and mourning; danger, disaster and deprivation. In G. L. Engel (Ed.), *Psychological development in health and disease.* Philadelphia: Saunders, 1962.

Fersch, E. A., Jr., & Vering, J. A. Divorce legal requirements vs. psychological realities. In H. Gruenbaum & J. Christ (Eds.), *Contemporary marriage: Structure, dynamics and therapy.* Boston: Little, Brown, 1976.

Freud, S. Mourning and melancholia. In *Complete works,* (Vol. 14), London: The Hogarth Press & the Institute of Psychoanalysis, 1953.

Friedman, S. B. The fatally ill child. In S. B. Troup & W. A. Greene (Eds.), *The patient, death and the family.* New York: Scribner, 1974.

Jourard, S. M. Marriage is for life. *Journal of Marriage and Family Counseling,* July 1975, **1**, 199–208.

Kubler-Ross, E. *On death and dying.* London: Tavistock, 1970.

Lederer, W. J., & Jackson, D. *The mirages of marriage.* New York: Norton, 1968.

Lindemann, E. Symptomatology and management of acute grief. *American Journal of Psychiatry,* 1944, **101**, 141–148.

Weiss, R. S. *Marital separation.* New York: Basic Books, 1975.

Part Three

Family Challenges

Chapter 12

Physical Illness in the Family

John Q. Griffin

Although any physical illness can assume a bewildering variety of forms, the usual context in which illness occurs and is resolved is the family. Since the family is an interdependent system, change in one member of the system is followed by change in other members. The family system therefore influences the course of illness in a variety of ways, just as the onset of illness alters the interdependent structures and functions of the family system. It is through the relationships of family life that processes such as making decisions, determining policies, acknowledging feelings, and providing support are implemented (Sedgwick, 1974). There is evidence that high levels of family transactions and interactions contribute to favorable prognosis and to the rehabilitation of the patient (Litman, 1966, 1974).

The established patterns of behavior within a family are disrupted by illness. The illness represents a change in one part of the family system which is followed by compensatory change in other parts. Flexibility and adaptability are essential to the maintenance of the system, and this is particularly true when illness intrudes. The interdependence of organizational structures and the nature of family functioning mean that no illness can be seen as an isolated event.

VARIABLES IN THE EFFECTS OF PHYSICAL ILLNESS

There are three general categories of physical illness: acute, chronic, and terminal. One way of distinguishing between the three types is the way in which the illness is resolved. Acute illness usually disables individuals for a temporary period, after which they recover all or most of their previous level of wellness. Chronic illness has no such hopeful resolution. There may be periods of relapse or remission, but the individual suffers or is disabled to some extent until the end of his or her life. Chronic illness may be progressively debilitating or it may have a prolonged but stable course. In some instances chronic illness restricts activity but does not shorten the life expectancy of the sufferer. Terminal illness is the phase of acute or chronic illness which ends in death, usually after a fairly predictable course. The onset of all three types of illness may be either sudden or gradual. Often the onset may appear to be sudden, but the disease process has in fact been insidious and hidden. The family must then deal with an advanced stage of illness of which there was no previous knowledge.

The intrinsic features of these three categories of illness influence the interventions of professionals helping the family to cope. In contemporary times, acute illness depends primarily on the physician for cure. Chronic illness depends for maximum recovery on the patient and family. While chronic illness needs sound medical treatment, the responsibility for the necessary dietary regimen, activity adjustments, and life modifications falls on patient and family, rather than on the doctor. The growing number of elderly people in the United States accounts for the prevalence of chronic illnesses such as cardiac, orthopedic, visual, respiratory, and mental disorders. It has been estimated that 22 million Americans suffer activity limitation, and over 6 million suffer mobility limitation due to chronic illness (Strauss, 1973).

Terminal illness may be the outcome of acute or chronic disability, and the response of the family is often affected by the characteristics of the onset. The transformation of chronic illness into terminal illness may find the family somewhat prepared. On the other hand, the preceding conditions of chronicity may have already depleted the physical, psychological, and economic resources of the family.

Every family reacts to physical illness in its own way, exhibiting different strengths and weaknesses, and using different methods of coping with stress caused by the illness. The ability of the family to use adaptive coping measures depends in part on attitudes and interactions that are already present in the home, on socioeconomic factors, and on the life stages of the patient and other family members. The ages of family members and the time in the family life cycle at which a member becomes ill greatly affect the system and the problems it must face.

The professional endeavoring to help the family cope with illness must be sensitive to the particular stresses which chronic and terminal illness impose. In chronic or terminal illness, the crisis model that is effective for acute illness must be augmented by other interventions based on appropriate theoretical concepts. Parsons (1951) defined the two major privileges and the two major obligations of the sick person. The privileges are: (1) the patient is exempt from the responsibility for being incapacitated, and (2) the patient is exempt from role obligations. The obligations are: (1) the patient has an obligation to get well, and (2) the patient has an obligation to seek help. Building upon the concepts of Parsons permits the inference that chronic illness requires a sick role unlike the one demanded by acute illness. Because victims of chronic illness are unable to discard the sick role entirely, they may find themselves in conflict with their family's expectations and the expectations of society.

The work of Weisman and Worden (1976) showed that some of the classic behaviors of "good" patients might be dysfunctional. In a study of cancer patients they found that patients who combined confrontation with redefinition and compliance obtained more successful adjustment than persons who used suppression, submission, and passivity. These data apply to the family as well, for it is not the patient alone who is engaged in the struggle to compensate for chronically impaired or diminished function.

THE EFFECTS OF ACUTE ILLNESS ON THE FAMILY

Onset of Acute Illness   How an illness is discovered or recognized can affect the family's ability to cope with it. Sometimes an illness which begins without warning, converting an apparently healthy person into a sick one, is easier for the family to accept. Often the crisis nature of the event causes the family to mobilize its energies and respond adaptively. In the case of an individual who suffers a myocardial infarction the life-threatening crisis is obvious. Regardless of ultimate economic and social consequences, the illness can neither be ignored nor immediately denied. There is at first no time for feelings of guilt or anger. In a sense the urgency of the problem defines the priorities: (1) obtain immediate medical care, (2) rearrange family functioning in order to maintain essential family services, and (3) reassure, support, and serve the sick member.

An illness, known or unknown to the family, which slowly and imperceptibly becomes acute presents different problems. The family still faces the need to make all the adjustments described above, but a sense of urgency and priority may be lacking. If the family has known that the illness was present for weeks, months, or years before becoming acute, there may be feelings of anger or guilt. If the illness has already caused role restriction for the patient, an acute phase may be complicated by negative feelings accumulated during earlier stages of the illness. A wife may feel that her husband knew he was sick but did not care enough for his family to take proper care of himself. The ill husband may feel that family demands were excessive or that his wife should have insisted that he seek medical care earlier. Each may displace feelings on the other that something should have been done to prevent the development of acute illness. Meanwhile the children may react with fear and confusion to the realization that the family provider is mortal and is in peril.

The course of illness is influenced by the family's ability to recognize and respond to early signs of poor health. A family's willingness to do this is a function of personal, ethnic, and social variables. Families who enjoy an adequate income are more able to pay for health maintenance, and to seek professional help at the first indication of illness. Such families are generally sensitive to changes in the health status of their members, and of the adverse effects of failing to act on early warning signals. At the other extreme are many marginal families who define health only as the ability to work, and ignore signs of illness until there is incapacity to continue working.

A well-insured family is better able to entertain the prospect of losing income and paying medical expenses than a family that can barely make ends meet. When the father's wage is the only income, he may deliberately misinterpret serious symptoms as something that is "going around." Then, as the symptoms persist, he may deny their importance by rationalizing that he has had them for weeks without serious consequences. In marginal families, illnesses which reduce earnings or increase expenses can destroy hopes and dreams for the future. Procrastination in getting medical help is frustrating for the professional but must be seen in the context of the family's limitations. Many families in lower socioeconomic groups may ignore illness as long as possible because they regard the health care delivery system as hostile and uncaring. There are also individuals in all socioeconomic strata who equate illness with personal weakness and fiercely reject the idea of ever being sick. The realistic and symbolic meanings of illness to the patient and the family will determine their response to any illness, whether acute, chronic, or terminal. The sudden onset of acute illness may temporarily disorganize a family, but the immediacy of the crisis helps the family to rally and to mobilize effectively.

Assessment and Mobilization of Family Resources   When a member has become acutely ill without previous warning, the family must immediately assess and plan its course of action. More often than not an acute illness follows a course that includes recovery, either complete or partial. The

249

nature of the illness and the strength of the family system influence the actions which will be taken. The more resources available within the nuclear and extended family, and the more imbedded the family is in the community, the easier it will be for them to manage. Finances are important in considering the effect of illness on a family. If the wage earner is incapacitated, will there be loss of income? If so, for how long? What is available in the form of insurance or unemployment benefits? Does the family have adequate savings to help it through the crisis? Have large financial outlays such as college or elective dental care for the children been planned for the near future? When a nonworking mother is the patient, family income continues but plans must be made to care for her and for the children so that the father can continue to work. Litman (1971) found that the negative consequences of illness were inversely related to family size. When persons suffering acute illness belonged to a family with more than five members, the family demonstrated greater resilience and fewer problems. There are generally fewer financial problems when the mother is the patient, but her illness deprives the family of the purveyor of cure and care. Illness of the father causes financial privation; illness of the mother tends to cause family fragmentation and disorganization (Hollingshead & Duff, 1968; Litman, 1971).

Regardless of the identity of the patient, acute illness demands some sacrifice from all members. If a husband or child is ill, the wife and mother is expected to provide care and attention. Siblings who are well find themselves giving up free time in order to assume greater responsibility in the family. Almost every aspect of family life undergoes change. If the father is ill, his tasks in the family may be performed by others, or not be performed at all. Even when the mother does not need to become a family wage earner, she may become a more active disciplinarian or decision maker. In the absence of their father, the children may have to provide psychological support for their mother. Members of the extended family become closer and may even breach the boundaries of the nuclear family structure by moving into the home for a time.

An individual suffering an acute illness who begins to recover may become anxious or depressed. Dependency may cause him or her to regress and to become demanding, or to become counterdependent and rebel against restrictions. The professional who is involved with the family must help all members deal with reactions to their obstreperous patient whose behavior merely reflects fear and concern. Acute illness may cause family disequilibrium, but the disturbance is usually temporary.

Strong community ties can be of great value, especially in the first phase of acute illness. However, in mobile America, neighborhood ties are often tenuous, and the family may be obliged to find its own supports. Community agencies try to offer the help once provided by relatives and neighbors. But this assistance may be impersonal, or the family may not know it is available. A health practitioner has an obligation to act as liaison between the family and community agencies, providing appropriate data as indicated.

The world of children is totally changed by family illness since neither parent is fulfilling the accustomed role. If the mother is ill, the father or other relatives may be caring for the home and children. If the father is ill, the mother may try to be both father and mother to the family. A wife who is accustomed to depending on her husband may unconsciously resent his convalescence while so many demands are being made on her. It is a time when the health professional must be cognizant of psychological stress as well as physiological impairment. What is most helpful for the family is a sense of unity and purpose. There are certain advantages to encouraging the family to look for help within its own system. Family competence and cohesion may be enhanced by the process of problem solving and collaborative action.

A distinction should be made between marginal families and disorganized families who face illness. In marginal families the parents attempt appropriate role enactment, even though they are living at a subsistence level. In disorganized families there is virtually no attempt at appropriate role enactment, and meager resources may be strained further by addiction, violence, impulsivity, and low stress tolerance. It is the disorganized family whose dramatic episodes bring the family to the attention of professional agencies. The marginal family is less visible, even in times of illness. Yet the marginal family, with little money and few connections to community or extended family, is subject to the greatest stress. Solving the everyday problems of buying food, paying rent, and just surviving consumes all its resources. When acute illness strikes the marginal family there is pressure on the patient to recover quickly so as to relieve the family of the burden of the illness. Since the marginal family, unlike the disorganized family, may have little knowledge of community resources, referral must be prominent in the work of the health professional.

Residual Effects of Acute Illness Because of the relatively short duration and the often successful resolution of acute illness, the family may emerge stronger, with a sense of solidarity and pride. There may be increased feelings of confidence and closeness. A common reaction is greater appreciation for the family member who was ill, although there may also be unexpressed anger about the difficulties caused by the illness.

Sometimes the recovered member must reduce previous levels of activity after the acute phase has subsided. The family may have to lower its expectations and even its standard of living if convalescence is prolonged. It is also possible that permanent role alterations will ensue. During an illness of the husband, the wife may gain a new sense of competence which will change the family system. Children who have accepted greater responsibility may become less dependent on parents, and less docile. The status of the patient may have declined in some respects while the status of those who coped may have risen proportionately. These consequences necessitate readjustments from every member of the system.

One of the most dysfunctional responses of the family is an unrealistic attempt to ignore the changes brought about by the illness, and to revert to previous patterns of behavior. A father who has suffered a heart attack may return to work and quickly resume his old position as instrumental or task leader of the family. He may interpret the increased competence of his wife and children as threats, ignoring the contributions they were making. The pretense on his part that nothing has changed is detrimental to his health, and thus to the health of the family.

CLINICAL EXAMPLE: MYOCARDIAL INFARCTION IN A 38-YEAR-OLD FATHER

Ed Mills, married and the father of three, suffered a heart attack while watching a football game in his own living room. He was rushed to a hospital and admitted to the intensive care facility. The reaction of Mae, his 35-year-old wife, his teenage sons, and his 10-year-old daughter was shock and disbelief, followed shortly by acute anxiety and depression. In many respects the feelings of Ed's family followed the same sequence as his own. Because the family had adequate health insurance and because Ed's job was not in jeopardy, the family had time to adjust to the first impact of the crisis.

The acute phase of Ed's illness initially focused on his medical status. Drugs, monitoring, and skilled nursing care made Ed comfortable and helped stabilize his condition. In addition, such professionals as the unit social worker and the family health nurse-practitioner assisted Ed's family in dealing with the illness and the problems related to it. An important task for the nurse-practitioner was to help Ed's family understand that the illness was time-limited, and that Ed would be moved from the intensive care facility as soon as possible. Ed's wife was kept informed of what was happening to her husband and of the rationale for his medical regimen.

After a few days in the intensive care facility it became apparent that Ed was going to recover, but that he was depressed about his situation. Since the heart may recover more rapidly than the psyche of patients suffering an acute myocardial infarction (Cassem & Hackett, 1973), the predictability of this emotional reaction was explained to Ed and his wife. This alleviated the situation somewhat, but a recommendation was made that Mae be scheduled for several counseling sessions with the mental health nurse-practitioner available to families of hospitalized cardiac patients.

Mae revealed to the mental health nurse-practitioner that Ed's illness had brought unexpected problems to a woman with little experience in problem solving. Mae had married just after finishing high school. Although she had developed into a capable housewife, she relied almost entirely on her husband for guidance. Ed had been a devoted husband and father, proud of his ability to take care of his family. Out of his own need for control, he had encouraged Mae in her dependency. The sudden illness had transformed the family problem solver into the family problem. Mae was frightened and dismayed because her active husband had become a withdrawn, morose, indifferent man. Although Mae did not have to become the family breadwinner, she nonetheless faced role reversal. She felt guilty for having depended on Ed so much and had vague fears that she had caused his illness.

Although confidentiality was maintained, the staff responsible for Ed's physical care knew of the counseling sessions. Mae was encouraged by the staff to express her feelings and cautioned about being overprotective toward Ed. Both Ed and Mae were given realistic, accurate information about his progress. Rehabilitation work was begun as soon as possible, and Ed was allowed to make some decisions about his care. Mae and the children were able to strike a balance between reassuring Ed about how the family was coping and telling him how much he was missed.

As time for Ed's discharge neared, he joined the mental health nurse-practitioner and Mae in their sessions. The involvement of both partners helped remove any tendency on their part to deny his illness, and helped Ed accept the idea of permitting himself some dependency. At the same time his importance in the family and his autonomy were upheld, because this mattered both to him and Mae. Since the couple was agreeable, arrangements were made to continue the sessions for a few weeks after Ed was discharged and to include the children if possible.

Assessment

Structure The husband's inability to fulfill his usual role because of his psychological reaction to illness caused him to withdraw from his wife. Through the years, her dependency and his counterdependency had created a stable family structure.

Function The prospect of role reversal frightened the wife, who was poorly equipped to assume a more active role in the family. The husband was experiencing depression as a reaction to his illness. Also it was difficult for him to accept the fact that his family could manage without him. He was worried about his reduced status in the eyes of his wife and children. He was also concerned about his sexual relationship with his wife, and was not reassured by the clinical statements of his physician. He needed to get some answers, but was afraid to ask.

Intervention

Counseling helped the wife to understand her husband's withdrawal as an indication of depression. During the sessions Mae was able to express feelings of being overwhelmed, but indicated that she was beginning to accept new responsibilities. The husband was given some decision-making power in his therapeutic regimen. Rehabilitation procedures were arranged to begin as soon as possible to help alleviate his depression. The husband and wife were informed of the realities of the illness, and of the husband's medical status and progress.

The husband was invited to the counseling sessions as soon as his condition warranted it. Sexual counseling was included in the sessions. The subject was introduced by the counselor but welcomed by the couple. Both of them had many concerns in this area but had been hesitant to bring up the topic.

Husband and wife were involved in discharge planning. Counseling was continued for a few weeks after discharge. The children were invited to join the postdischarge sessions, since the illness had been a traumatic event for them as well as for their parents. Ed's illness was treated as a family problem which required cooperative effort.

THE EFFECTS OF CHRONIC ILLNESS ON THE FAMILY

Onset of Chronic Illness By definition, chronic illness includes all conditions that require long periods of supervision, observation, or care. Chronic illness is more or less permanent, and is characterized by residual disability or pathological alterations. Because chronic illness is of a long-term nature, the privileges and responsibilities usually assigned to the sick role are not enforceable. A consequence is the conflict suffered by persons enduring chronic illness because of their inability to discard the sick role. Neither acutely ill nor completely well, the person with chronic illness must make daily adjustments in living. The dimensions of the chronic sick role are not clearly defined; the ambiguity that results is troublesome for both the family and the patient. Strauss (1973) listed some problems surrounding chronic illness, among them (1) preventing and dealing with medical crises as these occur, (2) controlling symptoms, (3) following a medical regimen, (4) normalizing interactions with others, (5) arranging payment for treatment, and (6) adjusting to recurrent patterns in the course of the illness.

Chronic illness makes excessive demands on the family system, and the demands are exacted for long periods of time. Even the most devoted family becomes weary when basic functions such as rearing children, maintaining a home, and earning a living must be performed in addition to caring for a member who is chronically ill. Klein and Dean (1967) reported an increase in role tension and physical symptoms on the part of patient and spouse when one member of the marital dyad was afflicted. The chronic illness of a child is painful for both parents, but there remains the comfort that the partners can share their grief with one another.

The occurrence of chronic illness may seem sudden, but in fact its onset is usually gradual. The major difference between acute and chronic illness is that chronic illness has no predictable short-term outcome. All that is certain is that the individual will be sick for the forseeable future, if not forever. In many cases the maintenance of optimum function can be the only realistic goal.

Chronic illness is far more than a medical problem to be treated by a physician. Medical intervention is of paramount importance, but even the implementation of medical treatment will eventually become the obligation of the family. After the medical program is outlined, it is the family who must see that procedures are followed sensibly, that medications are taken, and that diet and rehabilitation programs are observed. Family members quickly become experts on a chronic illness suffered by one of them, and their daily observations usually provide reliable data for health professionals in attendance. Family attitudes and actions are crucial in determining the course of the illness, and contribute to remission or exacerbation of symptoms.

Chronic illness, like all illness, requires that family members make sacrifices on behalf of the patient. However, when the illness is chronic, the sacrifices are not temporary; they become a permanent way of life. It takes strong family commitment to withstand the strains that inevitably result. A long-term debilitating illness which attacks a healthy family member brings hardship to the family. However, the family has known and loved the stricken member for a period of time. Sick or well, he or she has become an integral part of the family system. This is not true of the congenitally disabled child, who enters the family as a stranger. There is no greater tragedy than the arrival in a family of a child who has never been well. Because of the severity of this situation, the discussion of chronic illness in the family will deal with the birth of a congenitally disabled infant. In this case there is no residue of familiar love or trust on which to build. The imperfect child is an unknown element which introduces a problem of enormous magnitude into the family system.

THE CONGENITALLY DISABLED CHILD

Accepting the Diagnosis   The birth of a child is considered to be a time of joy and fulfillment, even for parents who embarked on the prospect with less than total enthusiasm. The birth of a flawed child is one of the worst disappointments parents can experience. Since denial of the unendurable is a common defense, it is not surprising that parents at first refuse to accept the diagnosis. Sullivan (1953) has described some prolonged defensive behaviors that may be used to avoid reality. Selective inattention is a process that can help families defend against accepting unbearable facts. Through selective inattention, grieving parents fail to hear or comprehend a diagnosis of congenital disability. Despite what they are told by professionals, parents continue to deny the meaning of the disability.

Even after acknowledging that there is a problem, some parents resort to a process known as *focal awareness,* which lasts months or even years. They have heard the diagnosis on a cognitive level, but still do not accept its implications. Hearing accounts of miraculous treatments available in distant clinics reactivates their hope for cure. Often they travel from doctor to doctor, from one medical center to another, always searching for the means to make the disabled child perfect. When verdicts are discouraging, the parents find reasons to discount them. Not only does their search create financial burdens, but also the denial of reality and false hopes place additional strain on the family system. Focal awareness allows parents to exaggerate tiny signs of progress in their disabled child and to ignore the child's actual limitations.

Consensual validation of their own observations with those of health professionals eventually enables most parents to accept the evidence of their child's condition. Only then can the family begin to cope effectively with the problem of congenital disability. If the parents arrive at consensual validation together, they form an alliance which serves the disabled child, their healthy offspring, and their own emotional needs. Should one partner accept the diagnosis but not the other, the attitudes of the parents toward the disabled child will be so incongruent that their relationship with each other will be drastically altered, and the family system will be impaired.

Assessment and Mobilization of Family Resources   A child with a congenital disability tends to become the central figure in the life of the family. All family activity is organized around the disabled child. As in an acute illness, the immediate crisis may draw the marriage partners closer through common suffering. In a few cases the birth of the disabled child may even unite partners who have been drifting apart. The birth of a seriously disabled child represents a permanent dilemma. In the long run it probably will not strengthen a weak marriage, and will test any marriage to the utmost.

Permanent structural and functional changes in the family system follow the birth of a disabled child. At the simplest level someone has to care for the child at all times, and the time this takes will have to be subtracted from other activities. Parents will have less time to spend with each other, with their healthy children, and with their friends, and less time to pursue their own interests. Furthermore, accumulated medical expenses will result in less disposable income for everyone. This means changed family eating habits, and reduced amounts of money for clothing or recreation. The need to care for the disabled child may mean that the mother cannot work outside the home unless foster care can be arranged.

The financial burden of chronic illness is hardest on the middle-class family. Wealthy families can care for their child with minimal material sacrifice. Poor families have access to public funds, but middle-income families may well be overcome by catastrophic illness of long duration. It is also likely that middle-class families with high ambitions for their children will regard the disabled child as a humiliation. Financial resources insulate wealthy families to some extent, while lower expectations of their children may offer some protection from disappointment in poor families, although this is debatable.

A family with a disabled child requires support over the years, the nature of which must change as child and family grow older. Friends and neighbors cannot be expected to alter their lives permanently to help the family of a disabled child once the immediate crisis has been met. A contribution which can be made through the years by friends and relatives is to offer diversion or child care to the parents. The parents of a disabled child tend to become so obsessed with their duties that they lose contact with friends, and rarely escape from the pressures at home.

It is difficult to predict the reaction of relatives to the birth of a disabled child. The disability may frighten relatives and cause them to seem cruel and distant. Some grandparents blame the disability on the in-laws, and feel that their own child has been unfairly burdened. Other grandparents may feel guilty, suspecting that their genes may have caused the defect. Relatives may be upset by the birth of a congenitally disabled child, wondering if they too will have defective children. These understandable reactions may restrict the amount of help that the stricken family can expect from relatives.

Because of the chronicity of the illness, good relationships between health professionals and the family are important. In addition to a physician, the family needs the services of a primary professional who can coordinate treatment programs, direct the family to specialists and agencies, clarify confusing instructions, and provide sustained, meaningful guidance.

In some communities there are established networks of parents whose children share the same disability. These groups are eager to help families with similar problems, and to give practical advice, answer questions, and offer emotional support. Most importantly these groups are living proof that parents can face problems which seem insoluble, and still survive. Community groups may be affiliated with national organizations devoted to education and research concerning particular diseases or disabilities. Such organizations provide additional resources for troubled parents. Many publish informative newsletters or journals, which convey practical help to the parents and a feeling that they are not alone in their trouble.

In a family with a chronically ill child, there must be periodic reevaluation of role effectiveness. Structural adjustments which once strengthened the family may later work to its disadvantage. In the first months after learning that the infant is seriously disabled, the mother may give all her time to caring for the child. At the same time the father may take on more work to reduce the family's indebtedness. The healthy children are called upon for assistance, and will respond to the best of their ability. These first adjustments are usually effective; the baby is cared for, income is increased, everyone is joined in a common goal. Over time these same adjustments may become maladaptive for the family. The mother finds she has become the sole caretaker of the child. Since she has been recognized as the expert, family members leave the infant in her charge. She feels overburdened, but at the same time is unwilling to allow her husband or the other children to take over her function. The father is already spending most of his time at work in order to meet his financial obligations. He is deeply concerned about the child, but his life is less dominated by the disability. As he sees his wife becoming more involved with the sick child he may feel jealous and excluded. Rather than make more demands on his wife, he may withdraw further, spending more time at work or looking outside the home for companionship. While the father is jealous of the close mother-infant relationship, the mother may envy her husband's life outside the family. In their zeal to meet the needs of the disabled child, the parents have caused their functions to be so sharply defined that they have little in common with each other. Meanwhile, the healthy children in the family are receiving insufficient attention from both parents and their early willingness to cooperate may have deteriorated into indifference or subtle rebellion.

Occasionally both father and mother assign the disabled child the central role in the family. In these circumstances all family life revolves around the limitations of the disabled child. The needs of all members are secondary to those of the sick child. By overprotection, the family inhibits the child's mental, physical, and psychological growth. The parents are so intent on coping with the disability that they lose sight of the real child. While single-minded attention to the sick child may create a strong partnership between the parents, it is unfair to the healthy children, and may prevent the disabled child from reaching his or her full potential (Gordon, 1975).

A paradoxical form of the sick role develops when the family "scape-goats" the disabled child. In this situation parents and siblings blame all adversity in family relationships on the child who is ill. Since the child is unlikely to get better, family problems need never be resolved. This behavior relieves a family of the difficult task of finding out what is really wrong and trying to correct it. The family establishes an unhealthy balance based on the child's illness; the sick child is blamed for whatever goes wrong. Simultaneously, the healthy children are not likely to have their needs met. Scapegoating the sick child allows all deficiencies to be rationalized. This may be the most pervasive distortion in families with chronically ill children, whether it is the maternal-sick child coalition or the parental-sick child coalition that dominates the family.

There may be secondary gains in a family with a chronically disabled child. A frequent secondary gain is that family relationships are simplified by the routine task of caring for the disabled child. Other gains result from recognition from friends and neighbors of the family's strength and courage. The mother, in particular, may feel pride in having met and overcome such a challenge. It is not uncommon for a mother, after learning to care for her own disabled child, to return to school and become a specialist in caring for others with the same disability. The professionalization of the mother is worthwhile if she is willing and able to give her husband and her other children the attention they need. Otherwise professionalization is only a signal of her total involvement with the disabled child, and her inability to give to other members of her family.

Residual Effects on the Family   The guilt that occurs after the birth of a disabled child can take many forms. Some parents who have produced a defective child feel that they are being punished for their sins. At times one parent may try to escape responsibility by blaming the other. Later, parents experience guilt because they cannot help the child by accomplishing the impossible. Devoted parents set standards for themselves which are unreachable, and this increases their feelings of inadequacy. As the child grows older, the parents may become ashamed to be seen with him or her in public, and at the same time they feel guilty for being ashamed. Siblings have similar feelings. They may be reluctant to bring friends home because of embarrassment, and feel guilty because their presence at home diverts parental attention from the task of caring for the disabled child. Conflicting emotions complicate the lives of every family member. One mother described her feelings as follows:

> I have an overwhelming sense of guilt about Andy. This is always present and diminishes all my pleasures. I will never be able to forgive myself for the frustrations and restrictions of his life. To the extent that I am responsible for that life, his handicap does become my responsibility. Additionally, because the experts told us so often that guilt is destructive, I feel guilty about feeling guilty (Behmer, 1976.)

The parent of two afflicted children recommended "keeping it clinical," and advocated using medical terms whenever possible in speaking of a child's disability. This simple tactic helped depersonalize the affliction by labeling it as a medical condition shared by others.

Parents of a congenitally disabled child go through a grieving process similar to the one experienced by parents whose child dies at birth. They mourn the loss of the anticipated perfect child who was not born. They grieve as well for the child they have, who must go through life handicapped. For many parents children represent a second chance. Parents strive to give their children advantages so that the children may accomplish what the parents could not. Since the birth of a disabled child frustrates these dreams, parents mourn the loss of their second chance.

Many parents admit to feelings of intense anger. They are angry with themselves for having conceived the child and at health professionals for being unable to cure their child. Parents may also be angry with the sick child whose existence makes so many demands and causes so many disruptions to family life. Some parents (Behmer, 1976; Katz, 1975) have described feelings of rage at the birth of defective children and the lessening of rage as their understanding and expertise grew. A typical description of one mother recalled feelings of frustration at her helplessness to stop the child's suffering. The response of some parents is to become as well informed as possible about the disabilities as well as about the methods and treatment prescribed. Parents who collaborated with and become an important part of the professional team find a measure of relief. Feeling effective seems to help parents to overcome sensations of helplessness and despair.

Chronic depression is another possible effect of the birth of a disabled child. Depression in the parents makes them less able to handle the disabled child. It also interferes with their ability to interact wholesomely with other family members, or to derive any personal enjoyment from life. The depression may be transmitted from one parent to the other, imbuing the family system with a sense of helplessness which becomes an additional source of tension and unhappiness in the home. When depression is evident, it must be addressed by the person coordinating treatment for the family, preferably by suggesting sustained family counseling.

To meet the challenge of dealing with a chronically disabled child is a task beyond the imagination of most parents. Buscaglia (1975) described some of the interventions which families of disabled children have a right to expect from health professionals. First, the parents must be offered an explanation of the problem in words which they can understand. The explanation may have to be given again and again. They also need continual reassurance that their conflicted feelings of guilt, anger, confusion, and depression are not abnormal under the circumstances. Definitive answers and predictions of the future are less important than repeated expressions of hope and confidence in the family's ability to survive. Approaching the family as a social system, the professional should be committed not only to the well-being of the child but to the creative growth of the family. In addition to helping with the practicalities of caring for the disabled child, the coordinating practitioner must help families sort out their misgivings, while permitting them some defensive behaviors as they move slowly toward comprehension and acceptance.

CLINICAL EXAMPLE: THE CHILD WITH CEREBRAL PALSY

Assessment

Structure   The Webb family consisted of George and Rose Webb, their 4-year-old daughter Louanne, and their 2-year-old son Joey, who was born with cerebral palsy. Joey showed several developmental lags, and had required constant medical care and personal attention since birth. Most of the responsibility fell on Rose. Her husband helped with household chores but not with the care of his son. In the last couple of years Louanne had been his joy and solace. Father and daughter were very close; George spent most evenings reading or playing games with his daughter. Louanne attended nursery school during the day, to provide her with playmates and relieve her overburdened mother.

Function   Although the family was coping, the distance between husband and wife was very great. Rose had become increasingly resentful toward her husband. George, for his part, was repelled by the services his son needed, and could not bear to watch the boy eat. Rose sensed this, although it was never discussed, and she became reluctant to ask George for assistance in caring for Joey. She also felt excluded from the happy times that George and Louanne shared in the evenings. In her loneliness Rose began to feel that she and Joey were both rejects. The family was visited regularly by a nurse-practitioner from the local chapter of the Cerebral Palsy Association. It was to her that Rose turned for help.

Intervention

The first intervention the health professional made was to provide practical advice. As an expert in cerebral palsy, she was knowledgeable about special chairs, feeding aids, suction machines, and other labor-saving devices. Rose had some equipment, but Joey obviously could use more. By arranging to visit in the evening, the health professional was able to involve George in helping to simplify the care of Joey.

Noting that George's relationship with Louanne excluded Rose, the health professional commented on Rose's need for company other than that of Joey. She suggested that the couple might plan some recreational activities together, and presented them with a list of qualified baby-sitters endorsed by the local cerebral palsy chapter. Because George resisted the idea of joining a group of parents with children like Joey, and needed more time to work through his feelings, the health professional put only Rose in touch with a parents' group. Rose needed to meet with other parents who might alleviate her feelings of isolation. The primary objectives of intervention were: (1) to reduce Rose's preoccupation with Joey and simplify his care, (2) to modify the relationship between George and Louanne in order to include Rose, and (3) to strengthen the marital partnership by encouraging communication and shared activity between husband and wife.

THE EFFECTS OF TERMINAL ILLNESS ON THE FAMILY

Onset of Terminal Illness   Terminal illness is defined by its resolution, which is the death of the person afflicted. The inevitability of the final outcome is a factor that affects family members in several ways. As in acute and chronic illness, the onset of terminal illness may seem sudden or gradual. In one sense all terminal illness has a sudden onset, for there is a time when the truth must be accepted, and the family must admit that the illness will end in death. The shock of this realization may temporarily stun the family so that effective reorganization must wait for the first impact to abate.

Like acute illness, terminal illness usually lasts for a limited period of time. Like chronic illness, terminal illness has a poor prognosis. Many of the issues mentioned in the discussion of acute and chronic illness are applicable to the terminal process. For example, if the early onset is unnoticed, the discovery of the illness and its consequences may cause family members to react with anger or guilt. When the family becomes aware of the prognosis, feelings of hopelessness and helplessness may appear, just as in chronic illness. As with an acute illness, a major short-term reorganization of the family must be made in order to care for the sick person. There must also be long-term changes in the family such as are needed in cases of chronic illness.

The immediate problems that confront a family with a terminally ill member resemble those which must be solved when acute illness is present. They include practical concerns such as obtaining medical treatment and providing care for the patient. Thus, a family's economic condition, its closeness with friends and relatives, and its stability in the community all affect its adjustment to terminal illness. The essential difference, which will alter the behavior of everyone involved, is the knowledge that there will be no recovery. Although economic factors are important, emotional support from significant others may be more crucial than any other factor.

Here again, the identity of the patient affects the kinds of adjustments which must be made. In a study of male and female colostomy patients, Dyk and Sutherland (1975) compared the behaviors of the patient's spouse. They found that when men became ill, their wives were the principal providers of nursing care. Although subjects selected the marital partner as the most desired provider of care, women who became ill were not always cared for by their husbands; care was sometimes provided by their daughters or sisters. This may reflect the bias of society that nursing is an activity best left to women. Whenever a mother is ill, special problems arise, partly because the mother is often the emotional leader of the family. Even with the increase in the number of working mothers, and greater sharing of household tasks, the family looks to the mother for affection and nurturance. Terminal illness of the mother may be especially difficult for young families in which children are still very dependent on both parents. The pain of the young mother who is dying is excessive, for she must turn over the care of her children to others. She must either see herself replaced by another, or have her children divided among relatives.

As the family realigns itself to support the terminally ill member, healthy members may find compensation in their shared objective of preserving the family system. When terminal illness strikes, some family members are able to define themselves through service. By reallocating tasks and roles, strong family systems can keep the terminally ill member as part of the system. This realignment eases the terminal process for the patient and the family, but may not prepare the family for the final moment of loss.

A terminally ill person usually goes through several stages before accepting the inevitable (Kubler-Ross, 1969).

Denial   The first tendency is to deny that the illness is terminal. The patient refuses to believe this illness will be different from other illnesses. Family members, too, may deny the illness, reinforcing the patient's denial and clinging to the hope that the family circle will be unbroken.

Anger When the reality of the illness and its nature become clear, the patient renounces denial and becomes angry. There is anger at God or fate for allowing the illness. The patient also becomes angry at family members because their lives will go on. There may be anger at health professionals who cannot help and at medical science for finding no cure. The anger may be focused on a few persons, or may include everyone who is not terminally ill. This is a time when overwrought family members require help in dealing with the irrational anger of their loved one.

Bargaining Bargaining in an attempt to obtain a few more years of life is a common phenomenon among the dying. Promises are made to God, to childhood saints, to caretakers, and to family members in a futile attempt to purchase life.

Despair This stage is one of depression and submission. It may take the form of remoteness and detachment from family members. Despair may manifest itself in a wish to die or in the expression of feelings of futility.

Acceptance In this last stage, which some patients do not reach, the patient accepts the nearness of death. A parent may find renewed pleasure in children who symbolize immortality. Sometimes a conscious decision is made to enjoy what time is left, to draw closer to family members, to make what the ancients called a "good" death.

These stages are not invariant, and the sequence may never be completed. A patient who has accepted imminent death may revert at times to anger or despair. Another may never move beyond the stage of denial. Since an already burdened family may find the moods of the patient incomprehensible, professionals who interpret the psychological stages of the dying can do much to mitigate family pain. The more the family understands what the patient is going through, the easier it will be for members to interpret and accept behaviors sympathetically.

The family of the dying, especially the children, may pass through the same stages as the patient. At times they may hope the patient will die so the ordeal will be over, or wish to die with the patient rather than endure separation. At other times they may be angry at the dying patient for abandoning them. Such conflicted feelings engender guilt in family members, and inhibit their ability to offer support. A therapeutic response is to assure family members that their feelings are not evil or selfish, but normal under the circumstances.

Once a person has been able to accept the idea of death, there may follow a time of disengagement from the spouse and children, which allows the patient to prepare for the approaching death. This anticipatory disengagement may be partly the result of waning energy, but may also represent an effort by the dying person to prepare the family for future loss. By encouraging the family to look to others or to find strength within its own members, the dying person may be offering one last gift.

During the last days of a terminally ill patient, the health professional tries to help the family and the patient understand each other. Since the professional is less involved emotionally, efforts can be made to help the family adjust to changes in the physical and psychological status of the patient. The patient offers cues as to the treatment which is desired from the family and from professionals. As far as possible, the health professional must follow these cues and let the dying patient indicate what is acceptable and what is not. In the absence of such messages some family member is usually able to determine what actions are necessary to prepare for the approaching death.

Even when time has been spent preparing a family for the death of a member, the actual impact of the loss is overwhelming. Shortly after the death, however, the family may experience feelings of relief that the long ordeal has finally ended. This reaction is human and understandable, but it contributes to excessive feelings of guilt. The process of mourning may last a year or more, but the most intense grief occurs during the first 6 weeks after the death. There may be feelings of anger at being abandoned, or of remorse for not having done more for the lost one. Family members may feel distant and strange with each other as a result of the drastic alteration in family structure. Those who sought self-definition by caring for the dying person may feel that they have lost their reason for living. The family system had reorganized to cope with the impending death of one of its members. With the member removed, the family must now consider how reconstitution will take place.

CLINICAL EXAMPLE: DEATH OF A
YOUNG MOTHER WITH METASTATIC CARCINOMA

The Ward family lived in the same lower-middle-class neighborhood where Bob Ward had met and married his wife, Betty. Their two children, Roberta, aged 11, and Richard, aged 6, attended school a few blocks from the neat frame house where the family lived. Until the last 6 months Betty Ward had been an energetic wife and mother. She was a conscientious housekeeper and had worked 4 days a week in a real estate office. Betty began feeling ill early in the spring, but attributed her symptoms to fatigue. When she did not improve, she was referred by her family physician for other tests. A few days in the hospital and a barrage of tests confirmed the suspicions of the family physician that Betty had an abdominal mass, probably malignant. Exploratory surgery was done and the surgeons found advanced carcinoma of the pancreas and liver which was inoperable. Betty's prognosis was very poor; Bob was told that his 33-year-old wife had less than a year to live. The distraught husband made two decisions immediately. The first was that Betty would want to know what her condition was and should be told soon. The second was that the children would stay with their grandmother for a few weeks while Bob took Betty to a quiet, sunny place where she could recuperate from the surgery. Once there, he intended to break the news to his wife so they could plan for the months ahead. The children were told only that their mother had had an operation and that Daddy was taking her on a vacation so she would get better and return to them soon.

Bob and Betty had 12 days together in their quiet retreat before Betty became much worse. She was rushed by ambulance to the hospital where her surgery had been done and in less than a week she was dead. The children were still with their grandmother and Bob had seen them only briefly in the week before Betty died. Ten-year-old Roberta found it hard to believe that her smiling, pretty mother was gone but she seemed able to understand Bob's incoherent, tearful explanation of what had happened. Richard heard the news of his mother's death with no outward emotion. Roberta and her father wept together, as Richard, without tears, held on to them both. The same behaviors continued throughout the funeral services, as relatives marveled that Richard bore his loss so calmly. The children remained with their grandmother a few days longer, while their father removed all Betty's belongings from the house so that when they returned home nothing would remind them of their mother. When the children were brought by their father and grandmother to the home, there were no traces of Betty. Although there had been no previous discussion of the arrangement, the children were then told that grandmother would now be living with them. Their father urged them to be good children and to do everything they could to help their grandmother.

Roberta returned to school saddened by the loss of her mother, but rather enjoying the sympathy she received from teachers and her friends. She and her grandmother were close, and although Roberta thought about her mother sometimes, she found her grandmother a good substitute.

Richard had always been shy and insecure at school, but now became even more withdrawn. At first his teacher made allowances, but Richard's behavior did not improve. He began wetting the bed at home, which made the grandmother angry. Richard remembered that his mother had never been angry about his occasional "accidents." He wanted to talk about his mother, to find out what really happened to her, but he was afraid his questions would only make everyone feel bad. While Richard worried, and tried to make sense out of everything, his behavior regressed further. He became taciturn and distant both at home and in the classroom. Some of the children began to taunt him. His academic performance deteriorated badly because he seemed unable to complete his work. After some months of this

behavior the school psychologist suggested a family referral for conjoint counseling. Because the grandmother was present in the home,
she was included in the referral.

Assessment

Structure   Before Betty's terminal illness, the family had been
warm and close. At 11, Roberta was beginning to move toward
independence, but 6-year-old Richard was caught up in possessive
feelings toward his mother and competitive feelings toward his father
just at the time Betty died. The suddenness of his mother's illness, followed by his parents' abrupt "vacation," left Richard wondering if his
feelings about his parents had contributed to his mother's death. He
and his father had been good friends, but after his mother died his
father did not pay much attention to him. He had so many questions
and no one wanted to answer them. Richard felt confused and worried
all the time but did not know why. Even with Roberta and his grandmother around, Richard was lonely.

Function   The suddenness of Betty's illness and the knowledge
that it was terminal caused Bob to think only of himself and his wife.
He saw that his children were cared for physically, but he deserted
them when they needed him most. He had expected to take Betty
home after a week or two, planning then to bring the family together
so that Betty's illness could be told to the children gently. However,
he had not taken into account the precarious state of Betty's health.
    After Betty's death, Richard suffered a pathological grief reac-
tion brought on by the suddenness of his mother's death, and by his
father's reluctance to prepare the children.
    Richard's bedwetting was an indication of regression and anxi-
ety. It made his grandmother impatient with him. Feeling unloved, he
missed his mother more than ever. Grandmother's constant admonition that he should be a big boy made Richard grieve even more for the
mother who loved him still when he behaved like a little boy.

Intervention

    1   Father and grandmother were encouraged to talk about Betty.
It was important for Richard to hear how Daddy felt when he learned
that Betty was dying, and to hear why Daddy and Mommy had gone
away instead of returning to Richard and Roberta.
    2   Grandmother was helped to understand why Richard resumed
bed-wetting, and to be more tolerant of this behavior.
    3   Roberta and Richard were reminded of what they both had
lost and encouraged to help each other to remember their mother.
    4   Bob felt guilty about how Betty had died. He realized that his
foremost thoughts had been of himself. Betty's terminal illness

should have taken place in familiar surroundings, giving Bob, Betty, and the children time for leave taking. Because he regretted that he had deprived the children of the last few weeks of their mother's life, Bob pulled away from them. This was interpreted by Richard as further punishment and loss. Bob was urged to move closer to the children, and allow all of them to share memories of Betty. With help in grieving, Richard was in time able to accept the loss of his beloved mother and establish stronger bonds with his father, sister, and grandmother.

SUMMARY

The impact of physical illness on families was linked to three categories of illness: acute, chronic and terminal. Differences between the categories were noted as well as factors such as the age and identity of the patient. Assessment, planning, intervention, and implementation were discussed as part of an ongoing process applicable to all three types of physical illness.

Attention was given to the stresses caused by limited financial resources, role reversal, and residual impairment, which add to complications of physical illness. The capacity of the family to reorganize around a physical illness was recognized as an adaptive behavior which may become dysfunctional after recovery. The dangers of having family life revolve around the sick member were mentioned, as well as the secondary gain inherent in playing the sick role.

The work of Kubler-Ross on death and dying was part of the discussion of terminal illness. A clinical example, which included assessment and intervention techniques, was provided for each category of physical illness.

REFERENCES

Behmer, M. Children with disabilities. *The Exceptional Parent,* 1976, **6**(1), 35–38.

Buscaglia, L. *Counseling the disabled and their parents.* Thorofare, N.J.: Slack, 1975.

Cassem, N. H., & Hackett, T. Psychological rehabilitation of myocardial infarction patients in the acute phase. *Heart and Lung,* 1973, **2**, 382–387.

Dyk, R., & Sutherland, A. Adaptation of the spouse and other family members to the colostomy patient. *American Cancer Society Educational Publication,* 1975.

Gordon, S. *Living fully: A guide for young people with a handicap, their parents, their teachers, and professionals.* New York: Day, 1975.

Hollingshead, A., & Duff, R. *Sickness and society.* New York: Harper & Row, 1968.

Katz, K. J. Precious days. *The Exceptional Parent,* 1975, **5**(4), 19–22.

Klein, R., & Dean, A. The impact of illness upon the spouse. *Journal of Chronic Disease,* 1967, **20**, 241–248.

Kubler-Ross, E. *On death and dying.* New York: Macmillan, 1969.

Litman, T. J. The family and physical rehabilitation. *Journal of Chronic Disease,* 1966, **19,** 211–217.

Litman, T. J. Health and the family. *Medical Care,* 1971, **9,** 67.

Litman, T. J. The family as a basic unit in health and medical care. *Social Science and Medicine,* 1974, **8,** 495–519.

Parsons, T. *The social system.* New York: Free Press, 1951.

Sedgwick, R. The family system: A network of relationships. *Journal of Psychiatric Nursing and Mental Health Services,* 1974, **12,** 17–20.

Strauss, A. *Chronic illness and the quality of life.* St. Louis: Mosby, 1973.

Sullivan, H. S. *The interpersonal theory of psychiatry.* New York: Norton, 1953.

Weisman, A., & Worden, J. W. The existential plight in cancer: A significance of the first 100 days. *International Journal of Psychiatry in Medicine,* 1976, **1,** 7.

Chapter 13

Mental Illness in the Family

Carlos Frias
Ellen H. Janosik

The issue of mental illness in the family may be approached from an interactional or a systems point of view, while at the same time acknowledging that the existing classifications of mental disorders are for the most part based on an individual approach, specifically that of the "sick" person. This situation produces an intellectual dilemma familiar to those engaged in the process of acquiring or building knowledge. On the one hand, the systems theorist is concerned with holistic appraisal; on the other hand, the professional dealing with mental illness is constrained to separate the whole into its constituents for analysis, much as the pathologist resorts to the microscope to examine disease at its most minute level.

What is sometimes forgotten is that the clinician who analyzes discrete elements or components has an intellectual and pragmatic obligation to bring together by a process of synthesis the coherent whole which the system represents. This is accomplished by combining the previously separated components in the proper way.

The necessity of synthesizing separate components into a coherent entity was noted by Speigel (1971):

> We can no longer afford, in any science, to focus exclusively on one region and to leave the rest of the universe out of account until we complete our investigations. We never actually "complete" our investigations, the nature of science being a continuous process of inquiry. Completeness is an illusion; and if, in any one science, we forever keep the rest of the universe out of account, we will never be in a position to consider the whole (p. 38).

The analytic aspect of inquiry into mental illness constitutes the beginning of a dual process. It is justifiable for clinicians to use existing classifications of mental disorder that are primarily oriented toward the symptoms of the identified patient, but clinicians must also use a larger perspective in order to understand these symptoms in the context in which they are exhibited. The dichotomy of analysis and synthesis is clearly acceptable in diagnosis (assessment) and treatment (intervention) which include the individual and his or her family. Thus the clinician refers again and again to a model of an alive, dynamic, interacting family system which perhaps generates—but may also contain within its boundaries—psychopathology that causes suffering and malfunction for all members.

If one accepts the concept of synthesis, it may not even be enough to focus on the family. Such a focus represents a distortion of the analytic process, since it ignores the fact that the family is only one system interacting with larger systems. There are, however, practical limits to what may be included in the clinical picture, and by focusing on the family the clinician enlarges the field of vision and maintains a position equidistant from the identified patient and the other family members, who are also suffering. It is important that the clinician maintain equidistance because the biological and physiological status of the patient must be assessed in conjunction with the social and situational context. Treatment planning and evaluation may be deficient if individual symptoms and situational factors are overlooked; however, exclusive preoccupation with social factors would also be detrimental.

One comprehensive solution to the question of the individual versus the family approach to psychopathology is supplied by Erikson (1963) who suggested that the clinician (1) begin by assessing processes inherent in the individual; (2) next consider the organization of experience in the individual ego; and, finally, (3) include the social groupings (family, class, community, and nation) of the afflicted individual. This triad composed of the biological process, the ego process, and the social process is within the legitimate purview of the clinician. For the purposes of this chapter and at the present level of understanding psychopathology, the family of the identified patient can be considered the primary social unit suitable for assessment, intervention, and evaluation.

Any practitioner who is endeavoring to help an emotionally disturbed family must have a basic knowledge of the accepted classifications of mental illness and of their behavioral manifestations. Therefore, a description of various types of mental illness is a necessary frame of reference, particularly since most existing psychiatric typologies are essentially descriptions of behaviors (symptoms) presented by the person experiencing some form of psychopathology.

TYPES OF MENTAL ILLNESS

Classifications of mental illness are helpful in spite of their deficiencies, because they facilitate professional communication and the understanding of psychiatric literature. Based on a large body of data accumulated from similar cases, these classifications permit a phenomenological identification (diagnosis) of the psychopathology being observed. Some inferences can then be drawn with respect to personality characteristics and possible precipitating causes (somatic, psychological, and social). The severity of the problem may also be assessed. Classifications also offer guidelines for data gathering. Based on appropriate information, decisions can be reached regarding what interventions should be made, and how and by whom they should be made.

A classification of the principal mental disorders which a clinician may encounter would include the following:

1 Affective disorders (depressions, hypomania, and mania)
2 Schizophrenic disorders
3 Organic mental disorders
4 Anxiety disorders (obsessions, phobias, etc.)
5 Hysterical disorders
6 Antisocial personalities
7 Adjustment reactions (adolescent, adult, mid- and later life)
8 Drug and alcohol addiction
9 Psychosomatic disorders

Mental retardation, which ranges from mild to moderate to severe and causes varying degrees of incapacity, is another classification which the family clinician should keep in mind. For instance, below certain intelligence levels transactions between parents and offspring are inadequate. Proper acculturation is therefore not accomplished and the family tends to become isolated and be unable to cope with social environments.

The affective, schizophrenic, and organic disorders can at times reach psychotic proportions. The term *psychosis* is used to indicate a profound disturbance of the personality with serious alterations in the perception of reality. Psychosis is often accompanied by irrational beliefs (delusions), hallucinatory experiences (sensory perceptions without external stimulus), and more or less pronounced impairment of everyday functioning. The popular, common sense perception of "madness" as irrational, irresponsible, unpredictable behavior is a fairly reliable way to identify psychosis. Anxiety and hysterical disorders, as well as some depressive reactions, are usually considered *neuroses.*

The term *neurosis* attempts to describe a partial disorder of the personality in which the individual shows good perceptual contact with reality (absence of hallucinations, delusions, or deep confusion), has a subjective awareness of being dysfunctional (insight), and is haunted by recurrent anxiety (deep apprehension or fear without apparent cause), all of which interferes with the ability to establish meaningful relationships and to achieve success in proportion to one's intelligence and ability.

Personality or *character disorders* are present in otherwise normal persons who show ingrained patterns of behavior which generate repetitive conflicts with others. The affected individual accepts these adverse behavioral characteristics as a natural way of being and does not recognize them as problems or symptoms to be treated. Based on the dominant characteristic of these maladaptive behavioral patterns, several types of character disorders have been differentiated. For example, persons with some typical disorders have been designated as *explosive, dependent, passive-aggressive, sadomasochistic, compulsive, paranoid, schizoid,* and *antisocial* personalities.

It may be inferred from this typology that some, if not all, of these maladaptive behavioral patterns are actually interactional in nature. By employing communicational-interactional terms, the psychiatric classification of mental disorder moves away from an exclusively intrapsychic and/or organic consideration of the presenting patient, thereby placing at least part of the psychopathology in the realm of interpersonal transaction. For instance, it is only in terms of social interaction that a passive-aggressive or sadomasochistic personality structure can be explained or understood.

Additional comprehension of the personality disorders may be obtained by examining in some detail the antisocial or *psychopathic personality.* Individuals with such a personality are generally young and often male, and present themselves as apparently healthy. They tend to be both charming and disarming, and are expert in manipulating others. Their judgment of reality shows no indication of serious distortion such as is evident in psychosis. It is only the observation or experience of their transactional conduct which reveals disturbance. Pathology is demonstrated by a persistent pattern of dishonesty, irresponsibility, and callousness, without sign of remorse or motivation to change. Rarely is there an awareness of dysfunction or suffering such as is seen in neurosis. As in any other psychiatric disorder, there are degrees of severity to the problem ranging from minor to moderate to extreme. For diagnostic purposes it is crucial to note that the disturbed transactional pattern must be entrenched in the personality. Isolated episodes of the described behaviors are insufficient to warrant the designation of a psychopathic or antisocial personality.

Psychopaths operate as if they cannot be influenced by the rules or moral values of their sociocultural group. Their orientation is egocentric rather than sociocentric, and they show little concern for the standards of either the "significant other" (Sullivan, 1953) or the "generalized other" (Mead, 1934). In one sense the old notion of "moral insanity" retains descriptive validity, for sociopaths are unable to respond to the needs of others or to develop internalized loyalties. Their behavior lacks the self-control one needs to act in a socially responsible manner, and they are impelled by a wish for personal gratification. The existential posture of the sociopath is expressed by the phrase "I'm O.K. You (and everybody else) are not O.K.," which was coined by the transactional analysts. With this egocentric existential attitude deeply ingrained in the self from early childhood, the antisocial personality becomes impervious to social attempts to inculcate norms and to therapeutic efforts to produce change. Disdain for others (the "not O.K." people) may explain the aggressive and destructive patterns of psychopaths. Sometimes the origin of the patterns can be traced to experiences of excessive punishment (the battered child), or to experiences of deprivation (the rejected, neglected, or abandoned child). It is noteworthy that approximately a third of these antisocial personalities relax their rigid, ungiving existential posture in the third decade of their life, as if an urge for relatedness finally overwhelms their egocentric posture.

SITUATIONAL OR ADJUSTMENT REACTIONS

The adjustment and situational disorders have been singled out from the other disorders previously discussed because of their intrinsic differences and because, for the purposes of this chapter, they will be the subject of more extensive discussion. The concept of adjustment reaction will be utilized as a point of entry to the psychiatric classifications by which the processes already mentioned may be approached from the vantage of an interacting family system.

Classifications of the personality disorders implicitly recognize the interpersonal or interactional factors in determining the locus of psychopathology. In the categories of situational and adjustment reactions, one moves still further from an individual or intrapsychic approach. Here the cause of psychopathology is placed squarely in the situation, and in the circumstances surrounding the identified patient that seem to be causing stress. The reaction of adjusting to a difficult or stressful situation produces symptoms which are interpreted clinically as a dynamic response to the problem. Symptoms in this paradigm may be regarded as understandable psychological or psychophysiological reactions to stress. The symptoms represent adjustments within the capacity of the individual involved.

Based on the magnitude of the precipitating factor, the psychiatric classifications permit the classical symptoms of mental illness—even psychotic symptoms—to be seen as stress reactions. Included among these *reactive* symptoms are depression and guilt, identity confusion, hostility and anger even to the extent of paranoia or violence, and excessive anxiety and tension. Physiological concomitants which are common in adjustment reactions include anorexia, headache, insomnia, and gastrointestinal and cardiorespiratory disturbances. Frequent behavior manifestations are drug and alcohol abuse, change in moral attitudes, and deterioration of levels of performance. Distortions of reality and perception can lead to delusion or hallucination, or to other phenomena of a similar nature. At this point it may be suggested that, if classical psychiatric symptoms can develop in obviously stressful situations, it may be possible to interpret most psychiatric disorders as stress reactions, even when the traumatic circumstances are not readily apparent. It must be remembered that only functional symptoms are being discussed, not psychiatric symptoms which are related to organicity or toxicity. In addition, the concomitance of both functional and organic symptoms, such as depression in senile persons, should not be overlooked.

The conceptualization of psychiatric symptoms as meaningful responses to situational stress has clinical merit because it suggests that symptoms may be altered, improved, or eliminated by introducing change into various aspects of the situation. Stress may be produced by any of the biological, psychological, cultural, economic, or ecological circumstances surrounding the individual and his or her family, which is the immediate social field. A systematic review of these circumstantial factors may be found in other chapters of this book.

The interconnections of individual and family are so complex that it is difficult to visualize any situational stress affecting one member which does not also affect the others. Even when individuals have no visible ties to home or family, their social adjustment remains to a great extent the reflection of reactive patterns, role modeling, and role expectations learned in the original family.

To understand the individual situational or adjustment reaction from the reference point of the family, one must consider several parameters simultaneously. These are:

1 The family as an interacting system
2 The family as a historical and developing system
3 The adaptive or maladaptive individual as a component of the family system

Situational reactions may be understood fully only in terms of the unique family system in which the situation evolved and the reaction took place. These interrelations are less apparent but still applicable to many other psychopathological conditions which develop in family systems, each of which possesses its own idiosyncratic climate of reactivity. It has already been suggested that any mental disorder is to some extent a coping reaction to stress. This relationship becomes more apparent when one differentiates acute and chronic situational reactions, observes vulnerability to mental illness, and reviews the concept of circular versus linear causality.

In general, situational reactions imply an acute change or crisis to which the individual and the family must respond. The onset of the change is usually rapid, sudden, and unexpected. Since the change is perceived by the individual and the family as a crisis, the theory and techniques of crisis intervention discussed in Chapters 14 and 15 are applicable. Depending on the proportions of the crisis and the resources of the individual and family, the situation may be resolved without professional involvement. Often, however, the persons involved are so overwhelmed that their resources must be augmented or mobilized by therapeutic intervention. In any case, the crisis event may prove to be a turning point which either introduces new coping methods or reinforces maladaptive behavior patterns. Maladaptive responses to situational crisis may exacerbate existing psychopathology in a family member, precipitate the appearance of psychopathological symptoms, or increase the susceptibility of individual members or of the family to future stress.

If the stressful situational factors which precipitated the crisis continue, coping behaviors will need to extend over time. Persisting adaptive or maladaptive mechanisms constitute manifestations of a *chronic situational reaction.* Prolonged maladaptive coping behavior creates additional stress on the family system. This stress is sometimes alleviated by the malfunctioning of one family member. The original crisis is thus resolved, but the maladaptive reaction engendered by the crisis is perpetuated by the family. For example, the family's maladaptive response to a situational crisis may contribute to the appearance of an acute psychotic episode in a family member for the first time. Tension and anxiety in the family system become centered on the afflicted member, creating a family response to the psychosis which will tend to sustain the psychopathological symptoms. The person displaying psychiatric symptoms becomes the identified patient and the scapegoat to whom all the pressures of the family system can be transferred. Perception that the original crisis actually involved the entire family is lost, while the symptoms of the identified patient are brought sharply into view. Even though the inherent unpredictability of psychotic behavior generates new problems for the family these may prove less distressful than admitting to deficiencies in the system as a whole.

The stress of having a family member with psychotic symptoms almost invariably produces intense feelings of guilt, fear, and shame. For the identified patient there is the experience of being pushed into the "sick" role, and of being discriminated from the rest of the family. Even when psychotic symptoms subside, the identified patient remains for an indeterminate period a marked person whose impulses and behavior cannot be fully trusted. The interactional behaviors between the identified patient and family tend to show this distrust, which only compounds the anxiety and the "sick" behaviors of the identified patient. The identified patient is seen by the family as the weak link which will probably break if another crisis occurs, and the self-fulfilling prophecy sometimes operates.

Some families unknowingly maintain the homeostasis of the system by preserving this state of affairs. By scapegoating the identified patient, the family fosters this patient's vulnerability, since the breaking of the weakest link preserves other links from unbearable strain. Numerous studies done with families of schizophrenics indicate that family members, particularly parents, keep themselves functional despite their own serious psychological problems, through the presence of a "sick" son or daughter who decompensates into psychosis when stress in the family reaches a certain point. Through his or her symptomatology the identified patient diverts family tensions that might otherwise compromise the functioning of a psychologically impaired parent or parental subsystem. Another reason for scapegoating is that caring and providing for the "sick" child may become the primary existential justification of the parents. Thus, the mental illness of the identified patient safeguards and preserves the family by permitting family members to function despite their interpersonal and intrapersonal limitations.

A SYSTEMS MODEL

The situational reactions of individuals and families frequently generate maladaptive behaviors which become chronic pathopsychological responses if stress persists over time, or if new stresses develop as a result of maladaptive coping. Abnormal behavior that appears in one member as a result of stress may be reinforced by the family system, and even become a justification for the continuation of the family.

The suggested explanations of the causes of acute and chronic situational reactions have some validity for all forms of mental illness, since it can be argued that any mental disorder is to some extent an adjustment reaction. This is a point of view which can be adopted profitably by the clinician dealing with mental disorders. A systematic attempt to establish the identity and the source of the stressors can bring into view the various factors in the interactions of the family which tend to precipitate and perpetuate psychopathology.

Adopting this therapeutic strategy produces two types of benefits. First, pressure is removed from the family scapegoat who is often the identified patient. Second, there is a lessening of guilt suffered by other family members as they realize that no particular member, but rather the interaction of the family system, is to blame. Placing responsibility in the realm of family interaction not only deemphasizes the sick role of the identified patient but indicates the direction the therapy should take.

Therapeutic intervention in the family should offer the identified patient the opportunity to assume a transitional role, since this will give the entire system time to assimilate change. Attempts to treat the identified patient as an isolated individual through chemotherapy or individual therapy alone, without some attention to family dynamics, may crystalize the sick role and immobilize the identified patient in a dysfunctional family system. From the systems point of view, lack of attention to family interaction permits previous feedback processes to remain operative, thereby counteracting therapeutic intervention. Consideration of these concepts underscores the importance of early family intervention prior to the decompensation of one member, so that the series of interactional events which reinforce psychopathology can be diminished.

Applying systems concepts alters the classical, scientific view of linear causality which considers that A can affect B, causing changes in B. According to systems theory, dynamic interactions based on feedback processes will include change in B produced by A, but will focus also on changes that A will experience as a result of feedback from B during their interaction. Simply expressed, the systems model proposes that all parts are related in such manner that change in one part generates change in all the others. Because of this feedback or return process, the systems concept of causality as opposed to traditional linear causality has been termed *circular causality*. The therapist using a systems approach is inclined to seek the causality or etiology of the mental problem mainly in the stresses produced by maladaptive family interaction.

A therapeutic corollary of the idea that change in one part of a system produces change in all parts is that an intervention in one aspect or stage of an interaction may be powerful enough to cause changes in all aspects of family interaction. The expected change will persist only if the natural inclination of the family to return to the status quo (homeostasis) is placed under therapeutic control, thus enabling the family to reconstitute at a higher level of functioning.

Vulnerability to Mental Illness

Family interaction and situational stress may precipitate and maintain mental disorders. It must be remembered that these psychosocial factors act upon a developing, maturing, vital organism of variable physiological and psychological vulnerability. In tracing the etiology of psychiatric disturbance Erikson (1963) urged consideration of a triad of factors, specifically, ego organization, and biological and social influences. It follows from this that the individual cannot be regarded as an abstract concept of "mind," or "psyche," lacking biological substrata.

From what is currently understood of the etiology of mental dysfunction it can be assumed that some individuals suffer a degree of biological predisposition or vulnerability which may be inherited or at least familial. This seems particularly true of persons who develop schizophrenia or serious affective disorders. It may also be true of persons with certain personality or addictive disorders. Vulnerability to mental illness should be understood only as a potential predisposition or precondition. A biochemical defect or a birth complication which damages neurological integrity may interact with adverse life experiences, negative family interactions, situational crises, or environmental trauma to produce psychiatric dysfunction. Appropriate therapeutic intervention at moments of distress or crisis may operate to inhibit or alleviate the appearance of psychiatric symptoms.

Vulnerability to mental illness can be mitigated in several ways. In certain individuals the avoidance of negative experiences and the fostering of positive cognitive and affective events may not only avert psychopathology, but also transform vulnerability into a force that heightens sensibility and creativity.

THE PSYCHOPATHOGENIC FAMILY

Since the late forties and early fifties family theorists have tended to trace the origin of certain psychotic processes, particularly schizophrenia, to certain aspects of family life. The names of Lidz, Bowen, Ackerman, Bateson, Haley, Jackson, Satir, Spiegel, Wynne, and Singer, among others, are associated with fundamental studies in this field. Theorists who have approached the psychopathogenic potential of family interaction from different vantage points, in different places, and at different times have reached similar conclusions that appear to have universal validity. For instance, there is general agreement on the value of clear generational boundaries between family subsystems, and between the nuclear and the extended family. In addition, the importance of gender identification based on parents who are confident in their roles is widely upheld. Systems of communication which are essentially irrational and whose meanings are detached from reality make consensual validation extremely difficult, and are therefore maladaptive.

Most of these studies indicate that often schizophrenics come from families bizarre enough to drive anyone "crazy." A lengthy study of fifty schizophrenic patients (Lidz & Lidz, 1949) led to the conclusion that all of them had been subjected to destructive elements within the family which appeared to be major determinants of their maladaptive personality development. A later investigation of seventeen families of schizophrenics (Lidz, Fleck, & Cornelison, 1965) included several families chosen because the parents and the family seemed quite healthy. Upon further study even these families proved to be as disturbed as the others, with the added dimension that they had camouflaged the incongruities of the system so as to produce the superficial impression of normalcy. Other researchers (Wynne & Singer, 1963a, 1963b; Singer & Wynne, 1965a, 1965b) became interested in the hypothesis that disruption due to communication distortion might be a precipitant of schizophrenic regression. The findings did not posit that disturbance in families in itself caused schizophrenia but that certain interactional patterns prevailed in families of schizophrenics. The point was made that, while parental influence operated in the children's direction, the children influenced their families as well. Maladaptive parental attitudes, feelings, and behaviors such as overprotection or domination may have been secondary to disturbances already present in a child. The marital relationship was often marked by severe conflict or characterized by the aggressive dominance of one spouse and the submissive passivity of the other. Intergenerational boundaries were not clear. Gender role enactment by the parents was generally blurred, and family interpretation of events was distorted in order to conform to the egocentric purposes and restricted role performance of the family. Family history, past and present, was rewritten according to parental preferences. The child's ability to validate his or her perceptions of reality was impaired by parental insistence on the irrationality that was essential to maintaining the system. No conclusion was reached by investigators that any one etiological factor was pathogenic. It was speculated, however, that if a specific x factor existed, it was potentiated by the adverse climate within the family. If parental neglect of a child's physical welfare predisposes to physical illness, it is possible that neglect of psychological needs predisposes to mental illness.

The marital relationship constitutes the matrix for family development, but it is not just the child who must be warmed and nurtured by the family. The two spouses, each of whom once sought completion in the other, must fulfill their basic emotional needs within the same matrix if the family system is to be viable. An effective parental coalition not only strengthens and supports the parents, but maintains generational boundaries which prevent the encroachment of one subsystem on another. Appropriate gender role enactment, fostered by effective parental coalition, permits individuation of members and promotes positive identifications by the children. The nonexistent or destructive parental coalition is frequently masked by verbal and behavioral distortions which cause flawed communication. The children's cognitive and language development is then inhibited as they search for coherent, validated meaning.

Dysfunctional Interactional Patterns

Two interactional patterns were discerned by Lidz (1958) in the families of schizophrenics, but their value and applicability far exceed the limits of this particular type of psychopathology. One pattern consisted of a dominant spouse whose erratic ideas on what a family should be were accepted by the more acquiescent partner. Families showing this pattern demonstrated a surface harmony which actually concealed irrationality and hostility. Their disguised structural-functional characteristics caused these families to be described by Lidz as "skewed." Other families were openly contentious and disharmonious in their interactions, and these families were termed "schismatic." At times the skewed family abandoned the charade and became schismatic, while the schismatic family occasionally developed "skewedness." Overall, however, one pattern usually prevailed over the other.

It was also noted that the skewed family is the more common manifestation in families with a schizophrenic son. In the skewed family the mother appears to be excessively intrusive in the lives of her children, especially in the life of a son, and insensitive to needs for individuation. Apparently self-sufficient, the mother actually lacks self-esteem and seeks gratification not in her husband but in the male child she has produced. The father is usually unable to provide positive role modeling for the son. He either accepts the symbiotic relationship between mother and son, deferring to it, or else he adopts a sibling role and competes with the son for the mother's attention. The inadequacy of the father and the intrusiveness of the mother create strange tensions in the child. To be like his father is to be powerless, and to become like his mother is to experience loss of self. Since the child must accommodate in some way to the family system it is not surprising when his personality development suffers the consequence of relating to this unhealthy parental subsystem.

In the schismatic family there is open warfare between family members, and especially between the parents, with one child becoming the special victim of the parental struggle. In a certain type of schismatic family, daughters are particularly affected. In this type, both parents may be narcissistic but it is the father who dominates and the mother who conveys an impression of emptiness and detachment. Although the mother may appear solicitious, her attachment to a daughter is often antagonistic and inconsistent. Since it is difficult to identify with her mother, a girl in this situation may turn to her father for love. In this she is often encouraged by her father, whose relationship with his wife is unrewarding. Conflict between the parents is such that the girl cannot receive affection from one without being rejected by the other. Developmentally, she is unable to surmount the oedipal crisis, for there is no incentive for her to renounce her father in order to identify with her mother. She is caught between two hostile parents, unable to please one without enraging the other. Seeking a way out, the girl may allow herself to be scapegoated as delinquent or mentally ill so that parental strife can be disguised through joint concern for a disappointing daughter. A schismatic pattern is diagrammed in Figure 13-1.

Figure 13-1 The schismatic family.

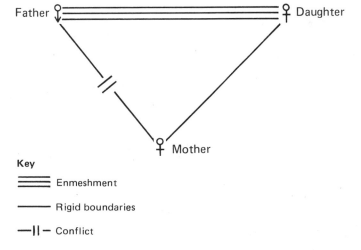

Key

═══ Enmeshment

──── Rigid boundaries

──‖── Conflict

Since there are similarities in skewed and schismatic families, one must search further to attempt to explain the apparent vulnerability of boys in skewed families with passive fathers and of girls in schismatic families with paranoid narcissistic fathers. A partial explanation can be found by comparing the developmental tasks of adolescent boys and adolescent girls. In order to achieve male identity a boy must turn from his mother, his first love object, and identify with his father. Becoming independent of his mother is necessary if the boy is to become capable of forming an attachment to another love object. Since the mother is dominant in the family and is symbiotically tied to her son, it is difficult for the son to break free. Therefore, the boy remains dependent on his mother, and does not develop the ego strength necessary to renounce her and identify with his father. The poor role enactment of the father does not persuade the boy to emulate him, and makes male prerogatives questionable in the mind of the boy.

Conversely, a girl normally resolves the oedipal struggle by identifying with her mother in order to win a love object who resembles her father. When the mother must contend with the domination and derogation of the father, there is little to encourage the girl's identification with her. If the father is seductive toward his daughter but actually denigrates women, the predicament of the girl is compounded. Feelings of helplessness cause the girl to identify with the aggressor father rather than with the mother, making the girl incapable of successfully resolving the oedipal triangle.

In both skewed and schismatic families the schizophrenic member is exploited to meet parental needs. In skewed families the child is used to fulfill the narcissism of an overinclusive, egocentric parent, usually the mother. Developmental tasks are not completed and the child's energy is depleted to augment the life of the mother. In schismatic families both parents are egocentric, and are therefore caught up in a perpetual struggle. The child is a pawn in the contest, and may sacrifice normal developmental progress in order to preserve the parents' relationship. What both family types have in common is the fulfillment of egocentric parental needs at the expense of the child's personality integration. For the skewed family it is usually the mother's egocentricity which is the locus of pathology. For the schismatic family the locus is the conflicting egocentricity of both parents.

The parents in these families have an overwhelming advantage over the child. While the interactions of the parents are destructive, their egocentric needs help them to remain functional, even though this is accomplished at the child's expense. The egocentricity of the parent or parents forces the child to view the world not from his or her own perspective but from that of the parents. In their attempts to remain integrated the parents have barred the child from individuation. During childhood, children make attempts to live their own life and validate their own perceptions of reality. However, the onset of adolescence with its many adaptational conflicts may be overwhelming for a child in a pathogenic family system. In some instances the result is the onset in a young person of a process of alienation and regression that may reach psychotic proportions even to the point of the disorder called schizophrenia. The clinical example below and Figure 13-2 illustrate a skewed family pattern.

CLINICAL EXAMPLE: MENTAL ILLNESS IN A SKEWED FAMILY

When the husband and father in the Lyons family died of a coronary attack at age 45, the sympathy of friends and neighbors was tempered by their confidence that Ruth Lyons and the four children would be able to cope. A capable woman who had been a legal secretary before marriage, Ruth Lyons had given up work to manage her household. At the time of Joe Lyons's death, the only son and two of the daughters were attending local colleges. Beth, the youngest girl, was a high school senior. A common belief in the family was that the three girls took after their competent mother, but that Joe Lyons and Joe Junior would not get very far without Ruth's drive and ability. When Joe was alive there was little difference in the way Ruth treated her husband and her son. She was meticulous in attending to their clothing and meals, but her manner was frequently condescending. Although she rarely expressed her wishes directly, Ruth was usually successful in getting her own way. She liked knowing every detail of the lives of her family, and was particularly proud of and interested in the accomplishments of Joe Junior. When he was alive, Joe had found it less troublesome to go along with his wife's decisions, and in fact considered it an admirable arrangement. The family was close; vacations were spent together, and holidays were always family affairs. Everyone knew that Ruth Lyons lived for her family and that the children would be a great consolation to her after Joe's death.

Figure 13-2 The skewed family (Lyons family).

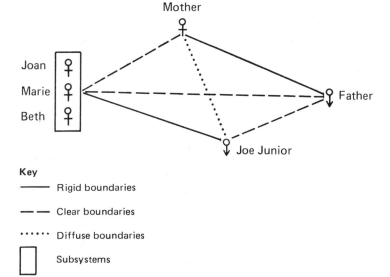

Key

——— Rigid boundaries

— — Clear boundaries

· · · · · · Diffuse boundaries

Subsystems

The oldest girl in the family was engaged to be married. Postponement was considered after Joe's death but Ruth insisted that the wedding take place as planned. "After all," Ruth said, "It's not as if I'm alone. There are your two sisters and Joe Junior is the man of the house now."

In the first weeks after his father's death, Joe Junior could not do enough for his mother, and Ruth, in turn, felt that no one else could help her. She commented often on Joe Junior's resemblance to his father and said repeatedly that her husband would never be dead as long as she had her son to help her. When their father was alive, the three older children attended a local college and lived on campus, although Ruth was always disconsolate if they failed to come home on weekends. After the funeral there was a conference about expenses and Joe Junior found himself agreeing to live at home and commute to school in order to save money. Since campus social life was more important for girls, it seemed selfish to insist that they come home as well. Ruth said she could manage room fees for two children but not for three.

Joe Junior's father had been a quiet reserved man, and the two had never enjoyed many father-son activities together. After his father's death, Joe had a strong sense of bereavement, which seemed to deepen as the grief of his mother and sisters lessened. What Joe could explain only to himself was that he felt a sense of great abandonment and of being smothered in a household of women. He missed the noise and commotion of the college dorm even though he had not made many friends before leaving. He worried about his mother, felt angry toward her, but did not know why. There were times when she seemed to see him not as a 19-year-old son but as a 45-year-old husband. He found this upsetting. His sisters seemed to function just as they always had, but Joe Junior sometimes felt that he was wearing the mask of a boy, and living the life of someone who was really much older.

Insomnia began to be a problem for him, although he really did not mind being awake during the night when everyone else was sleeping. It was a good time for thinking and reflecting on what had happened during the day. During the night Joe's father seemed very near. At times his father seemed to be speaking to him but the messages were very confusing. Sometimes Dad gave quite sensible advice about how to handle Mother; at other times he seemed to be laughing at Joe Junior. Dad was free now, but Joe Junior had inherited the job of pleasing Mom.

The family became increasingly concerned about Joe Junior's behavior. They knew he had trouble sleeping after his father died but there were other changes in him. Often he did not answer when anyone spoke to him. He stopped attending classes and seldom came out of his room except at night. At first the strange actions were attributed to grief and sleeplessness. Ruth wanted Joe Junior to see a physician but her suggestions went unheard. He slept a great deal during the day, but soon stopped going to bed at night. The nighttime hours were used for walking aimlessly. He seemed to feel his father's presence and to be able to talk with him. Because the conversations with his father were so important, Joe Junior began visiting the cemetery at night. The messages from Dad were clearer then. Dad seemed to be trying to help in some way. He had been visiting Dad's grave every night for quite a while before he thought of taking along a pillow and blanket. This made everything a lot better. The pillow fitted nicely against the headstone and the blanket kept him warm. Sleeping on the grave made Joe less confused. It didn't seem to matter whether he had become part of his father or just felt close to his father. The cemetery, furnished with a simple headstone and inhabited by Joe and his father, who seemed to be one and the same, was safe and reassuring. Joe would lie under his blanket and stare up at the stars, listening to Dad and sometimes answering. He was lying there, hovering between sleep and wakefulness when the police found him.

Structural Assessment

Ruth Lyons was a dominant mother who lived vicariously through her family. Joe Lyons was a well-meaning but passive man who died as his children were approaching adulthood. Joan, the oldest girl, was 21 years old, and engaged to be married. Joe Junior was 19 years old. Marie was 18, and attended the same college as her brother and older sister. Beth was the youngest child, and a high school senior.

Within the family the three daughters formed a strong subsystem. There had been a weak, tentative alliance between Joe Junior and his father, but this was not durable enough to be called a subsystem.

The marital coalition was weak. As mother and task leader for the family, Ruth ruled husband and children firmly. If she had a family favorite, it was her son.

Functional Assessment

Beneath the facade of family happiness, Ruth was a tyrant. Her weak, ineffectual husband gladly allowed his son to supersede him in Ruth's affections. Because of their strong subsystem the daughters in the family were able to wrest some autonomy from their mother, and in this they were assisted by Ruth's preoccupation with Joe Junior.

Attending college and living on campus had been a major achievement in Joe Junior's attempt to separate. But the death of his father and Ruth's connivance had pushed him back into his mother's iron control. The personality integration that Joe had accomplished was seriously threatened by the events surrounding the death of his father. His ego boundaries proved insufficient. Receiving no help from his self-sufficient sisters, and foreseeing no escape from his intransigent mother, Joe found a measure of relief in an acute psychotic episode.

Intervention

Individual therapy was indicated for Joe, and family therapy was indicated for the system in which Joe's symptomatology had
developed.

The objectives of family therapy were:

1   To establish boundaries between Joe Junior and his mother
which would weaken the closeness between them
2   To reopen the subsystem of the daughters so as to admit Joe
Junior to it
3   To allow the daughters to express feelings about the favoritism shown toward their brother
4   To help the daughters recognize that Joe Junior had been exploited by the parents and by them, as well
5   To help Ruth accept the inevitability of separating from all her
children
6   To teach Ruth and the children to interact in ways which
recognized that the children were adults with a need for autonomy
7   To encourage Ruth to search for gratification in ways other
than living for and through her children

SUMMARY

In the first part of this chapter classifications of mental illness were discussed. These classifications are directed essentially toward the individual,
but the additional perspective of a systems-oriented approach which centers
on family interaction was introduced. Special attention was given to acute
and chronic situational reactions, and an attempt was made to explain the
classic psychiatric symptomatology at least in part as an adjustment to
stress. This approach accepts the possibility that benefit can be derived
from the therapeutic manipulation of various circumstances which appear
significant.

The second part of the chapter presented structural and functional concepts based on theories postulating the family genesis of psychosis, particularly of schizophrenia. The scope of the chapter did not permit detailed
discussion of the psychodynamics underlying the disjunctive behavior of
family members, nor the crucial importance of language and cognition in
personality development. Enough was presented, however, to aid in the
formulation of a theoretical framework for analyzing mental illness in the
family.

An important objective of this chapter was to inspire additional study
of the psychopathological potential of the dysfunctional family organization, and of its positive counterpart—the importance of sound family
organization and interaction in fostering and preserving mental health.

REFERENCES

Erikson, E. *Childhood and society* (2nd ed.). New York: Norton, 1963.

Lidz, T. Intrafamilial environment of schizophrenic patients: II. Marital schism and marital skew. *American Journal of Psychiatry,* 1958, **114**(3), 241–248.

Lidz, R. W., Fleck, S., & Cornelison, A. *Schizophrenia and the family.* New York: International Universities Press, 1965.

Lidz, R. W., & Lidz, T. The family environment of schizophrenic patients. *American Journal of Psychiatry,* 1949, **106**, 332–345.

Mead, G. H. *Mind, self, and society.* Chicago: University of Chicago Press, 1934.

Singer, M., & Wynne, L. Thought disorder and family relations of schizophrenics III. Methodology using projective techniques. *Archives of General Psychiatry,* 1965, **12**, 187–200. (a)

Singer, M., & Wynne, L. Thought disorder and family relations of schizophrenics IV. Results and implications. *Archives of General Psychiatry,* 1965, **12**, 201–212. (b)

Speigel, J. *Transactions: The interplay between individual, family and society.* New York: Science House, 1971.

Sullivan, H. S. *The interpersonal theory of society.* New York: Norton, 1953.

Wynne, L., & Singer, M. Thought disorder and family relations of schizophrenics I. A research strategy. *Archives of General Psychiatry,* 1963, **9**, 191–198. (a)

Wynne, L., & Singer, M. Thought disorder and family relations of schizophrenics II. Classification of forms of thinking. *Archives of General Psychiatry,* 1963, **9**, 199–206. (b)

Chapter 14

Consequences of Sudden Disaster and Unemployment for the Family

Betty Jane Kinsinger

There are probably few situations that create greater disruption in the total family system than those which threaten the safety and/or economic welfare of family members. Unfortunately, however, few empirical studies have dealt directly with the effects of natural disasters or unemployment on the structure and functioning of the family. In this chapter an attempt will be made to explore the way in which these two very different situations create changes in the family system which have consequences for the system as a whole, as well as for individual family members. It is hoped that contrasting and comparing the effects of these two situations will provide the reader with greater insights than if the situations were discussed separately.

Because role concepts will be used to describe and analyze the stresses of natural disasters and unemployment, this chapter begins with a definition of basic concepts and terms. This is followed by a discussion of some general factors that influence responses to external stress and, more specifically, a discussion of the structural and functional changes likely to occur within the family. The remainder of the chapter deals with factors which influence the strategies families employ in attempting to cope with stress. The implications of studies of disasters and unemployment for health professionals will also be presented.

ROLE CONCEPTS AND THEORETICAL PERSPECTIVES

The utility of a role systems approach to the study of family behavior during natural disasters and unemployment seems clear. Viewing the family as a system of roles has the distinct advantage of allowing family phenomena to be interpreted in terms of interpersonal processes. Family members can be identified as occupying certain positions in a semiclosed system of interacting members of a group (Turner, 1970). The concept of *social role* is central to this perspective of the family as a group and implies that family members share perceptions and expectations concerning the behavior of persons occupying well-defined positions within the group. For example, family systems have positions defined as mother, father, son, and daughter. For each of these positions there will be common expectations concerning the rights and obligations of the person who occupies the position, as well as common expectations concerning that person's behavior. Some role expectations will, of course, be based on shared societal and cultural definitions. In addition, a system of informal roles will tend to develop within the group structure itself, and it is usually possible to identify members of the family system who assume roles such as leader, follower, aggressor, peacemaker, etc. It is important to keep in mind that all social roles must be considered in relation to other social roles, so that one can properly begin to think of the family as a social system and to analyze the systematic relationships of its members. Dyadic relationships, such as parent-child and husband-wife relationships, or more complex relationships involving all the members of a family system can be analyzed within this framework provided that the problem under study is sufficiently formalized and the relevant concepts can be operationally defined.

Another useful concept in the analysis of external stresses on the family system concerns the meanings people attach to events that disrupt their established patterns of interaction and normal activities. The concept *definition of the situation* as it is used in the framework proposed by Hansen and Hill (1964) to study families under stress seems appropriate here. These authors have suggested that the perception of stress and the meaning that is attributed to a stressful event may differ from one family to another. That is, what becomes a crisis situation for one family would not necessarily be considered a crisis by another family in a comparable situation. The development of family crisis is represented as an interplay of variables in which A (the stressor) interacting with B (the family's stress-meeting resources) interacting with C (the definition the family makes of the hardship) produces X, which is the crisis. This is not to suggest that the personal meaning that the family gives to a stressful situation will be the only factor that influences the response, since undoubtedly a number of variables will be involved. However, the inclusion of this concept has value in that it forces researcher and professional alike to look more closely at the less objective and less obvious factors that are operating to maintain the family system.

Influences from outside the family as well as from within the system need to be taken into account when analyzing the family's response to unemployment and disaster. The concept of *reference group* is important because it calls attention to other groups and individuals that the family is using as a frame of reference in assessing its predicament. A reference group can be defined as any group which sets guidelines for what is believed to be appropriate behavior or which functions as a comparison group in setting guidelines for evaluating personal outcomes (Kelley, 1968). Like the concept definition of the situation, this concept is difficult to operationalize. Nonetheless, both are valuable sensitizers to the variations that may be present in family systems.

Role conflict is another concept that has frequently been used to describe the stresses of disasters. This concept can be defined as the ambivalence and consequent strain that individuals experience when they are confronted with a situation that forces them to choose between what they perceive to be their obligations in one role and what they perceive to be their obligations in a different role. An example of role conflict is provided by Killian's (1954) study in which he described the conflict experienced by persons who had to make choices between remaining on the job or going home to the family at the time of a community disaster. *Role strain* is a concept that is closely related to role conflict. It is a broader term which implies that persons unable to meet the obligations they associate with a given role, due to conflicting role demands or a lack of role clarity, will experience feelings of guilt or inadequacy (Secord & Backman, 1974).

GENERAL FACTORS INFLUENCING RESPONSES
TO DISASTERS AND UNEMPLOYMENT

The term *disaster* is used in this chapter to refer to situations in which unfavorable changes or conditions in the natural environment produce destruction to property and, in some instances, personal injury or death. No attempt is made to describe the effects of various types of disaster. The term *unemployment* is also defined broadly and refers to situations in which many members of a community are out of work. Variations in unemployment situations are not dealt with here. The focus in discussing both situations will be on the stress and social disruption that events of this nature produce in the family. It is assumed that the family system will be in a steady state prior to either event.

When families are confronted with external stressors such as disaster or unemployment, some general factors will influence their responses to the situation. Although the two situations are very different, they are similar from the standpoint that the stress imposed on the family system originates from an outside source. In both cases the family becomes vulnerable to disorganization and may become dysfunctional. That is, roles which had become stabilized over time in the course of continuing family interaction are susceptible to change. How great a change will occur cannot be predicted from the type of event—unemployment or disaster—since a number of different factors operate in both situations to influence the equilibrium of the family.

When a disaster occurs the entire family system as well as the immediate surrounding environment will be disrupted. There is evidence from the literature of disasters to suggest that the decisions made just prior to a disaster tend to be based on collective definitions of the situation rather than on individual assessments (Bates, Fogleman, Parenton, Pittman, & Tracy, 1963; Dynes & Quarantelli, 1976; Hill & Hansen, 1962; Moore, 1963). Whether this has any direct influence on the behavior of family members immediately following the event is not known. It has been observed, however, that widespread panic and disorganization following the initial reaction of disbelief and shock are not characteristic in disaster victims. Contrary to common belief, individuals do not become immobilized but instead display unusual signs of courage in helping themselves and those around them. Of interest here is that only recently has research on disasters been directed toward analyzing the stresses of disasters from the perspective that disasters will not always produce a crisis for the families involved. In fact, some data suggest that variations in adjustments to the stresses of disaster are not unlike variations in adjustments to other conditions of stress. What is important to this discussion is the identification of the factors that determine differences in family adjustment.

From the perspective of the family's preparedness for a crisis situation, it is obvious that a distinct difference between disasters and unemployment is the suddenness with which each of these events occurs. Even though modern technology has made sophisticated warning systems available to most communities, in most disasters there are seldom more than a few hours, or days at the most, between the warning and the event. This is unlike the unemployment situation in which workers generally hear rumors of a strike before it occurs, or, because of a declining national economy, anticipate impending layoffs from work. In each of these situations, however, the period that precedes disaster or unemployment will be significant. Past experiences with similar events will undoubtedly play an important role in the family's perception of threat to the system and will be a factor in subsequent behavior. For example, Bates et al. (1963), in a longitudinal study of hurricane Audrey, reported that many persons in the impact area had expected the brunt of the storm to hit elsewhere. Like those who thought themselves on safe ground because water had never risen very high in their respective areas, these persons based their evaluations of the impending threat on past experience. In this disaster, as in some others which have been studied (Hill & Hansen, 1962), it was found that families tended to define their situation by seeking information from relatives rather than relying upon reports from official weather agencies. Apparently, collective definitions of the situation have a major influence on the course of action that families decide on prior to the disaster.

Unlike the disaster situation, the unemployment situation tends to be of crescive nature. That is, the period between the warning of the impending event and the actual occurrence is seldom short. Even when no formal communication has been made regarding layoffs, rumors usually serve to warn workers that they may be unemployed in the near future. Since there may be a great deal of ambiguity toward threats of unemployment, one can anticipate that preparations for the event will vary. Previous experience with unemployment, especially when it has involved a long period of time or has necessitated a change in life-style or residence, helps determine how the family defines the impending threat and prepares to deal with it. The occupation and marketability of the family member who assumes the provider role will undoubtedly have affected a family's past experience with the stresses of unemployment.

The family's composition and its stage of development in the life cycle are additional factors that may influence responses to unemployment or disaster situations. The number of children will probably be less of a factor than the ages of the children, since the dependency of children undoubtedly increases the degree of role strain for the adult members of the family.

Conceptualizing the family as a system open to transactions with other social systems facilitates the assessment of the role played by the community in assisting the family to adapt to unexpected crises. Dynes and Quarantelli (1976) pointed out that the mediating effects of the family and the community become apparent when the family is viewed within the context of the larger system. From their research, these investigators conclude that behavior during disasters tends to be goal-directed and adaptive rather than maladaptive and dysfunctional. They suggest that individuals are better able to cope with loss when it is evaluated in relation to the *relative deprivation* of others within the same social context. For example, when others within a community experience similar traumatic events they become reference persons for evaluating personal losses. While there is no empirical data on which to base the assumption, one may conjecture that similar mechanisms operate in an unemployment situation to influence the degree of stress experienced by persons involved.

Examples of mutual sharing and the assistance individuals provide for one another during disaster situations can be found in the literature. There are numerous accounts of people who continued to help others even after they themselves had suffered great personal losses, including the death of family members. The links which exist between the family and the community when mass unemployment occurs are extremely important. Examples of such supporting links are the credit which local banks and merchants extend to unemployed workers, and the increased services provided by public health and social service agencies. It seems likely that economic hardships are easier to accept under conditions of common stress. Personal losses can be compared within the community, and personal responsibility for economic hardships decreases. Moreover, economic hardships are less likely to be attributed to the role inadequacy of a particular family member.

STRUCTURAL AND FUNCTIONAL CHANGES

In a disaster situation the family is suddenly forced into behavior directed toward the survival of its members. After the initial impact, old roles will be disrupted, and must be reorganized or in some cases abandoned. Less obvious, but of no less importance to the family, are the role changes which occur when the family has to meet the crisis of unemployment. In both situations, a period of disorganization is followed by a recovery period in which family members attempt to deal with the new circumstances in the best way possible.

In the period immediately or shortly after the event (which will be referred to as the stressor) the family generally does not have adequate knowledge of its personal resources nor of available outside resources. In addition, family members are generally not clear about what is expected from them nor about their respective roles in meeting the new demands imposed by the stressors. The ability of families to reorganize roles and, thus, to resist threats to the integrity of the system will vary according to the resources available to them and to how they define their situation.

In disaster and unemployment situations alike, it is apparent that changes over time must be considered. In catastrophic disaster situations the immediate role demands upon the family usually involve dealing with the trauma of injury and with losses of members or property. The family's behavior immediately following the initial shock of the disaster will probably influence later stages of recovery, for it is at this stage that decisions must be made concerning role priorities. For example, a father whose job involves law enforcement may feel obligated to fulfill the commitment to his occupational role even when he cannot be fully assured of the safety of his family. While much has been written about the role conflict that arises when individuals cannot meet the expectations of two roles and as a consequence must choose between them (Bates et al., 1963; Dynes & Quarantelli, 1976) little attention has been given to the resolution of the role strain that is produced by the conflict. How individuals resolve role conflict would seem to depend upon a number of factors specific to the situation and to what is perceived to be a part of a family role. Some data from disaster studies (Dynes & Quarantelli, 1976) suggest that at this point collective definitions of the situation serve to mobilize individuals toward common goals aimed at recovery and restoration from loss. What is probably most important to the future functioning of the family is how behavior at or immediately following a disaster influences the later reorganization period of adjustment to the crisis situation. When interpersonal and/or group conflicts begin to emerge as a result of recrimination against a member of the family for earlier behavior, it is unlikely that the family will become sufficiently organized to restore or maintain its equilibrium.

Because of the crescive nature of an employment crisis, the normal role patterns of the family are not, as a rule, subjected to the sudden or total disruption that characterizes a disaster situation. When the event does occur, however, the family is forced to face the reality of economic loss, and decisions must be made regarding alternative sources of income. The immediate responses of family members may be of optimism and hope that the situation is temporary and will have positive future outcomes. As mentioned earlier, one factor that may influence the response to an economic crisis is the family's interpretation of the event as stressful. When family stress is evaluated in relation to the stress of others within the same social context, the situation takes on a different meaning than when a reference group of others experiencing similar stress is lacking. This will become clearer when role relationships within the family are examined.

Role Changes within the Family

Under the conditions of stress created by disasters or unemployment one can expect to find changes in the system of role relationships. These role changes will have implications for the stability of the family, since the adjustments to stress will be largely determined by how adequately family members are able to modify old roles and take on new ones.

Although the stresses of disaster or unemployment are greater for some families than for others, the outcomes in terms of adjustment depend to a large extent upon three factors: (1) the integration of the family, (2) the flexibility of the group structure, and (3) consensus regarding family goals and values. As mentioned previously, other interrelated factors which play a role in how the family responds are: (1) prior experiences with stress, (2) the composition of the family, and (3) the social context in which losses from a disaster or unemployment are experienced.

Although the effects of unemployment do not include personal injury, death, or destruction to property, families who have experienced this stressor event must nonetheless cope with the problems of role loss and the feelings of role inadequacy and role strain that accompany loss. Angell's (1936) study of the adaptations families made to the economic crises of the Depression revealed that highly integrated families were best able to adapt to strains associated with a decrease in income. Highly integrated families tended to be characterized by feelings of mutual affection, unity, and economic interdependence of its members. Members of poorly integrated families, on the other hand, were generally reluctant to give up old roles associated with authority and control. Some members also wished to hold on to familiar life-styles even though this resulted in marital conflict and discord in the family.

The significance which the loss of a vital role has for family relationships was borne out in Komarovsky's (1940) study. The study found that in families in which authority was based largely upon the husband's control of economic resources rather than upon affective relationships the loss of the provider role resulted in a decline in the husband's authority. The prestige which the wife attributed to her husband was lowered as a result of his loss of earning power. This led to marital conflict and sexual problems as well as to impaired parent-child relationships.

Findings from studies of unemployment have illustrated how the loss of a vital role can bring about a change in the system of role relationships. Because of the interdependency of family roles, the loss of the provider role not only creates role strain for the husband, who cannot adequately fulfill the provider role, but also alters his relationships with other family members. However, these studies also noted that roles can change within a family without disturbing the equilibrium of the group. For example, it was found that the strain which accompanied the loss of the husband's earning power was offset by the affection and sentiment which served to maintain close family bonds.

The strain that results from the inability of a family member to perform a role is likely to be augmented by the strain produced by the individual's loss of self-esteem. Thus, when expectations associated with a role can no longer be met, it is not unusual for a family member to experience feelings of despair and depression. An example of the role strain that is likely to be experienced after several months of unemployment can be found in the words of a copper miner who stated:

If I didn't have my kids here, I wouldn't have stayed one minute after the shut-down. . . . I can't get food stamps for my daughters, only for myself, so I'm going to have to make every penny stretch. I'd do anything to keep my kids from starving (*Phoenix Gazette,* September, 1977).

When faced with a situation such as this, a family may attempt to adjust to the loss of the provider role by having other family members assume this role. The flexibility of the group structure will be an important factor in determining the responses of the family. A highly integrated family seldom has a problem when other members of the family become involved in roles that were formally allocated to the husband/father. However, when the roles of family members have become rigid over time, or when roles within the family are based on traditional cultural values, it may be very difficult for other members of the family to assume new roles. For example, family members may not be able to work out an arrangement that enables both husband and wife to share child care responsibilities and take on part-time jobs if the attitude of one or both partners regarding appropriate sex role behavior is inflexible. Abandoning a role, even temporarily, creates additional role strain and role stress for a member who has traditionally held a role that served to sustain the unity of the family.

Since verification of data on family adjustments to role changes after a disaster is lacking, one can only speculate that factors similar to those that operate in the unemployment situation influence adjustment to economic losses from disaster. The major differences between these two situations lie in the numerous role demands a disaster situation imposes on the system and the amount of information that is fed into the system from outside sources. Some data from disaster studies suggest that collective definitions of stress may serve to reduce the stress and strain that follow a disaster (Bates et al., 1963; Dynes & Quarantelli, 1976; Siporin, 1976). The altruism and value consensus which emerge in the social context in which the loss is experienced appear to mediate stress. That is, family values and goals are likely to be influenced by mutual assistance, and by communication with others in the same situation. A major point to consider is that communication with others outside the family boundaries is almost certain to increase communication within the family. This could have either a positive or negative effect for the members (Siporin, 1976). When increased communication assists family members to redefine their values and goals, or serves to reinforce or validate existing beliefs and values, consensus and solidarity among family members is likely to increase. The effects of increased communication are apt to be negative when communication from the outside is interpreted as interference by some members of the family, or when new information coming into the system creates disharmony and conflict among family members.

Although longitudinal studies are lacking, evidence from disaster studies suggests that affective relationships within the family become closer as a result of a disaster (Taylor, 1977). It is reasonable to assume that value priorities will be reassigned, at least temporarily, when members of a family have been confronted with a life-threatening event, especially when increased communication with persons or groups outside the family has strengthened existing bonds within the family. For some families the opportunities that members are given to assume new roles under disaster conditions have lasting effects. A husband and wife, for example, may find that they are more capable of taking on the role of the other partner than they had thought. The consequences for them may be a more egalitarian relationship in the future. Role expectations regarding the children are also likely to change when their parents take on new or additional roles. For some children, this may mean becoming more involved in household tasks or giving up certain recreational or school activities. In families where economic losses have been great the children may help to lessen the economic burden on the family by obtaining part-time jobs. Involvement in decision making is likely to increase when family members work toward meeting common goals.

Adjustment to disasters is undoubtedly made easier by the fact that the situation is amenable to a common interpretation by members of the family. That is, blame for the event cannot be associated with any one family member. This is unlike the unemployment situation, in which members may be resentful because the husband/father lacks the education or skill necessary for seeking alternative job opportunities.

Because a disaster event involves natural forces, it may be given a religious interpretation by some families. This will have a positive effect on family relationships if it helps members to accept the reality of their situation and to take steps to resume as many of their previous functions as possible. Religious belief may also be a factor influencing the family's adjustment to bereavement and grief. Accounts of individual reactions to the death of family members have described the intense pain and grief families experience when faced with the reality of a disaster (Civca, Downie, & Morris, 1977; Perry, Silber, & Bloch, 1956). In situations such as this it seems likely that values which served to bond individuals may continue to operate to mediate stress. Negative influences on the system may be felt when strong consensual beliefs prevent members from seeking or utilizing sources of assistance from the outside community. Although it is likely that adults will in most instances play supportive roles in times of intense stress, a study of the Vicksburg, Mississippi, tornado (Perry & Perry, 1954) revealed that in some cases children assumed such roles. For example, it was found that the children of some mothers who became immobilized with fear and anxiety took on the role of comforting and reassuring other family members, in-

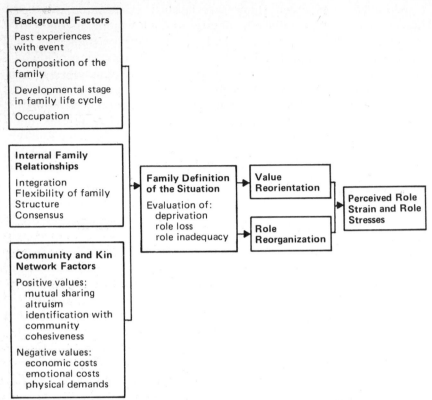

Figure 14-1 Variables related to family adjustments to external stressors.

cluding the mother. The important point is that the energies within the family were utilized to meet the role demands of the situation and to maintain family equilibrium.

A model is presented in Figure 14-1 for the purpose of delineating the variables that have been identified in this chapter as most likely to influence the family's responses to the external stressors, disaster and unemployment. In this model the family's definition of the situation becomes a key variable in determining how the family adjusts to stress. Adjustments to external stressors are conceived as being dependent upon both environmental and family resources.

IMPLICATIONS OF STUDIES FOR HEALTH PROFESSIONALS

Although they are lacking in scope and depth, data from studies of families suffering external stresses due to disasters and unemployment have some implications for health professionals. For the purposes of this chapter, only findings related to the stress of disaster and unemployment are summarized.

The findings of relevant studies showed that families confronted with external stresses generally experienced an initial period of disruption followed by a period of role reorganization. Health professionals should recognize the family's need for accurate information and for support from others to help them define their situation. This is especially important during the initial period of adjustment when feelings of role inadequacy and role strain are paramount. Flexible role assignments during noncrisis periods enhance the ability of family members to empathize with one another and to adjust to role changes necessitated by crisis.

It should also be acknowledged that the family's perception of impending threat to the family group and its individual members will depend largely upon the social context in which it occurs. Decisions may be made during this early period which will affect relationships between family members at a later stage in adjustment. This is especially true of disaster situations in which decisions to take a particular course of action may have resulted in the death or injury of a family member. Feelings of depression and despair may be mediated to some extent by definitions of the event within the community setting. The meanings that individuals within the community attach to a situation can serve a therapeutic function by substituting common responsibility for personal responsibility.

There is also evidence from disaster studies that individuals may experience role conflict or feelings of inadequacy, unsure that they can perform a role in ways that meet their own expectations or the expectations of others. During times of disaster or mass unemployment, collective definitions of the situation may serve to reduce role strain by increasing communication between family members. It is also possible that factors which perpetuated a stable but not necessarily reciprocal relationship between family members in the past may influence the future stability of the family system.

When working with families which are experiencing unemployment it should be kept in mind that, even though economic crises do not directly involve injury and death of family members, there is a problem of role loss. Health professionals must be aware of the family's need to attach blame to an external source and must allow family members to be angry, unless, of course, the anger is directed towards a family member. In that case, the family may need help in redirecting the anger until such time as its members are able to channel their energies more constructively.

Health professionals must also realize that the boundaries of the family should be respected. This means that the independency as well as the interdependence of families should be maintained as far as possible. One problem that may occur when families are suffering stress from disaster or unemployment is that helping agencies may unintentionally rob the family of the potential to be resourceful in adjusting. The mutual sharing which tends to be characteristic of the earlier stages of disaster declines when individuals find that the new roles they have assumed are being taken over by others outside of the family. In such cases, individuals are not only deprived of learning new roles but are also made to feel inadequate about meeting the expectations of the roles that they have assumed.

Finally, symptoms of depression and despair are commonly found in both disaster and unemployment situations. In disaster situations there may be anxiety about a possible reoccurrence of the event. Worries about injury and death may dominate the thinking of disaster victims long after the event has occurred. In addition, despair and feelings of hopelessness may accompany the loss of the provider role. A primary concern of a family confronted with this situation is likely to be uncertainty regarding the future. It is important for health professionals to recognize that the loss of a customary role may create strain for the family member who previously fulfilled that role. For this individual, the strain of not being able to meet the obligations associated with his or her position is likely to be compounded by feelings of bereavement and grief over having to give up cherished family possessions or of having lost the family home. The grief process must be recognized as a phenomenon that may be present whenever a family experiences a marked change in its structure or function as a result of external stressors. While losing a family home or relinquishing the various rituals which family members have established over time may not seem significant compared with losses incurred as a result of a disaster, all losses have an impact on the role relationships between members of the family. Loss of an important family role means changes in the entire role system that previously sustained the boundaries that identified the family as a unit.

CLINICAL EXAMPLE: FAMILY REACTIONS TO UNEMPLOYMENT

The Frys were a happy and stable family until Ted Fry lost his job along with 200 other workers following a fire which completely demolished the company for which he worked. Ted, aged 45, had been a salesman for 15 years; he had taken pride in his work and in his ability to be a good provider for his family. His wife Ada, 20-year-old son Grant, and 17-year-old daughter Mary respected Ted's role as controller and source of economic resources for the family. Ada's role was to cook, clean, and see that the household ran smoothly. Grant was at college and Mary kept busy with high school activities.

The immediate response of the 200 families who were affected by the fire was one of optimism and hope, since the situation seemed to be a temporary crisis which would be remedied by a new building. Many of the families visited one another following the fire and were mutually supportive; however, tensions began to rise after 6 months when it looked as though the company would never operate again. Ted hunted for a new sales position, but to no avail. Family relationships began to deteriorate as Ted sat around at home not knowing how to help. Ada felt the extra burden of having Ted home during the day, but was unwilling to have him do any housework. As family savings decreased, quarrels occurred more frequently than usual and family members seemed to withdraw emotionally from one another. Mary often stayed out late, and letters to Grant nearly ceased.

Ted felt depressed and tired, was unable to sleep soundly, and often suffered from headaches. He sought help from his health care provider who asked the entire family to come and discuss their situation.

Assessment

1   The family's definition of the situation was that it was a disgraceful one that made all family members feel helpless. In addition, Ted felt as though he had failed his family and that he could never regain his authority.

2   Ada and Ted had difficulty sharing roles and assuming new roles.

3   Worries about finances, family prestige, and self-esteem led to conflict between family members and to emotional isolation.

4   Family boundaries were open to supportive sharing with friends.

Intervention

The results of intervention were as follows:

1   The family reoriented their values so that they were less dependent upon financial resources for self-esteem and family esteem. The situation was viewed as a time when family members could band together.

2   Ada, Ted, and Mary reorganized their roles in the home so that Ada and Mary were freed to obtain temporary employment while Ted searched for a job and helped with chores in the home.

3   Family members learned to express their feelings and talk to one another without conflict.

SUMMARY

This chapter has explored the effect of external stresses on the family system. Literature regarding the stresses of disaster and unemployment has been drawn upon for the purpose of identifying some of the major factors that influence a family's adjustment to external stressor event. A discussion of the implications of the studies and a clinical example conclude the chapter.

REFERENCES

Angell, R. C. *The family encounters the depression.* New York: Scribner, 1936.

Bates, F. L., Fogleman, C. W., Parenton, V. J., Pittman, R. N., and Tracy, G. S. *The social and psychological consequences of a natural disaster.* Washington, D.C.: National Academy of Sciences, National Research Council Publication, 1963.

Civca, R., Downie, C., & Morris, M. When a disaster happens. *American Journal of Nursing,* 1977, **77**(3), 454–456.

Dynes, R. N., & Quarantelli, E. L. The family and community context of individual reactions to disaster. In H. J. Parad & H. L. P. Resnik (Eds.), *Emergency and disaster management.* Bowie, Maryland: Charles Press, 1976.

Hansen, D., & Hill, R. Families under stress. In H. T. Christensen (Ed.), *Handbook of marriage and the family.* Chicago: Rand McNally, 1964.

Hill, R., & Hansen, D. Families in disaster. In C. W. Baker & D. Chapman (Eds.), *Man and society in disaster.* New York: Basic Books, 1962.

Kelley, H. Two functions of reference groups. In H. Hyman & E. Singer (Eds.), *Readings in reference group theory and research.* New York: Free Press, 1968.

Killian, L. M. Some accomplishments and some needs in disaster. *Journal of Social Issues,* 1954, **10**, 66–72.

Komarovsky, M. *The unemployed man and his family.* New York: Dryden Press, 1940.

Moore, H. E., Bates, F. L., Lyman, M. V., & Parenton, V. J. *Before the wind.* Washington, D.C.: National Academy of Sciences, National Research Council, 1963.

Perry, S. E., Silber, E., & Bloch, D. A. *The child and his family in disaster: A study of the 1953 Vicksburg tornado.* Washington, D.C.: National Academy of Science, National Research Council Publication No. 394, 1956.

Schanche, D. The emotional aftermath of the largest tornado ever. In R. H. Moos (Ed.), *Human adaptation: Coping with life crises.* Lexington, Mass.: Heath, 1976.

Secord, P. F., & Backman, C. W. *Social psychology* (2nd ed.). New York: McGraw-Hill, 1974.

Siporin, M. Altruism, disaster, and crisis intervention. In H. J. Parad & H. L. P. Resnik (Eds.), *Emergency and disaster management.* Bowie, Maryland: Charles Press, 1976.

Taylor, V. Good news about disaster. *Psychology Today,* October 1977, pp. 93–94; 124–126.

Turner, R. H. *Family interaction.* New York: Wiley, 1970.

Chapter 15

Family Crisis Intervention*

Ida M. Martinson
Ellen H. Janosik

GENERAL CONCEPTS OF CRISIS WORK

A crisis is a stressful event in the life of a family or an individual which disrupts the ability to function effectively. Crisis intervention is a circumscribed treatment modality concerned with the management of the crisis situation. A state of crisis begins with a hazardous event which threatens the equilibrium of the system. Such an event represents a change, or turning point, which becomes a crisis after the usual coping measures of the individual or the system have failed. Since crisis is time-limited in nature, some form of reequilibrium is always established, but the restitution may not always be advantageous for the persons involved.

Psychological distress may or may not occur in the crisis situation. A high level of anxiety is usually present as individuals experience the failure of their usual coping measures. At times the hazardous event is immediately apparent, as in separation or terminal illness. At other times it is more difficult to identify the hazard. If the defense mechanism of denial has been

*This chapter was supported in part by Grant Number CA 19490, awarded by the National Cancer Institute, Department of Health, Education and Welfare.

used, the hazardous event must be traced back in time. Not infrequently a family mistakes a recent precipitant for the actual hazard, which took place earlier.

The outcome of a crisis situation is uncertain, since potential for change is inherent in crisis. The change may be for the better or for the worse, or there may be a return to the previous level of adaptation. An example of possible outcomes to crisis can be found in the predicament of a drug addict whose supply has suddenly been curtailed. The unavailability of illegal drugs causes a crisis to which several responses are possible. The addict may attempt to find a new source of supply, or resort to theft if the price exceeds his or her resources, and be apprehended. These behaviors represent maladaptive problem solving. Failing to obtain illegal drugs, the addict may turn to alcohol, replacing one addiction with another. Here the addict uses coping measures which are neither better nor worse than the precrisis behavior. Finally, the addict may use the crisis as a time to renounce addictive substances and make a commitment to a rehabilitation program. If this happened, the level of coping would be appreciably improved.

Crises may be classified as developmental or situational. As described by Erikson (1963), *developmental crises* are periods during the life cycle when change takes place at comparatively rapid rates. The identity crisis of adolescence and the generative crisis of adulthood are experienced by everyone. *Situational crises* originate in specific life events which happen at a particular point, and which arise unexpectedly or with little warning. The birth of a child or the death of a loved one are hazardous events which for some families become the precursors of crisis. Natural disasters such as hurricanes, earthquakes, and floods are prototypes of crisis events that affect communities and even nations.

The major concepts of crisis theory came from Lindemann (1944) and Caplan (1961). Lindemann worked with individuals who had suffered losses in the Cocoanut Grove fire in Boston. He found that for survivors the first 6 weeks after bereavement were crucial in determining the course of the grief reaction. In normal grieving there was preoccupation with the memory of the deceased, some disorganization of daily routine, and vague feelings of fatigue and confusion. There were verbal expressions of loss and of longing for the lost one, followed ultimately by acceptance, which released energy for new relationships and plans. Through these normal, time-limited grief reactions, attachment to the lost one was loosened. Lindemann found that pathological grieving was more prolonged. It was characterized by greater denial or distortion of the loss, identification with the deceased to the extent of acquiring similar characteristics, and severe somatic and psychological dysfunction. Differences between normal and pathological grieving were largely differences of degree.

Basic to crisis theory is the idea that crises are part of the human condition. Although the parameters of crisis theory are broad, problem solving is a common dimension, as is the urgency of the problems. The predictable nature of crisis has permitted the formulation of generic and specific approaches to crisis intervention. The concept of *generic* or *nonspecific crisis intervention* is based on Lindemann's observations that adaptive forms of grief differ from maladaptive forms, and that intervention in the early weeks following loss may mitigate or prevent pathological grief responses. Caplan elaborated on the work of Lindemann by identifying the sequential stages of the developing crisis. These are:

Stage 1   Tension arises as usual coping measures are tried in response to a life change or hazardous event.

Stage 2   Lack of success in coping leads to greater tension, which then produces disorganization of the system.

Stage 3   The failure of usual coping measures creates a need for alternative solutions and receptivity to change.

Generic crisis theory permits the care provider to focus on the event, and not on the particular persons involved. For this reason, theoretical expertise is not a prerequisite, although the care provider must be familiar with the coping means that are appropriate to the crisis event being confronted. The worker adopting a generic approach to crisis intervention begins by assessing the proportions of the crisis and reviewing previous efforts to deal with the hazardous event. Next, the boundaries of the crisis must be defined, and distortions produced by overwhelming anxiety must be corrected. Only then can a family begin to move toward effective planning, which will introduce new coping stratagems. The role of the worker in generic crisis intervention is an active one, but is restricted to the situation. A family or individual is mobilized toward problem solving; the environment may be manipulated when this seems appropriate. The nonspecific nature of generic crisis intervention allows for rather wide application of its principles; however, lack of specificity in the intervention may also be an impediment. What is generally helpful for most families will not be acceptable to all, although crisis theory is a useful framework in many situations.

Growth-oriented crisis intervention takes account of the unique features of the event as they impinge upon a particular individual or family. Because this type of crisis intervention makes dynamic connections between the event and the persons involved, it provokes more anxiety than the generic approach. Therefore, it requires considerable expertise and sound knowledge of psychodynamics and family theory. Clients should be involved in deeper crisis work only if they possess enough ego strength to tolerate exploratory interventions while the crisis is being resolved. This type of crisis intervention can be tolerated only by responsive and motivated persons, and even they may find it difficult after customary coping measures have failed and emotions are intense. Still, there are times when the failure of previous coping measures creates a climate of growth. It must be emphasized that a more intensive approach to crisis intervention should be undertaken only after anxiety has fallen to tolerable levels, and then only by qualified professionals working with selected clients.

The emotional or symbolic meaning of the hazardous event is extremely important. A birth, a marriage, or a separation may be a source of gratification for some families but a crisis for others. The same may be said of all events which alter the structure or function of the family. Within a family, the death of a loved one often represents a crisis for which intervention is required. Grief is a painful emotion, even though it is regarded as a normal response to an inevitable life event. Engel (1961) argued that many elements found in grief could be contained within the medical paradigm of disease. From this it can be postulated that all human grief is deserving of professional attention, which at present is reserved for abnormal grieving states. In 1977 Engel reexamined grief as a pathological condition and proposed a conceptualization which was applicable to crisis theory. Grief is viewed in this biopsychosocial model as a potentially morbid problem which must be faced at various times. An advantage of this model is that it implies that individuals need not suffer unassisted merely because their grief reaction is within normal limits. Grief-stricken persons should not have to be labeled physically or mentally ill before they can obtain help.

Aguilera (1978) outlined four phases of crisis intervention which are suitable for generic and growth-oriented crisis work. These are: (1) assessing both the individual and the problem; (2) planning interventions based upon available strengths and support systems; (3) implementing planned interventions; and (4) resolving the crisis and planning for the future. Interventions may include helping clients gain intellectual understanding of the crisis, bringing feelings into the open, exploring coping methods, and removing precipitating factors, if possible.

The last component of any crisis intervention is termination. If further work is indicated, it is advisable to refer clients for other forms of treatment. Because crisis work is confined to the presenting difficulty, it should not be extended beyond that. The inherent value of crisis intervention is its limited nature, because the time limitation causes clients to work actively at resolving the crisis. Motivation is diminished, dependency increased, and results jeopardized when crisis intervention encroaches on other treatment modalities. Since a state of crisis usually lasts from 4 to 6 weeks, extended therapy around the event is seldom indicated. If individuals or families might benefit from additional help, the methods should be changed or the clients should be referred to other professionals. Crisis intervention provides a supportive buttress during the event; once the event has passed, the principles of crisis theory need to be replaced with other modalities of treatment.

There is probably no stress greater than that endured when a family member is diagnosed as having a fatal illness. This is especially true when the illness is cancer. Giacquinta (1977) proposed a four-stage model for health professionals to use with families of cancer patients. Stage I is *living with cancer.* Within this initial stage families learn the diagnosis. They must begin to deal with the diagnosis and the implications for the family. If the cancer patient goes into remission, feelings of shock and disorganization lessen. Interventions directed toward solving the everyday problems of life are useful at this stage in order to reduce the family's feelings of helplessness and confusion.

When it becomes apparent that the stricken member will not recover, a second crisis appears, termed Stage II, *restructuring in the living-dying interval.* This stage was described as follows:

> But if the condition of the ill family member progresses gradually toward death, family members slowly get in touch with what is happening. They begin to recognize the defeat and loss they feel, the strain of carrying additional role obligations, and their need to change sights, to find satisfactions with life as it is evolving, and to plan more realistically for their life together. Grieving usually begins at this phase (Giacquinta, 1977, p. 1587).

During Stage II the family has two major tasks. The first is to reorganize family life to meet the crisis of dying. This requires new role distributions and collaborations within the family. The second is to go through a process called "framing memories," which means that the family recalls memories of the dying person from happier times. In this way the dying person remains a beloved family member rather than a symbol of mortality and disease. Through conscious processes of recollection, the presence of the dying person remains in the collective family memory even as life ebbs.

Stage III, *bereavement,* is the stage which brings physical separation and loss to the family. Active mourning is the only route toward the acceptance of loss and the internalization of the person who has died. Avoiding a sense or a realization of loss is dysfunctional, since mourning must be experienced in order to move on to the next stage of renewal.

Stage IV, *reestablishment,* has been reached when the family shows signs of overcoming tendencies toward isolation. In this period the family begins to return to ordinary activities and reenter social systems abandoned during the earlier stages of extreme crisis.

CRISIS INTERVENTION IN THE FAMILY OF A DYING CHILD

When a diagnosis of cancer has been made and the stricken person is a child, the effects on the family are particularly traumatic. In the following section three separate time periods in the disease chronology will be discussed, each of which represents a crisis in its own right (Martinson, Armstrong, Geis, Anglim, Gronseth, MacInnis, Nesbit, Kersey, 1978b). The first crisis comes at the time of diagnosis and early treatment; the second crisis occurs with the failure of treatment and the approach of death; the last crisis arises as the family grieves and struggles to adjust after the child has died. The principles of crisis intervention can be applied to many illnesses, but childhood cancer was selected as an example since it is an especially difficult crisis for a family to endure.

Physical aspects of patient care often cause the family to be preoccupied solely with the patient. This is equally true of health professionals, who may overlook the suffering of all the family members. Parents often need more assistance than is available to them. It must be remembered that family-focused interventions are a way of aiding the patient. Usually it is less effective for professionals to provide supportive intervention directly to the child. What is more useful is to assist the family so that their improved coping will be reflected in their interactions with the sick child.

Crisis during Diagnosis and Treatment

Assessment   The impact of childhood cancer on family members is multidimensional. Hopkins (1973) pointed out that, while any diagnosis of life-threatening illness is overwhelming, the possible loss of a child through disease completely disrupts family functioning. Children with malignant disease and poor prognosis certainly face a dismal future. Nevertheless, these children have the support of their parents, who may have no one to whom they can turn. Many times it is the parents who suffer the greatest psychological distress, since children are protected for a time against complete awareness of their plight. With improvements in medical treatment, children may survive for a number of years, while parents and siblings endeavor to adjust to periods of illness, remission, and relapse. One mother stated:

> Well, it was really me that was labeled because we got into terrible conflicts over it. And the more angry I got, the quieter my husband got and the more we went apart. So the times our daughter was hospitalized were really difficult for our relationship because of that. I felt my husband thought I was crazy.

Apparently the distraught mother projected her own fears of "going crazy" to her husband, but during the period of crisis the two parents never talked about their feelings. Each bore the anguish alone, whereas a health professional might have opened avenues of communication which would have made the way less lonely for both.

When a child is diagnosed as having cancer, the family system is immediately faced with medical, psychological, economic, and logistic problems. Regardless of its previous competence, the system will be taxed to its limits. It is not surprising that malfunction generally ensues. As soon as the diagnosis is made, treatment, which usually includes hospitalization, must begin. As a general rule, cancer treatment is concentrated in highly sophisticated facilities scattered geographically throughout the country. Therefore, just as the grim news is communicated, the family must be physically separated in order to obtain the required treatment. At a time when closeness and mutual support are most needed, the child is removed from the home. Since treatment facilities are often several hundred miles away, the mother usually accompanies the child. Subsystems within the family structure must adapt to the change, which for many families means that they can no longer interact in accustomed ways.

In some respects the first crisis is the hardest to endure. Siblings may not be able to visit the sick child; fantasy and guilt may distort their understanding of the problem. The well children feel bereft as parents interrupt usual family patterns in order to serve the sick child. Removal of the mother and the sick child to another city may be expedient from a treatment point of view, but it reduces the interdependence which has made family life meaningful. Even when the sick child is not removed from the home, life changes for the family, as parents and child embark on a medical odyssey which will end only with the child's death. While all this is happening, the attention of health professionals may be limited to treating the ill child. Even though the child is entitled to the best treatment that can be offered, the psychological effects of the diagnosis on the whole family warrant attention to them as well.

Depending on the responses of the parents, early planning sessions can be held at which feelings are expressed openly, even as solutions for medical problems are being sought. Siblings may have secret fears of having caused or been infected with the illness. These fears will not be verbalized unless an opportunity is provided to do so, since well siblings are reluctant to add to the problems of their parents. Often parents do not know what to tell the patient or what to tell their other children, and will need help with this. Frequently patient and siblings cannot comprehend the seriousness of the situation. All that is perceived is that a brother or sister is in a frightening new environment being subjected to painful procedures masquerading as treatment. The assessment stage of crisis intervention in these circumstances should include building a professional relationship on which parents can depend in the months ahead. At first the family needs to meet as a dyad or unit. Later parents may be helped by other couples facing the same problems.

Intervention   The relationships established with families in the initial crisis of their long ordeal should include friendship as well as treatment for the child who is ill. The established supports of the patient should be altered as little as possible, especially the child's interactions with parents and siblings. Sibings need to understand that it is important for the mother to help care for her hospitalized child since she was the primary care provider when the child was well. Relatives and friends may be asked to help with the children who are well or, better still, the children can be encouraged to help and sustain each other.

The presence of parents may be inconvenient for hospital staff at times, and may generate more work for the professionals. However, the psychological importance of parental involvement has positive value for both parents and the sick child.

At the time of diagnosis there is a great potential for therapeutic intervention. Friedman, Chodoff, Mason and Hamburg (1963) described emotions parents manifest upon hearing the diagnosis. One is a feeling of shock or disbelief. Parents speak of being "stunned," and it may take several days before the meaning of the diagnosis is fully comprehended. Even so, the disease does not wait for the shock to pass. Decisions must be made immediately for which the parents need complete information. Thus an early intervention should be a clear, understandable description of the situation and of alternatives open to the parents. Because of their mental state, explanations may have to be reiterated several times.

The oncologist in charge of treatment usually spends some time with the parents, but the primary commitment of this specialist centers around the patient. It is essential that other health professionals such as nurses or social workers assume the responsibility of providing information and offering appropriate assistance to the family. Professional nurses can answer questions about the disease process, and should spend whatever time is necessary to help parents understand what is happening. At the same time the coordinating or primary nurse should extend him- or herself to involve the parents since it is they who will be responsible for care between hospitalizations. Building trust entails processes which have little to do with direct care. Assistance may take practical forms such as helping out-of-town parents find places to eat or stay. By enabling parents to deal with mundane problems, professionals free parents to direct their energies toward helping each other and their child. To learn how to handle the rules and procedures of the hospital during this period of severe crisis, families need the help and support of persons who are an integral part of the system. Nurses are eminently suited to give this help, since they are more accessible than the physician. Their work is known and necessary; they are able to show concern without excessive emotionalism and can act as liaison persons between the family and the health care delivery system.

Family organization is fragmented by the child's hospitalization. Reliable subsystems become disorganized and function with minimal efficiency just as a formidable parade of professionals begin to enter the life of the family. These persons are necessary, but imply family dependency and loss of autonomy. As the child suffers, the parents suffer also, and feel powerless because their pain cannot mitigate the suffering of their sick child. Side effects are unbearable for parents to watch. Parents, siblings, and the stricken child are locked together in shared suffering and common helplessness. A mother described the experience of her little daughter.

> I didn't feel a stigma, but my daughter had a lot of psychological problems at school because of losing her hair. She just got razzed and if she would go with a wig, people would try to pull it off on the playground. If she would go without it when her hair first started to grow back, they would call her "Baldy." It really got so bad she hated to go to school.

In commenting on the same experience, the father shared his observations.

> That was part of the kind of shell she built around herself. Her only way of coping with other children at school, in particular, was to ignore them. They could call her anything that they wanted to and she walked down the hall and she looked straight ahead and she wouldn't respond at all to them.

Coping was achieved but at considerable cost for parents and child.

Planning for the Future   After the child's initial treatment, provided it is effective, there may come a period of months or years when the disease is under some control, and family functioning is partially restored. Even during this period when crisis is not acute, shifts in family organization will take place. Benoliel (1972) described the newly protected position in which the child with cancer is placed. Parents are inclined to be overly concerned, to restrict activities, and to favor the ill child over other siblings. Solicitious parents may encourage absences from school, or deny the child opportunities for sports or games with peers. The mother may even become the child's principal playmate and source of entertainment; this development interferes with closeness between parents and with closeness between parents and their healthy children.

At this stage parents are able to benefit from sustained or organized interaction with other parents of children with cancer. Parents have a strong need to talk to others like themselves, as evidenced by the intimate conversations between parents waiting in hospitals or outpatient rooms. Inviting parents to join parent support groups led by various professionals is a valuable way of extending their support systems. These support groups give parents understanding, practical advice, and information, as well as a sense of universality. Support groups convey the message that the troubled family is neither unique nor alone (Martinson & Jorgens, 1976). The group experience may also help prepare the parents for what awaits them—the approaching death of their child.

The number of parent support groups varies in different communities, but such groups are multiplying rapidly. *Candlelighters* is a national foundation made up of laypersons, the majority of whom have had children with cancer. It is a prototype of such groups, and the strength derived from such organizations helps stabilize families which are operating under conditions of extreme stress.

Crisis Surrounding Dying and Death

Assessment   The dying and death of the child, the second great crisis after diagnosis, are particularly poignant experiences for the family. There comes a time in the course of the disease when cure-oriented treatments are no longer helpful for the cancer-stricken child. These treatments may continue for a while, but a time usually arises when a decision is made that only palliative measures will be used. This is a crisis that has been dreaded since the day of diagnosis. Over the course of the illness the family may have been reconstituted, incorporating the illness, the treatments, the professionals, and the support groups into daily life. Now, with the prospect of death imminent, the latent crisis becomes manifest. While the family may have already accepted the prospect of death on a cognitive level, the reality of death must be faced on an affective level.

Planning the Intervention   There is much that can be done to alleviate the experience of the family, but the medical system as it functions at present may be quite unresponsive. The health care delivery system in the United States is geared toward curing disease and restoring health. The way death is approached, especially when the victim is a child, represents a notable failure of the health care system. Realization of this has prompted the inauguration of alternative programs for the dying and their families. Palliative units have been developed which substitute human warmth and caring for the technical efficiency of intensive care facilities. Hospices and home care plans have brought a measure of dignity into the world of the dying, although these resources are still largely restricted to adults.

Research on home care for children dying of cancer has shown this new approach to be both feasible and effective (Martinson, Armstrong, Geis, Anglim, Gronseth, MacInnis, Kersey, & Nesbit, 1978a). The success of the innovation rests upon changes in relationships between health professionals and the family, as well as changes among the professionals concerning role flexibility. Professionals involved in home care activities should work with the family to coordinate the resources of the family system and those of the health system, so that the most advantageous use may be made of both.

Intervention   The success of home care during the crisis of dying depends first on creating the least possible disruption of family life. The worsening child is in familiar surroundings, comforted by loved ones. Although the system is strained to the utmost, all existing coping behaviors of the family are called into use. The home care worker, usually a professional nurse, ministers physically to the child and emotionally to the family. During home care the parents remain the primary care providers, with the attending nurse coordinating the regimen and the physician being available as consultant. What is accomplished is that health professionals help the family to help the child in the home. Instead of dying in a hospital cared for by strangers, where parents are treated like interlopers, the child ends life in a familiar environment, lovingly tended by the family. As few or as many visitors as the child can tolerate are permitted. Even the child's friends may be permitted to visit for a little while.

One mother related the meaning of such a visit to herself and her dying child.

> Her classmates were just incredible. You see, she had her tenth birthday about 6 days before she died—and the kids in her class spent the whole morning making a birthday cake for her and then they all came over to the home, and brought the cake and cards. You wouldn't have believed it—that bedroom with 22 kids crowded around the bed. Although she didn't feel well, she thought it was so nice of them to come.

Since the parents are the primary care givers, they are active participants, not spectators, in the child's final days. Although they cannot halt death, they are in control of the child's environment. The effects of feeling helpless are deleterious; it is physically and psychologically debilitating to be in a situation in which nothing can be influenced or predicted (Seligman, 1975). The home care program gives the parents work to do which cannot change the eventual outcome but can help keep the child comfortable and peaceful.

In this terrible phase, families may feel hostile and bitter toward professionals, who worked valiantly but failed to arrest the disease. Some of this hostility is displacement of anger, or a projection of feelings of helplessness. The parents are reacting to their own inability to work a miracle. It is their beloved child who is dying; nothing they can do will avert the outcome. Professionals who should be able to help can or will do nothing. This seeming ingratitude must be interpreted as what it really is—the efforts of the family to deal with overwhelming emotion.

Some aspects of the home care program deliberately encourage decision making by the parents. It is the parents who request visits or assistance
from the home care worker, when these are considered necessary. By offering home care, the health worker is able to interact with the family as an
understanding, reassuring, and available human being, thus becoming more
than just a purveyor of technical care. Another mother whose child died at
home reported on her own feelings about the experience.

> That's another thing about home care. Somehow, even though you don't get a
> lot of sleep, the sleep that you do get is better sleep than when they are in the
> hospital. Because I always had visions of being called in the middle of the night
> to rush over there and then being thrown out of the room so that they could do
> a trach and put in fifty thousand tubes just to maintain her life for 5 more hours
> . . . you know. And I think the home care program really alleviates all that kind
> of worry and hassle because you know you are right in the next room and then
> if you are needed you can get there fast.

An interesting finding about deaths which take place at home is the
variability among families of practices immediately after death. There is an
inference to be drawn from these behaviors which can be applied to hospital
deaths. Rigidly defined cultural patterns of behavior seem to be ignored for
an interval immediately following the child's death. When families were
allowed to do whatever they wish after the death, some, within a very short
period of time, allowed the home care worker to wash the child, change the
clothing, and cover the body, just as would have been done in a hospital
after a death. However, many families simply embraced the child's body for
an extended period of time. If the child who had died was a baby, the little
body might be passed from one family member to another and held. Some
families bathed and clothed the child's body without assistance. Others
took the child's body to the mortuary in the family car, cradling the child in
their arms. Families were not required to do any of these things but were
allowed to do whatever assuaged their grief. Some of these practices
shocked professional health workers, and the behaviors were alien to accepted hospital practice. To the family members, however, the activities
were natural and meaningful, and seemed a source of comfort.

The interventions of the health professional after the death were
limited to notifying the attending physician. The goal of the home care
worker was to encourage the family to grieve without unwarranted interrup-
tion. In some cases the family indicated a wish to be left alone in order to
grieve in private. In others the family welcomed the presence of the worker,
whose behavior was dictated by the family's apparent wishes.

The Crisis after Death

The death of a child leaves a void in the structure and functioning of a family. The member who was the object of so much care and attention is gone. Immediately after the death friends and neighbors come to visit. The extended family gathers together for the final ceremony, but these rituals last a very short time. Even the most sympathetic mourners must return to their normal lives as the family begins the grief work that must be accomplished if adaptive living is to be resumed. The weeks following death are resolutely ignored by most health professionals, many of whom are glad to leave the scene. In addition, family members rarely seek prolonged contact with professionals in the belief that, with the sick child gone, the family has no claim to professional attention. A unique feature of the home care program is the continuance of professional concern during the early weeks of grieving.

Their common experience of tending the dying child makes families susceptible to strong bonds with the home care worker. It seems reasonable not to break this bond abruptly or prematurely. Health professionals and the family have been joined in a common purpose, and the weeks following the death are a poor time for the family to be separated from their closest allies. The fact that the health professional, whether working in the hospital or the home, has witnessed the family's struggle equips the professional to help with the grieving process. The alliance of family and health professionals should not be broken until it is no longer needed.

In some instances, the parents of a child who had just died stated that the last few days were more endurable than the previous period before hope was fully abandoned. The protracted nature of the illness mitigated the ultimate pain of separation. It is also possible that the home care program provided opportunity for anticipatory grieving. This seemed true in the case of one dying child who asked her family to pray with her. They all came and stood around her bed to pray. Then they opened her birthday presents for her and she thanked each one for the gifts. She drank a little water. There was no longer a strong grip in her hands. Her father held his child's hand and said later, "She just went to sleep. There was no suffering. We wouldn't have been with her if she had been in the hospital." They were surprised that she had died so quietly.

Planning for the Future

The grief crisis may be overcome in a matter of weeks, but grieving lasts much longer. The first year after the death of their child is very difficult for the family, especially for the parents. Still, they must continue with household and employment responsibilities so that family equilibrium can be reestablished. Recreational and social activities which have been abandoned may not be resumed for a time, but parents may need to be encouraged to resume them. Many parents become motivated to engage in leisure time activities for the sake of their surviving children. Occasionally parents sublimate their grief by working to help cancer research or participate in support groups for other parents of cancer victims. Such a reaction is wholesome if performed appropriately, but excessive involvement with cancer-related work to the exclusion of other pursuits may indicate an unhealthy determination to hold on to the dead child. In one sense the family is never the same after such an ordeal, but if the grief is worked through the family will be stronger as a system and the parents closer as marital partners. Melancholy may pervade the family for a time, but grief can be resolved with the timely application of the principles of crisis intervention. Denial of grief or refusal to mourn predispose to pathological grief reactions. A fundamental contribution of the home care program is not that it protects the family from pain, but that it allows the family to experience sorrow fully, while dispelling feelings of total helplessness. Caring for the dying child at home makes the whole experience less solitary. In the weeks after the child has died, the professional may facilitate grieving by encouraging a life review of the family. Reminiscing and life review are steps which move the family from morbidity toward renewal of family life.

SUMMARY

In this chapter fundamental tenets of crisis theory based on the work of Caplan and Lindemann were reviewed. Engel's conceptualization of grief as a condition which need not be labeled pathological in order to merit assistance was considered within the framework of crisis intervention.

Terminal illness was viewed according to the model of Giacquinta, which addresses family tasks in a four-stage sequence following the diagnosis of cancer in a family member. Stage I, *living with cancer,* deals with daily problems which must be faced along with the overwhelming situation. In Stage II, *restructuring in the living-dying interval,* family members begin the dual task of role redistribution and of "framing memories" of the patient in happier times. Stage III, *bereavement,* is the period when the actual loss takes place; the deceased must be actively mourned, and the pain experienced and endured. Stage IV, *reestablishment,* is a time of renewal or growth after the period of profound sorrow.

The crisis of terminal illness was illustrated through case examples of cancer-stricken children. Professional help offered to caring family members improved their ability to minister to the child. The importance of providing therapeutic support to parents and siblings was borne out by the testimony of stricken families whom Martinson encountered in her work. Grieving parents described their own experiences with death and told of measures which had brought a degree of comfort. The long-term involvement of caring professionals was advocated, as was the possibility of alternative home care for the dying child. The involvement of professionals in assisting the family was recommended, and reference made to support groups which might ease the ordeal of the child and the family.

REFERENCES

Aguilera, D. C., Messick, J. M., & Farrell, M. S. *Crisis intervention: theory and methodology* (3rd ed.). St. Louis: Mosby, 1978.

Benoliel, J. Q. The concept of care for a child with leukemia. *Nursing Forum,* 1972, **11**, 194–204.

Caplan, G. *An approach to community mental health.* New York: Grune & Stratton, 1961.

Engel, G. L. Is grief a disease? A challenge for medical research. *Psychosomatic Medicine,* 1961, **196**, 129–136.

Erikson, E. H. *Childhood and society.* New York: Norton, 1963.

Friedman, S. B., Chodoff, P., Mason, J. W., & Hamburg, D. A. Behavioral observations on parents anticipating the death of a child. *Pediatrics,* 1963, *32*, 610–625.

Giacquinta, B. Helping families face the crisis of cancer. *American Journal of Nursing,* 1977, **77**(10), 1585–1588.

Hopkins, L. H. A basis for nursing care of the terminally ill child and his family. *Maternal-Child Nursing Journal,* 1973, **2**, 93–100.

Lindemann, E. Symptomatology and management of acute grief. *American Journal of Psychiatry,* 1944, **101**, 141–148.

Martinson, I. M., & Jorgens, C. L. Report of a parent support group. In I. M. Martinson (Ed.), *Home care for the dying child.* New York: Appleton-Century-Crofts, 1976.

Martinson, I. M., Armstrong, G. D., Geis, D. P., Anglim, M. A., Gronseth, E. C., MacInnis, H., Kersey, J. H., & Nesbit, Jr., M. E. Home care for children dying of cancer. *Pediatrics,* 1978, **62**(1), 106–113. (a)

Martinson, I. M., Armstrong, G. D., Geis, D. P., Anglim, M. A., Gronseth, E. C., MacInnis, H., Nesbit, Jr., M. E., & Kersey, J. H. Facilitating home care for children dying of cancer. *Cancer Nursing,* 1978, 1(1), 41–45. (b)

Seligman, M. E. P. *Helplessness: On depression, development and death.* San Francisco: Freeman, 1975.

Part Four

Family
Interventions

Chapter 16

Planning the Therapeutic Process with the Family

Joan E. Bowers

DEFINING THE PROBLEM

The first stage in formulating a plan for the therapeutic process with the family will of necessity be the development of a comprehensive data base. When the identified patient is already receiving treatment for a physical problem, the family health professional may be asked to intervene because of attendant family difficulties. These difficulties may have originally contributed to the development of the illness; they may be related to the event of the illness; or, while not directly related to the patient's illness, they may be a hindrance to the treatment and/or rehabilitation of the identified patient.

Regardless of the origin of the problem, family members may find it difficult to accept the need for a family approach to intervention. A thorough familiarity with the circumstances surrounding the event of the illness, including previous treatment experiences for both the patient and the family will provide a baseline for exploring family structure.

The family health professional, with the support of the health team members who are recommending family intervention, will be in the position of having to convince the family of the wisdom of this type of intervention. By exploring with each family member his or her relationship to the identified patient and involvement in the illness process, both the health professional and the family will begin to collect the necessary data on which to base an appropriate decision about this treatment approach. In addition, the health professional will bring to this process knowledge of the developmental needs of the children in the family as well as an understanding of family concepts such as boundary issues, hierarchical issues, enmeshment, conflict, and disengagement. Without using diagnostic labels, these concepts can be incorporated into the preliminary discussions about the need for the proposed treatment, so that emphasis is placed on the family's potential to function at a higher level and on the capacity of individual members for further growth and development once family problems are resolved.

The nature of the problem for which help is sought—i.e., whether it is acute or chronic—will influence the receptivity of the family to seeing it as a problem for the family system rather than for the identified patient alone. An acute health problem, regardless of its origin (e.g., physical illness, accidental injury, etc.), by definition brings a state of disequilibrium to the family system in which it occurs. The crisis nature of the event can be useful in helping to make the family more amenable to a system intervention. On the other hand, a chronic problem in the identified patient around which the family has developed a homeostatic balance is likely to be viewed by the family as requiring treatment exclusively for the identified patient.

The health care setting through which intervention is sought can also play an important role in determining the nature of the contract to be developed. When a family member is hospitalized, either for acute illness or for the exacerbation of a chronic problem, the family is likely to be more accessible to the intervention of the health professional in the family problems attendant on the illness process.

Should the request for intervention in a health problem occur in an ambulatory health setting, the greater autonomy experienced by the family in this environment may impose limits on the health professional's ability to define the problem as one that involves the family system rather than just the identified patient. This will be particularly true when the presenting problem involves "only" the physical health of the individual patient. These circumstances are in some respects similar to those in an outpatient mental health facility when the original problem is defined by the family as residing only in the identified patient. In this setting, efforts to view the problem as one which involves the entire family rather than the identified patient in isolation may be met with resistance from the family. This resistance may result in the family's seeking treatment elsewhere, or even withdrawing from treatment until the occurrence of the next acute episode for the identified patient.

Because traditional medical care has been focused on the individual, the family health professional must be skillful in exploring ways in which the symptom or illness of one member affects other family members. Analogies such as those presented in detail in Clemens and Buchanan (1975), can be invaluable in helping the family accept the need for more than individual intervention. Analogies should be selected that fit in with the specific family's interests or cultural expectations. One family may respond to an analogy describing the work of a baseball team; another may see more meaning and application in the masterful organization of a symphony orchestra; still another may achieve insight when a health professional describes the interaction processes associated with making a favorite cake.

DEVELOPING A CONTRACT

To help the family to accept an expanded approach to treatment, it is crucial to focus on the problems which they have presented for attention. It is necessary that both the health professional and the family have a clear and explicit understanding of what these problems are and, further, that they realize that the problems can be realistically resolved through the contract as it is developed and defined (Seabury, 1976). While the health professional may regard a child's behavioral problem as symptomatic of a marital conflict, this family structural diagnosis should be kept in reserve until the family is able and ready to accept it. Nevertheless, the unexpressed assessment will in large measure influence the health professional's choice of interventions. If the presenting problem is being resolved by these interventions, the more basic problem of marital conflict will eventually emerge as a major factor. At that point, the therapy contract may need to be renegotiated if the marital dyad is to become the focus of therapy. In some families resolution of the presenting problem is all that is desired, and therapy will be terminated by them at that point. This decision, even when premature, must be respected and accepted by the family health professional. Such acceptance may leave the door open for future work should the problem reappear or a new symptom arise. In response to a freely granted acceptance of their decision, the family is often more willing to engage in therapy at a later time. Precipitous movement into covert dyadic conflicts could serve to alienate the family, to disrupt balance further, or to prejudice the family against therapy even before the presenting problem is resolved.

In defining the problem with the family, the health professional must be sensitive to extrafamilial systems which may be contributing to the current disequilibrium. A child who is failing in school may be the symptom bearer for a family in conflict. The child may also have a heretofore undiagnosed learning disability which brings conflict into the school situation. On the other hand, the child may legitimately be in conflict with some aspects of the school situation. The child's manner of meeting his or her needs in the classroom may mobilize a countertransference reaction in the teacher and thus place the child in further jeopardy. For example, a dependent child who makes bids for attention from the teacher may be gratified if his or her behavior is boisterous and amusing; a child with a similar need for attention may antagonize the same teacher by a behavioral repertoire that includes sulking, withdrawal, or angry acts. If the assessment of the problem indicates that problem solving must include the school setting, the health professional may elect, with the family's agreement, to move the locus of treatment into this extrafamilial system. In the example given, therapy could fruitfully be conducted in the school with the teacher as an integral member of the process (Aponte, 1976). Similar involvement of the suprasystem has been used with impressive results in the treatment of chronic schizophrenic patients (Speck & Attneave, 1973).

The health professional and the family need to view the contract as flexible and dynamic; as family needs change, so must the contract. Regardless of the health care setting in which treatment takes place, all parties to the process will be helped by having an established time limit within which the goals and objectives of the contract can be reasonably achieved. Goals and objectives should be stated in behavorial terms for the family (father changes jobs, daughter enrolls in college, mother resumes her participation in church activities, etc.). These goals will need to develop gradually, with the family's motivation and ability to accomplish specific goals being major criteria in their selection and pursuit. The order of priority of treatment goals must be congruent with the family's expressed values and wishes.

In essence, then, the goals developed are those which the family desires, i.e., change directly affecting the presenting problem. Such explicit goals will, in many cases, be buttressed by less explicit goals which the health professional may choose not to share immediately with the family. One example of an implicit goal is intervention in an enmeshed family system consisting of a mother and son. Resolution of the presenting problem—the son's fearfulness and inability to develop friendships with peers—could be dealt with by encouraging the mother to help her son engage in activities which free him from their close relationship. An implicit and unstated goal will require that the mother develop more appropriate peer relationships for herself. Essentially, the presenting problem can be viewed as a metaphor for the system's disequilibrium. The resolution of the presenting problem may lead to necessary changes in other dyadic relationships within the system. When this does not occur, redefinition of the objectives and renegotiation of the therapeutic contract will be necessary.

In some families, commitment may be only to symptom relief in the identified patient and, thus, to a return to a previous level of homeostasis that the family finds acceptable. The family of a truant junior high school student who has been failing in school might have as an explicit goal a return to a previous level of functioning, which means a successful school career for the student. Through the health professional's therapeutic maneuvers, family members may be induced to commit themselves to a higher level of equilibrium, that is, the achievement of a more satisfactory relationship between the parents. At this new level, the son would no longer need to work at keeping the parents' marriage together by being disordered himself. Only if the therapist has been successful in broadening the diagnosis to include members other than the identified patient who are having similar difficulties, or to include additional problematic aspects of family functioning, will system changes become crucial goals for the family. It is, however, of critical importance that the presenting problem that brought the family in to therapy remain a primary focus of the therapeutic process. All too often, families have sought help for a specific problem only to be confronted with the revelation that the whole family is dysfunctional. In fact, when confronted in this manner, a family which is more or less seriously disordered will almost inevitably become defensive and turn away from whatever help could be given (Haley, 1976). In summary, the proposed goals must be syntonic with the family's request for help with the presenting problem. Only after some relief of the original symptoms has been obtained is it likely that the family will become willing to renegotiate the therapeutic contract and define a further set of goals.

FAMILY EXPECTATIONS OF THE HEALTH PROFESSIONAL

The expectations which the family is entitled to have of the health professional should be outlined in detail during the preliminary sessions. The family may need to have access to the health professional between sessions should uncertainties or questions arise. Such access should be allowable at the outset. Only after problems arise should limits on access be set.

Discussion of fees, where appropriate, should take place as early in the contact with the family as possible. Billing departments often take care of financial arrangements with families, but if this service is not available, the health professional will need to discuss with the family whether or not fees can be collected through a third party. Since nurses and other health professionals who are not physicians or psychologists cannot collect third-party payments directly, the formal or informal arrangements made with a physician or clinic to collect such fees should be shared with the family. If the family is being seen in an acute health care setting (for example, when the identified patient is receiving treatment for a medical problem as a hospitalized patient) discussion of fees for this service would be inappropriate. If contact with the family health professional is to continue beyond hospitalization, fee arrangements will need to be negotiated at that time.

If the identified patient is a student, or if the family has had previous therapy contacts, arrangements should be made, and formal written permission obtained, to have contact with the appropriate agencies. This may be for the purpose of obtaining information, or, in the case of schools or courts, to share information about the family's current therapy.

If audio or video taping is to be used, whether for the purposes of education or supervision or for more accurate assessment of process and progress, adequate explanations to the family, as well as formal written consent, are necessary.

Finally, in situations in which medication of the identified patient may be indicated, the family should have information about the arrangements which the health professional has made or may make for consultation, prescriptions, and follow-up.

HEALTH PROFESSIONALS' EXPECTATIONS OF THE FAMILY

The health professional's expectations of the family begin with the initial contact. It is the family's responsibility to bring to the sessions all the family members who have either direct or indirect bearing on the presenting problem. This may include all household members, other relatives who do not live with the family such as grandparents, cousins, etc., and, when indicated, a single parent's new partner. In addition, the family should be made aware of their responsibility for attending the sessions, as well as the requirement to notify the health professional in advance if an appointment cannot be kept.

Beginning with the initial interview in which verbal contact is made with each family member, the health professional conveys to the family the expectation that each member will play an important role in the process of therapy. As the therapy progresses, the health professional will need to emphasize to the family the importance of accomplishing tasks both within the sessions and in their everyday transactions. This feedback serves two purposes; it encourages the continuing involvement of the family in working towards stated objectives, and it places the responsibility for change on the family system. The latter is especially important, because it both prepares the family for inevitable termination and ensures that the changes within the system are more likely to continue after the termination is effected.

CENTRAL PHASE

In the actual conduct of the therapeutic process, treatment modalities will be selected by the health professional based on the structure and configuration of the family and the manner in which presenting problems serve to maintain the family's homeostasis.

Because the health professional has contracted to meet with the entire family, sessions are organized in ways which provide opportunities for further exploration of difficulties that become evident in the family's structural alignment. Some of the cues to be looked for include the following: Who is the spokesperson for the family? Can the health professional, in the course of the initial interview, direct questions to other family members, or is it necessary to go through the spokesperson in order to address all other members of the system? What kinds of transactions, either in the family or between family members and the health professional, activate the identified patient? Are other members of the system activated in diverse ways that reinforce dysfunctional transactions?

As the health professional works with the family to define the problems, the family begins to reveal itself in the presence of the outsider. This provides the opportunity for the family health professional to begin to make what Minuchin (1974) calls "experimental probes." Asking the identified patient to sit next to the father instead of the mother may be one such probe. Requesting that the mother not work so hard in the session, but instead allow the children to speak for themselves, is another example. The family *system* reaction to such probes provides additional data on the role the illness or symptom plays in maintaining the system's homeostasis.

If the presenting problem represents a health crisis for one of the family members, the therapy will need to progress through several phases. The initial assessment will include a determination of the ways in which the family can be helped to cope with changes in role assignment necessitated by the incapacity of the ill member. Various resources outside of the family system may be drawn upon, for example, hospitalization of a parent. If a child is the ill member, the parents may need assistance in caring for the other children in order to devote themselves to the needs of the patient. Strains placed on the marital relationship by this crisis may become the focus of therapy and supportive interventions.

While working with the family to deal with the acute phase of disequilibrium created by the illness, the health professional will have the opportunity to further assess the family structure. Eventually, the family can be induced to recognize that the disequilibrium precipitated by the member's illness is symptomatic of other preexisting strains on the system. Planning for follow-up care, as in a family with an aged family member or a chronically ill person, may necessitate prolonged intervention.

When the presenting problem is one of psychiatric illness or of behavioral problems in one family member, the acute nature of the problem can be used as a springboard to develop goals for basic system interventions. Preliminary and later interventions are planned and implemented through a systems framework. Contrary to traditional, individually focused psychotherapy, the presenting problem is viewed as a systems problem with its locus in the family structure, rather than in the individual identified patient. Changes in the system rather than changes in the symptom bearer are considered critical to the achievement of the therapeutic goals. In the event that hospitalization or temporary placement are deemed necessary for a member, these maneuvers need to be framed as systems interventions and must be congruent with the overall goals of *family* therapy.

When family disequilibrium results from conflict with external social systems (school, welfare agency) the health professional will involve self and the family in dealing with these suprasystems. The family whose child is manifesting behavior problems in school as a consequence of a learning disorder will need active assistance from the health professional in dealing with the school system. Thorough diagnostic procedures to determine the child's learning needs will be a first step. Contact with appropriate personnel in special schools, or in some cases active intervention with the child's current school, will constitute useful steps. The health professional must be informed about supportive arrangements available to families with special children. Throughout this process, the family may need the health professional's support as well as tactful interventions with the appropriate external systems.

Additionally, family structure as affected by family composition will be an important factor in determining approaches used. For example, the single parent with an only child presents quite a different intervention challenge from the two-parent nuclear family or the extended family residing in one household unit.

When the initial goals, as determined by the health professional and the family, have been achieved, renegotiation of the original contract is often in order. The direction of such a renegotiation will be determined, in large part, by the family's willingness and ability to work toward further change in its structure. An important concept to be assimilated by the health professional is that equilibrium within the family is a highly subjective experience rather than an externally imposed ideal. In some families, achieving the resolution of the original presenting problem is all that the family hopes for. Following such an achievement, the family may be content either to terminate treatment or to be given a testing period in which to ''see how things go.'' In the latter case, it is important to finish on an open-ended note, encouraging the family to exercise its newly achieved or consolidated strengths in measuring its satisfaction with originally articulated goals.

In the event that the family desires to continue in therapy, new objectives for treatment must be worked out, in keeping with the family system's potential for change.

TERMINATION

As is true of all forms of helping relationships, termination of family therapy should begin with the first contact with the clients. In family therapy specifically, the maneuvers of the health professional should be directed to encouraging movement toward independence and autonomy. In the initial phase of therapy, this is accomplished by making family members active participants in determining what are the desired outcomes. As therapy progresses, the family should be continually involved in evaluating the accomplishment of various subgoals. When the subgoals are achieved, it is essential that the health professional allow the family to accept credit for having made the various changes. In this way, the health professional avoids a central role in the family and ensures that, once therapy is terminated, the family will have the confidence, skills, and motivation to continue the new behaviors learned through the therapeutic encounter. Maneuvers for achieving these goals include congratulating the identified patient and other family members for specific behavior changes. A focus on the work which has been accomplished, recognition of the difficulties inherent in making some of the changes, and the suggestion that the health professional or the clinic will be available for further therapy should the problem recur all serve to facilitate the health professional's exit from the family system. Final termination may include plans for one or more follow-up sessions in 3 to 6 months to assess the continued improvement of family functioning.

CLINICAL EXAMPLE: INSTABILITY IN THE FAMILY OF A LABILE DIABETIC CHILD

The Brown family came to the attention of the health professional at the time that Mr. Brown brought Annette, aged 8, to the hospital emergency service because she was in incipient diabetic acidosis. At the time of her initial discharge from the hospital, she had been in good control. Several months later, Mrs. Brown died as the result of in-

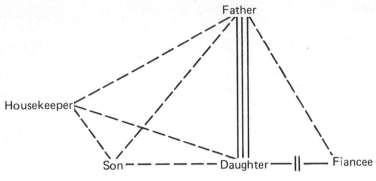

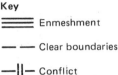

Key

≡≡≡ Enmeshment

— — Clear boundaries

—‖— Conflict

Figure 16-1   Unstable family structure.

juries sustained in an automobile accident. Mr. Brown, aged 35, assumed responsibility for Annette and her 6-year-old brother, Jeffrey, with the assistance of a part-time housekeeper.

At the time of this visit, Annette was rehospitalized to have her diabetes brought under control again. A family conference was planned to which Mr. Brown's fiancee, Lee Johnson, was invited. During this session, it became apparent that Mr. Brown and his children were overinvolved (*enmeshment*), with Jeffrey being less incapacitated by this process than his father and sister.

Assessment

Structure   The family structure was assessed as presenting an unstable configuration, which is shown in Figure 16-1. The proposed stable configuration toward which therapy would be directed is shown in Figure 16-2.

Function   Annette's behavior toward Ms. Johnson was one of anger and withdrawal; she was clinging and somewhat seductive toward her father. It was evident that her father's impending marriage to Lee Johnson had functioned as a precipitant in her most recent diabetic crisis. In addition, the threatened loss of the housekeeper, to whom she felt attached, added to her fears of loss and abandonment.

Intervention

Planned interventions directed toward the development of a more stable configuration within the family involved the creation of four family dyads: father-fiancee, father-son, fiancee-daughter, and sister-brother. Drawing firmer generational boundaries between the father-

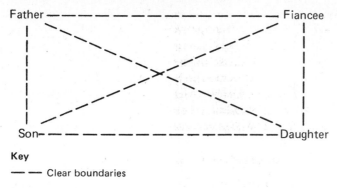

Key

— — Clear boundaries

Figure 16-2   Stable family structure.

fiancee dyad and the brother-sister dyad also played an important part in the interventions and facilitated the disengagement of the father-daughter dyad from its enmeshed state. Because the enmeshment existing in the family did not strongly involve Jeffrey, the father-son dyad was not worked on directly. Disengaging the father and daughter relationship resulted in changes in the father-son relationship, which enhanced further developmental progress by Jeffrey.

SUMMARY

The limits of therapy, including both its extent and duration, are determined by (1) the acute or chronic nature of the problem; (2) the relative intactness and inherent strengths of the system within which the acute problem arose; and (3) the initial and subsequent goals of therapy as determined by the health professional and the family members.

REFERENCES

Aponte, H. J. Family-school interview: An eco-structural approach. *Family Process,* 1976, **3,** 303–311.

Clemens, I. W., & Buchanan, D. The use of analogies in introducing the systems concept to families in therapy. In S. Smoyak (Ed.), *The psychiatric nurse as a family therapist.* New York: Wiley, 1975.

Haley, J. *Problem-solving therapy: New strategies for effective family therapy.* San Francisco: Jossey-Bass, 1976.

Minuchin, S. *Families and family therapy.* Cambridge, Mass.: Harvard University Press, 1974.

Seabury, B. A. The contract: Uses, abuses, and limitations. *Social Work,* 1976, **21,** 16–21.

Speck, R., & Attneave, C. Family networks. New York: Pantheon Press, 1973.

Chapter 17

Structural
Family Intervention

Dorothy R. Popkin

Structural intervention is concerned with individuals in the context of the family matrix. These individuals function as parts of a system as well as apart from the system. Every family constitutes a system which preserves its integrity by maintaining boundaries, whether intrinsic or extrinsic. The individuals who comprise the system must maintain selfhood through boundaries established between family members, just as the family system must rely upon certain boundaries to separate itself from external suprasystems. Essentially there are two forces or elements within the family system which are inherent in the processes of human growth and development. One is a sense of belonging and the other is a sense of individuation or separate self. A functional family system permits the coexistence of both forces.

The goal of structural intervention is to assist the dysfunctional family in changing its organization so that new patterns of behavior may evolve. Any living organism is dependent upon its external environment. This is true of individuals, for whom the family constitutes much of the external environment. It is equally true of the family itself which, like any group, is dependent for survival on the structural and functional relatedness of its members. According to Minuchin (1974) the structural approach to family intervention is based upon three axioms: (1) a person's psychic life is influenced by the context in which he or she lives; (2) psychic processes are changed through changes in family structure; and (3) professionals working with families become a part of the family system.

Whether a multi-model, or an analytic, systems, communication, or structural model is used, family intervention may employ cognitive as well as affective styles. While intervention through structural realignment will be emphasized in this chapter, there are commonalities between Minuchin's (1974) structural family intervention and Bowen's (1976) systems theory of family intervention. Both approaches view the family as an interacting system and postulate that it is the system that embodies the dysfunction. Both the structural and the systems theorists advocate guidance, modeling, and teaching in order to increase family problem-solving skills. But, while the structuralist joins the family to diagnose and intervene, the systems advocate maintains distance from the family and avoids becoming part of the emotional experience. Each approach is concerned with recognizing families in which one member receives an inordinate amount of attention.

BOUNDARIES

Emotions bind people together in relationships and help establish group boundaries around them. Group boundaries prevent excessive intrusion from persons or influences outside the family. Closed systems have impermeable emotional boundaries, and survival depends upon supplies within that system. In open systems, boundaries are permeable; information and energy are exchanged more freely, and survival is based on the regulation of transaction and communication across boundaries. Excessive, indiscriminate, confusing information flowing into a system leads to fragmentation and disorganization. This results in a dysfunctional condition, which is as inimical as the disorganization and stagnation resulting from lapse of communication and vitiated energy in a closed system.

Expanding the Field

Individuals do not easily give up old-established ways for those which are new, unpredictable, and different; the practitioner must nevertheless confront family efforts to maintain the system as it is. The family often reacts to such intervention by opposition, indifference, or rejection of therapeutic change. Its members are entrapped in unsatisfactory relationships, but are united against any breaching of boundaries which might introduce threats to the status quo.

A family fluctuates in its resistance to change. At times family distress is extreme enough to cause recognition of the need to alter family organization. The entry of the practitioner into the system is facilitated in the case of an emergency or crisis, the nature of which makes family boundaries more penetrable and the system somewhat less resistant to intervention. At such a point the family has identified a problem, or has accepted its identification by an agency or practitioner. This attitude of acceptance usually stems from the urgency of the family's distress and offers an opportunity for timely intervention. The crisis situation has created a climate of receptivity, at least temporarily.

Before intervening in the family, the practitioner must assess the environment in which the problem developed. This implies an assessment of the whole social field, including the structure and organization of the nuclear and extended families as well as their supportive network. Assessment also includes communication patterns, hierarchical structure, coalitions, and role differentiation and specialization. In making a family assessment, the importance of the comprehensive interview and psychosocial history cannot be overemphasized. The family diagram devised by Bowen and the family map devised by Minuchin provide schematic guides which help portray family structure and organization.

The family diagram establishes linkage with the past, provides an indication of continuity, and is a useful tool in assessment, not only initially but as intervention progresses. Being able to locate or trace illness or maladaptive behavior on the family diagram tends to reduce blaming and bias among family members, and helps family and therapist understand intergenerational perspectives. Diagramming also enables the practitioner to present to the family a cogent illustration of an active goal or objective. The family map (Minuchin) and diagram (Bowen) are tools that chart the organizational pattern of families, past and present, but they do not catch the tone or quality of family relationships. They are useful chiefly because they make it easier to cut through extraneous detail and to find a therapeutic direction.

The health professional is under pressure to diagnose and treat the member whom the family has labeled as the identified patient. Pressure may come from the family, and perhaps even from colleagues, to treat symptomatically rather than to attempt family realignment. If the health professional can convince the family that all involved family members are engaged in dysfunctional transactions, and that a change in any of them will impel the system toward improvement, he or she should be able to work toward realignment without intensifying family reactivity or defensiveness. This does not imply that the problem identified by the family should be ignored, merely that it may be symptomatic of other problematic conditions unrecognized by family members. Any family seeking assistance expects that the health professional will help the family deal with the identified problems. This expectation cannot be casually dismissed, even when other issues are discernible to the practitioner.

Isolation of one member in the system is a pattern frequently seen in dysfunctional families, regardless of whether the dysfunction is of long duration or a precipitated crisis. Through structural interventions, the practitioner discourages the labeling of one member as the symptom bearer or sole cause of dysfunction. In restructuring family organization, the practitioner actively sets the course of therapy, challenging rigid or diffuse boundaries, and interrupting fixed transactional patterns so that the family can begin to consider alternative transactions and accommodations.

Analysis of family structure provides insight into transactional patterns within the family. The practitioner may direct interactions so that the most responsible member is encouraged to delegate responsibility while the least responsible member becomes more so. The practitioner conveys the expectation that each family member will perform a fair share. Fixed transactions which isolated members from each other in the past are discouraged. Individuals who accept new responsibilities and functions are no longer removed from the enriching potential of diverse and flexible role enactment in the family.

When the practitioner moves into the family, the transactions which occur inevitably produce some restructuring and some reactive change. The therapeutic act of entering the family expands the interactional field and introduces new possibilities for instituting changes. Any practitioner who joins the family experiences the tensions of the system and responds affectively and cognitively. The spontaneous response of the practitioner is syntonic with the family system. As the practitioner feels the pain of being blamed or excluded by the family, or the pleasure of being praised and accepted, the experience of being a member of this particular family becomes real. Joining the family must be carefully monitored, for one must engage with members and at the same time observe their and one's own response. The practitioner who receives too many rewards in the form of praise or approval risks being rendered powerless. Fostering dependency in a family that is already dependent is another hazard that an active practitioner encounters and must regulate. It is essential that each family member feel confirmed and valuable; the health professional who enters the system to assess and intervene must project this value to every member.

Projecting individual value means outlining some simple rules which become part of the therapeutic contract. Family members are instructed that they are expected to listen and to respond to one another. They must talk directly to each other, not about each other nor for each other, and never through a third party. In early sessions the practitioner introduces and enforces these rules. It may be done simply by saying, "Since Mary was there, why not let Mary tell about it?'' or, "I would like to hear George answer the question.'' Regulating unclear communication is difficult at times, and it may be useful for the practitioner to describe how confusing it is when everyone speaks for everyone else. Clarification of incoherent communication patterns can become a means of clarifying boundary issues. The basic strategy of intervention is one of restructuring interactions, supporting some aspects of existing structure, and challenging others by presenting alternatives.

During periods of family stress aggression occurs. This aggression may be turned toward other members or be directed at the practitioner. Modulating aggression may mean accepting it at times and deflecting it at other times. Affective disturbance causes families to be less functional, but with therapeutic assistance affective disturbance may be translated into improved interaction. The family is an organization with infinite possibilities for realignment in structure and for redefinition of roles and alteration of positions. Fear of change or fear of further disequilibrium often immobilizes the family. These fears may be mitigated during the early interviews as family members move toward acceptance of the practitioner and experience the practitioner's acceptance of the family. As the practitioner joins the system, therapeutic goals begin to be outlined. Assessments are made and interventions based on assessment are planned, but the practitioner is limited by what the family is willing to accept at that particular time. Alleviation of an immediate problem may be all that can be accomplished, but successful resolution of the immediate problem may cause the family to return for help in the future. The practitioner may wish to deal with other sources of dysfunction in the family, but can address only the issues which the family is willing to explore.

ROLES

Systems operate in ways that maintain their functioning; family members accept roles that preserve family balance or equilibrium. In functional families there is flexibility and adaptability exemplified by family solidarity and tempered by a sense of individual separateness and autonomy. Role enactment emerges out of boundary maintenance, but also helps establish individual boundaries. A daughter acts as the child to her mother, but is parent to her own children; a father acts as parent to his son, but remains a son to his own father. Throughout multiple role enactments, individuals must retain an inner knowledge of who and what they are. Boundaries help set rules defining who is who and how each relates to the others. It is around boundaries that role specialization and role differentiation emerge. Role specialization refers to the tendency for one family member to assume a particular family function; for example, the mother may become the socioemotional or affective leader of the family. Role differentiation is a family group characteristic which permits different members to assume distinctive roles.

Each individual must have sufficient space and freedom in the family to learn the uses and limits of power. Boundaries may become blurred at times. In some families, roles become so rigidly defined that the individual is transfixed within the role; in others, roles become so blurred that there is neither individual nor generational difference in role enactment. Flexibility in role enactment is necessary to some extent so that the potential for growth and individuation can be realized.

Distance or disengagement may be so great between the members of some families that no recognition is given to supporting one another. When distances are very great there is no involvement or caring between members. Enmeshment of family members can be equally dysfunctional. When families are enmeshed there are no internal boundaries between the members or between the family subsystems. Without individuation every member gets caught up in the emotional responses of the others. Enmeshment and disengagement represent opposite ends of a spectrum. In the disengaged family there is insufficient nurture or concern and in the enmeshed family there is too much. Disengagement may be a characteristic of the entire family system, or it may be a phenomenon seen in the withdrawal of one family member who defends against excessive closeness or enmeshment with other members. In both types of families, enmeshed or disengaged, the practitioner functions as a boundary maker, clarifying diffuse boundaries and opening inappropriately rigid ones. Role enactment becomes flexible rather than rigid, as both parents assume instrumental (*task*) and socioemotional (*affective*) leadership in the family. Leadership resides in both parents, who do not assume rivalrous peer or sibling roles. When family members move toward appropriate assumption of roles, the strength of the marital alliance is affirmed; clear (neither *rigid* nor *diffuse*) boundaries are established around the parental and sibling subsystems.

COALITIONS AND ALLIANCES

The family system contains subsystems within its boundaries. Subsystems may consist of the two parents who form the parent subsystem and of the children who comprise the sibling subsystem. Occasionally the daughters of the family form one subsystem while the sons form another. In other families sibling subsystems may not be formed by gender or age, but by subtle attachments between certain members. When subsystems are based on attachments or on achieved rather than ascribed roles, they become coalitions or alliances. Coalitions or alliances transcend system or sub-system boundaries. A coalition may include a mother, a grandmother, and a favorite child, but exclude father and others. Alliances fulfill emotional needs and enhance the power of the members of the alliance, sometimes at the expense of others in the family.

The practitioner who joins the family has the opportunity to reshape previously existing alliances. This may be accomplished by strengthening a weak alliance or questioning a strong one. In the process of forming alliances or coalitions within the system, the practitioner must adapt to the family just as family members must adapt to the entry of the practitioner. Each coalition or alliance differs, and the entering practitioner must accommodate to members who have formed the alliance and be cognizant of the underlying needs which support it. The goal of the practitioner is to model role-appropriate behavior in order to establish boundaries and redefine roles. When a child has become her mother's friend and confidant in an alliance which excludes others, the practitioner interrupts this process by dealing with the marital relationship. Simultaneously, the practitioner will explore with mother and daughter the possibility of their replacing parent-child interaction with a peer alliance. Moving the marital pair closer to each other by reinforcing the parent subsystem and fostering the child's reentry into the sibling subsystem would be effective restructuring maneuvers. The child-mother alliance usually impedes healthy interaction between husband and wife. Removing the child from the inappropriate alliance with the mother decreases distances in the parental subsystem and encourages parental engagement in neglected issues which separate them.

The "sick" role of one family member affects the role performance of all other members. A family member who is ill and dependent may deplete the resources of the family, leaving other members with little time for socialization. Families can usually meet disproportionate demands if they do not become socially isolated. They need an infusion of energy from external sources to provide ongoing support and reassurance. They also may need corrective interpretation of reality. Without external feedback, patterns of response become habitual and family members respond dysfunctionally if no alternatives are in sight. They become trapped in designated but unrewarding roles. Labeling may become prevalent, with various members categorized as "the leader," "the helper," or "the shirker." The practitioner who enters the family system can begin to reduce family rigidity and immobility by the simple expedient of relabeling. A family leader can be encouraged to follow; the chronic shirker can be persuaded to help and the helper to allow others to know the joy of accomplishment.

The Restructuring Process

A practitioner who starts by taking the family history removes attention from the identified patient who personifies the problem. This is a crucial step in the process of redirecting and restructuring. History taking includes so many dimensions of the family that the presenting issue, which is emotion-laden and institutionalized, can then be perceived in a new perspective. History taking does not ignore the identified problem, but rather removes it from the foreground for a time. When there is an identified dysfunctional member, the family system becomes organized around the dysfunction or problem. An appropriate therapeutic goal is to enter the family in a way which illustrates a divergent viewpoint, through presenting new designations of roles and transactions. This might be done by redirecting communication. When comments are directed through the practitioner, one might say, "How about telling John directly?" The practitioner may ask members to move their chairs closer, to face each other, or to face away from each other. In some instances the practitioner may move physically between members in order to highlight an enmeshing or a disengaging phenomenon. In diverse ways the practitioner becomes the keeper of the process, enacting the definitive role as director, catalyst, or facilitator.

After entering the family, the practitioner may redirect family interaction by observing who speaks to whom, who interrupts whom, and who speaks for another. Structure can be discerned by examining who takes the lead or acts as family spokesperson. The nature of interaction can be analyzed through observing how family members respond to different styles of leadership and to nonverbal cues. As the practitioner experiences the family, the issues which are workable can be distinguished from those which the family is unready to admit. Limitations to the therapeutic contract begin to be apparent, and the practitioner working with the family begins to consider appropriate referral sources and readiness for termination. The future termination of therapy and appropriate disposition become topics for consideration and discussion, and the family will show its readiness or unreadiness to move responsively through the therapeutic process.

Outcomes

The art of the practitioner consists of moving into the family without becoming enmeshed in the emotional matrix of the system. Overinvolvement is evident when the practitioner becomes personally invested in urging the family to do what seems best to the practitioner. Although the structural practitioner joins the family and forms coalitions with various members, these are deliberative strategies based not on personal preference but on theoretical constructs. The health professional must know the tolerance of individual members and of the family system for confrontation or anxiety. Through therapeutic guidance the family begins to learn that conflict resolution is possible and that peace at any price may be a growth-limiting operation. Change in the family is introduced by encouraging autonomous stands, redistributing roles, and realigning coalitions. Learning that compromise is adaptive and that win-lose situations are maladaptive allows the family to change. Consistent modeling and reinforcing by the practitioner are needed initially; gradually the family begins to rely on the effective techniques it has learned to employ in problem solving. Boundary maintenance combined with expanded role performance may be the precursors of increased problem-solving ability.

Reinforcement of Family Solidarity

As a system, the family is constantly faced with demands to engage in routine daily activities, and to accommodate to nodal life events such as marriage, birth, entering school, going to college, and moving out of the family. While the practitioner deals with the present, there must be acknowledgment of the past. Knowledge and awareness of events of the past, and of the impact of family history on current family relationships, lend objectivity to the present. Through a shared historical perspective the family develops knowledge of its origins, which lends cohesiveness and a sense of family solidarity. Common family roots support the idea that the family is a system to be counted on, not disengaged from or enmeshed in—a network which helps us define ourselves.

The family practitioner must repudiate the myth that the family has no power, and that only the helper has the power to heal. This myth is dispelled by the way the practitioner joins family members in consultation around common issues rather than solving their problems for them. Entering the family is a maneuver which allows the practitioner to become part of structure, implicitly expressing trust and confidence in the family's ability to solve its problems. The resourcefulness of the practitioner in being the facilitator or director encourages family members to move toward dealing with answers and finding solutions. The practitioner is not totally responsible for making things better but combines with the family in a common search for alternatives.

The search for alternative behaviors may provoke considerable anxiety in some families, especially among members who have the most to lose by change. As immediate issues are resolved, the practitioner gauges how much anxiety and confrontation the family can accept. When family members experience confidence in their own strength and begin to trust the strengths of other members, they become less resistant to change. Learning to listen to one another, they recognize as if for the first time each other's differences and potential. Family members become more able to praise, to be generous and realistic in their expectations of other members. Fear of change is not experienced equally by all members; some may be more resistant than others. It may be necessary to assert repeatedly that change, while frightening, can be rewarding for all members.

Families do progress. Separation from dysfunctional structure does take place. As disengagement and enmeshment decrease, more effective subsystems and coalitions develop. Many families abandon, at least partially, the problematic interactions that produced dysfunction and distress. Some families learn new methods of communication, interaction, and structural realignment. The practitioner as participant-observer has taught the value of being specific in expressing needs and explicit in responding to needs. Diffuseness, overinclusiveness, and generalization have been pointed out by the practitioner as causes of family malfunction.

Family structural intervention is aimed at strengthening the family through structural realignment. Weakness in the family structure can be modified through careful therapeutic intervention. Task negotiations relative to family system maintenance that were inefficient may become more productive when family members are shown alternative methods of interacting. If successful, structural realignment markedly alters executive or parental function. In speaking of executive functions in the family, Minuchin (1974) wrote that, when the executive or parental role enactment in a family is weak, the practitioner entering the family may be required temporarily to take over the executive functions. The practitioner strengthens the parental alliance by modeling leadership roles and then relinquishing them, so that the reinforced executive functions are restored to the appropriate family members.

CLINICAL EXAMPLE: DYSFUNCTIONAL COALITIONS IN A TWO-GENERATIONAL FAMILY

The Granger family consisted of Lew and Julie Granger, a couple in their mid-forties, married for 25 years and the parents of three children. The oldest son was Ted, aged 24, who still lived at home but talked often of moving out. Steve, the third child, was 13, and Judy, the only daughter, was 16. Julie's mother, a wiry, talkative woman in her sixties, lived with the family. The identified patient was Steve, who was failing in school despite above-average intelligence and an excellent record in the early school years. After observing the interaction between Steve and his mother in the intake interview (which was marked by tension in the mother and defiant behavior in the child) the practitioner suggested that the entire family, including the grandmother, be present at the next session. This was resisted by Julie, but accepted after the practitioner explained that helping Steve involved getting to know the whole family.

The sessions revealed that Julie and her mother were locked in a struggle for control of the household. Their relationship was close, but marked by disputes and contention. Steve was caught in the center of the struggle between his mother and grandmother. Judy managed to avoid involvement in the struggle by handling her school and social life competently. Ted was working part-time and attending graduate school, and tended to disengage or distance from the family. Lew worked conscientiously at his job and found enjoyment in woodworking. He was involved very little with any family member, but showed more pride in Ted than in his other children.

The grandmother had been living with the family for 8 years, and her entry to the household had effectively weakened the marital relationship. There was intense friction between Julie and her mother, but Lew steadfastly refused to take sides with either woman. He felt that his mother-in-law was a help around the house and did not mean to be "so bossy."

Lew Granger was a phlegmatic man who said, "I don't let the arguing between my wife and her mother bother me. It really is up to them to settle things." Steve appeared angry at his father, but nonetheless seemed to yearn for his attention. Steve's efforts to get Lew's attention were expressed in negative ways. Frightened and beleaguered by the contradictory admonitions of his mother and grandmother, Steve confronted his father in an early session. "Yeah, you stay out of the fights but I'm the one who always gets yelled at by both of them." Steve's solution was to obey neither.

Julie was the central "switchboard" in the family, transmitting messages, talking for other members, directing, nagging, coaxing all of them in turn. She had feelings of wanting more from Lew, of not being needed by Judy or Ted, and of guilt for resenting her mother's intrusive presence. At the same time, the grandmother's assertiveness concealed her inner uncertainty about how welcome she was in her daughter's home. Her challenges to Julie's competence as mother and housekeeper were in fact an attempt to feel more accepted and valued by her grandchildren and son-in-law. The attempt was futile, since she was ignored by everyone except Julie. It followed then that her quarrels with Julie seemed better than being overlooked. Unless the grandmother asserted herself, no one in the family seemed to know she was present. The Granger family's relationships are illustrated in Figure 17-1.

Assessment

If an adult member of the family (Julie) continues to try to please and placate her mother, issues of control and dependency arise between the two. Transactions between Julie and her mother must be moved from a parent-child level to an adult-adult level. The assumption of adulthood would clarify the mixed messages Steve receives from the mother and grandmother. If Julie would stop trying to please her own mother by being "supermom," she might become less directive toward Steve and more accessible to Judy, who still needs her mother's counsel.

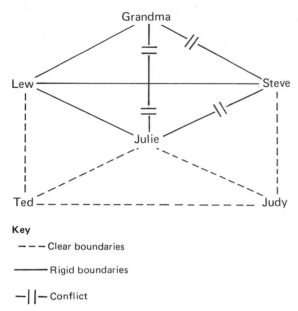

Key

— — — Clear boundaries

———— Rigid boundaries

—||— Conflict

Figure 17-1   Map of family structure.

Ted's peripheral role in the family is not inappropriate, but strengthening the sibling subsystem would be helpful to Steve, who needs male role models, and perhaps to Judy, to whom relationships with boys are already very important.

Lew has virtually abdicated role performance as Steve's father. This needs to be changed so that Steve can have the relationship with his father which he desperately needs. Julie, too, needs the support of an interested, involved partner. Lew's expanded role in the family should be a primary objective since it might effectively reduce dysfunction in the family subsystems. The withholding behavior of Lew can be modified through structural intervention.

Intervention

Appropriate intervention might consist of the following stratagems.

1   Remove Julie from her pivotal, but uncomfortable role as family "switchboard" by setting rules about communication.
   a   No one should be allowed to talk for anyone else or through anyone else.
   b   Shouting and yelling make it harder to receive messages. Therefore, these communication styles should be discontinued.

2   Strengthen the marital dyad, but include the grandmother as a contributing adult member of the household.
  a   Clarify the roles of Lew and Julie as executive leaders of the household.
  b   Reduce competitiveness between Julie and her mother by designating specific areas in which the grandmother is the household authority and limiting her authority to those areas.
3   Strengthen the sibling subsystem but encourage role differentiation between siblings.
  a   Foster interaction between Ted, Judy, and Steve. Each has the capacity to give to the others, but at present Ted and Judy are isolated, while Steve is trapped in the conflict between his mother and grandmother.
  b   Reinforce the developmental tasks of the siblings, each of whom is at a different stage.

The crucial figure in the family constellation is Lew. His greater involvement in family life is essential to improvement. If Lew moves closer to Julie, the following consequences will ensue:

1   Steve will have a mother and a father, both of whom he needs.
2   Julie will have an ally in her attempt to assume leadership as a family executive. She will then be able to reinforce Lew's greater involvement with the family.
3   Limit setting for the grandmother will be accomplished subtly. Lew's alliance with Julie will in one sense reaffirm the grandmother's right to be a family member. The grandmother needs reassurance regarding this.
4   A coalition between Lew, Julie, and Julie's mother will, by suggestion, place the siblings in the position of having to establish their own coalition, unless they are to remain solitary. The sibling coalition will effectively balance the parental coalition, which has permitted the limited entry of the grandmother.

SUMMARY

The practitioner first makes therapeutic contact with the purpose of gathering data about how the family functions and about the nature of its structure. Through modeling and interacting with the family, the practitioner defines his or her operational role, and some mutual goals of therapy. To achieve these goals, the practitioner utilizes elements within the family system to transform functional relationships. Structural intervention with families is based on the premise that they are systems and possess the following properties of systems:

1   A change or transformation in one part of the structure will produce change in other parts.
2   The family system is organized around energy exchange and action, support, socialization, and regulation of its members.

Families are motivated to come for assistance because they experience pain. They come with the expectation of having their discomfort diminished or removed. In the initial interviews, the family practitioner gathers data about the family's perception of distress and begins to examine family process and the patterns of transaction which contributed to the development of the presenting problem, and the resultant pain. The identified problem is not ignored by the practitioner, but may be assessed as indicative of more disguised problems. The willingness of the family to deal with other types of dysfunction will determine the amount of intervention which can be offered. Alleviation of the presenting problem and reduction of distress may cause a family to terminate early but to resume treatment at a later time. Families with dysfunctional transactional processes may be helped through a process of restructuring family organizational patterns. Effective structural family intervention requires that a practitioner join the family, experience family interaction cognitively and affectively, and function as a participant-observer-facilitator.

REFERENCES

Bowen, M. Theory in the practice of psychotherapy. In P. Guerin (Ed.), *Family therapy: Theory and practice.* New York: Gardner Press, 1976.

Minuchin, S. *Families and family therapy.* Cambridge, Mass.: Harvard University Press, 1974.

Chapter 18

Functional
Family Intervention

Elizabeth G. Morrison

Function refers to the operations undertaken by individuals and by families
to accomplish their stated and unstated goals. Some families, and the majority of individuals in those families, go through life having little apparent
difficulty in obtaining what they need and, in turn, in contributing to the
community in which they live. Other families, and individuals in those
families, require fairly frequent assistance and support from a variety of
community agencies. Most families fall somewhere between these two extremes. At some time during their life cycle, a number of families come to
the attention of a helping agency, very often a health care system. Usually,
help is sought because the family has some kind of distress which cannot be
satisfactorily resolved through its existing functional capacities.

One way to operationalize working with families in distress is to assist
them to improve the way in which they function. Function is a rather broad
term and covers a multitude of behaviors, both verbal and nonverbal, that
are observable to some but not to others. Observation and experience indicate that while improved function may be beneficial to some members of
the family, not everyone in a family may be interested in achieving it. For

some, maintaining the status quo, even though it is uncomfortable, is preferable to trying something new and subsequently living with the fear of the unknown.

Most people like to be able to predict what happens next, even if it is not going to be especially pleasant. However, experience has shown that if one influential member of the family is willing to accept change in the form of improved function, and can maintain that change, other members will react adaptively. For that reason, a family approach is essentially the one utilized by health care professionals, and one that may have nothing to do with the number of family members seen at any given time. This approach precludes the setting of arbitrary rules and regulations about who needs help, who deserves help, who should come for help, etc. The professional works with whoever in the family is willing to cooperate. An exception to this occurs when a family identifies problems with a child. Though the child may, in fact, be problematic, the parental subsystem is the one that has, or should have, the power and influence to do something about the problem. It is frustrating and eventually nonproductive to focus attention and energy on a child when the parents control the family system. The focus of implementation of planned functional change is on the member or members of the family who have influence and control, and are motivated to change.

REVIEW OF CONCEPTS RELATED TO FAMILY FUNCTION

Significant concepts related to family function include homeostasis, stress, anxiety, and differentiation. Any system, by definition, is committed to keeping itself going as a system. Thus, the major functional goal of any system is to maintain homeostasis or equilibrium. In one paradigm, family homeostasis involves "depicting family interaction as a closed information system in which variations in output or behavior are fed back in order to correct the system's response" (Jackson, 1970, p. 2). For example, Mrs. X. decides to get a job. She tells the family of her plans and notes disapproving looks from her husband and complaints from her children. On the basis of their feedback, she changes her plans and remains at home. Within families, the individual members become responsive to feedback which may or may not be noticeable to the outside observer. In this sense the family is a closed feedback system. It is on the basis of this feedback that behavior is modified and/or changed. When attempting to assist a family to implement change, the health provider considers the unique feedback system which evolves in every family. To the degree that the family takes other feedback into account, it is an open system. What the family tells you about its functioning, what you observe about its functioning, and how family members actually behave may be three different things. Maintaining equilibrium is not a conscious family decision; it is an automatic function of a system, and homeostatic forces work to maintain the status quo and to resist change. Regardless of the amount of change desired, it is difficult to overcome the system's tug for equilibrium. In the above example, had Mrs. X. proceeded with her plans to get a job despite perceived negative feedback from her family, she could have anticipated a period of increased tension and stress in the system before the rest of the family members adapted to her changed behavior. Systems work hard to maintain the behavior of each member in the context of that member's role or place in the family. Only through concerted effort can an individual change his or her usual way of functioning. This does not mean that changes in the system are impossible, but rather that change takes time and planned effort.

Stress

An external event can be labeled as stressful when the individual or family reacts to it with anxiety. For instance, a pedestrian may cross many traffic intersections every day without mishap and without even thinking about the behavior. The pedestrian walks on the green light signal and waits on the red light signal. However, one day an automobile enters the intersection and nearly collides with the pedestrian, who jumps back onto the sidewalk. The previously nonstressful event of crossing the street becomes a stressful event for this particular pedestrian. Based on experience, he or she reacts to the situation of crossing the street with increased anxiety and *perceives* the event as stressful. Events in themselves are not inherently stressful; it is the perception and subsequent reaction of the individual that make them so. Some events have evoked anxiety in enough families to become labeled as *anticipated* family crises. Examples of these events, well documented in the literature, include marriage, the birth of a child, the death of a family member, children beginning school, children leaving home, and retirement (Duvall, 1977). What makes these events crises is the emotional response of the family rather than the events themselves.

Anxiety

Anxiety refers to the butterflies in the pit of the stomach, the sweaty palms, or the trembling knee sensations with which every human being is familiar. All humans are born with the capacity to experience anxiety. It is an innate warning device which serves to keep people from getting comfortable with the status quo and, when attended to, provides motivation to change the status quo. Peplau (1963) described four levels of anxiety. The first level is the degree of anxiety that alerts individuals to their external and internal environments, stimulates heightened perception and awareness, and is necessary for learning. At the second level, there is increased focus on selected aspects of the environment, although the total picture is not attended to. The third and fourth levels preclude learning and rational thinking. Focus is extremely narrow, panic occurs, and behavior is instinctive and automatic, rather than rational or planned. Most individuals become aware of anxiety at or above the second level, when thinking becomes secondary to feeling better.

Since anxiety is unpleasant most individuals devote considerable energy to trying to avoid it rather than paying attention to it and utilizing it as a motivating force. An interesting thing about anxiety is that it can be transmitted from one person to another in almost indefinable ways. In families, children are extremely adept at "reading" anxiety in their parents, particularly in their mothers, since mothers are the major emotional caretakers in families. Children learn early to respond with anxiety of their own to events which evoke anxiety in their mothers, sometimes without ever having experienced the event firsthand. For instance, a mother cannot swim, as she has a fear of the water. Whenever swimming is mentioned, the mother changes the subject, does not take her infant child to the local swimming pool, and, when invited to the swimming pool of a friend, is careful not to get too close to the edge. The child senses this, and when the mother decides that it is time for her son, about age 5 or 6, to have swimming lessons so he will not be afraid, she finds that she has a terrified child on her hands. She cannot understand his fear, since, after all, he has seldom been near the water in his life. This process occurs in many areas of family living. Tension is both personally experienced and empathically communicated by important others.

Families function at a fairly productive and successful level when there is little perceived stress in the system, that is, when the system is calm. Some families continue to function effectively even when perceived stress and tension begin to escalate. All families have a point—a level of stress—beyond which they can no longer function effectively. What makes the difference?

Differentiation of Self

Bowen (1976) has proposed a set of theoretical constructs which have proved to be useful in studying family functioning. These constructs were discussed in Chapters 3 and 6, but a review of differentiation is germane to this discussion of functional adaptation. Basic to the discussion is the distinction between individuals as thinking beings and emotional beings. According to Bowen (1976), it is their emotional responses or reactivity that prevent people from using their thinking skills to solve problems and to deal with day-to-day living. This emotional response (anxiety) is a part of the human condition and when it becomes operative, it impairs rational thinking. Therefore, in working with families in the health care system, one can assume that they are to some degree caught up in their emotional responses to a problem or situation and are not always able to distinguish their alternatives. They are functioning on automatic circuits and little logical decision making or planning is taking place.

Each human is born into an emotional field called a family. The family is in existence prior to the birth of any one member and is affected by the birth of each member. The member influences the family emotionally and is, in turn, emotionally influenced by it. Some families are very concerned with "sticking together" as a family. They believe they all need to think the same way, feel the same way, and present a united front to the outside world. Other families are less concerned, and allow for more individual differences. However, all families have emotional boundaries, or limits, beyond which individual members may not go and still be considered acceptable to the family. In general, the more flexible the emotional boundaries, the more differentiated or individuated the members of the family have a chance to become. It is impossible to be completely independent emotionally of others: every individual needs to be in touch with other people in order to survive. It is also impossible, given an intact physiological and neurological system, to be completely dependent on others for survival. Everyone approaches life with a certain degree of both emotional dependence and emotional independence. It is interesting to note that the families who go through life with a minimum of problems in living seem to be those who are more differentiated, that is, their members are emotionally mature and can function as individuals even under stress. What are some characteristics of more differentiated and of less differentiated people?

One characteristic of differentiated persons is the ability to discern between thoughts and feelings (Bowen, 1976). It is common in American culture (and possibly in other cultures) to use the words *thought* and *feeling* as if they were synonyms. They are not. Pick up any professional journal or article and scan the pages for the use of the word *feeling*. You will note that, in a majority of instances, the words *thought, idea* or *belief* would have been much more appropriate to the context of the sentence. The ability to discern such differences, even though common usage may be inappropriate, indicates an awareness of the difference between thoughts and feelings. Some people are literally unable to tell the difference between these terms and will argue that the concepts are one and the same. Such people are so feeling-oriented that they do not discern the difference between what is felt and what is thought; therefore, they cannot make the distinction even when it is pointed out to them. Those individuals are not well-differentiated. To be feeling-oriented may mean that one is comfort-oriented. When a family is comfort-oriented (a concept sometimes referred to as the pursuit of happiness), it spends a great deal of time on trying to keep things "nice," trying to make people happy, and trying to avoid conflict or trouble. No time is left over for long-range planning because it takes a lot of emotional energy to try to make everything "go all right" every day, or to pretend that this is the case. In more differentiated families the energy goes toward setting goals, and happiness seems to be a by-product of accomplishing something worthwhile rather than an end in itself. The consequences of decisions are considered in light of long-term effects rather than of immediate comfort and satisfaction. A multiplicity of things "just happen" in relatively undifferentiated families, while planning and decision making are characteristics of more differentiated families.

The ability to differentiate between one's emotional and intellectual processes determines the degree to which one is differentiated from the family system or fused into the family system. Keep firmly in mind that we are dealing with degrees and not absolutes. We are talking about the pull toward getting along with the family or group at hand rather than making a decision which may temporarily alienate one from the group or family. Every individual has a core of *solid self* (Bowen, 1976) which is nonnegotiable in the relationship system. The solid self contains beliefs, principles, and values to which the individual will adhere no matter what the situation or its pressures. Every individual also has a *pseudoself* (Bowen, 1976) which is negotiable in the relationship system and which permits the individual to change his or her position, ideas, feelings, and statements to adjust to the conditions of the moment. The pseudoself is the part of the self that fuses with others to maintain comfort or the status quo, or to avoid rocking the boat.

An excellent place to observe the interaction of pseudoselves is a cocktail party or similar social gathering. By eavesdropping on almost any conversation, something like the following dialog will be heard. Mr. A. says to Mrs. B., "Did you see the latest horror movie?" Mrs. B. responds, "Yes, and I thought it was terrible, absolutely no redeeming social qualities, awful." Mr. A. states, "I thought the acting was terrific and the scenery beautiful, and I do think we ought to be aware of the presence of evil in the world." Mrs. B. (not wanting to hurt Mr. A.'s feelings) says, "Perhaps you're right, there certainly is a lot of food for thought in that picture." This kind of negotiation in a relationship is designed to avoid hurting or upsetting the other, or is conducted for the purpose of getting along with the other, and is evidence of pseudoself. Another instance of pseudoself can be found on first dates, when each individual is trying to figure out what the other wants and to play that role as opposed to acting naturally. "Making a good impression" is tantamount to negotiating in the relationship and demonstrates characteristics of fusion.

Fusion is most intense in important, intimate family relationships. When two people meet and decide to marry, they enter into another emotionally intense relationship and are socially sanctioned to "become one." Even though they are distinct individuals in their own right, the pressure for "togetherness" encourages them to think alike, feel alike, and present similar ideas to the world at large. This means that a great deal of compromise and adaptation is going to occur in the relationship with not all of it mutually satisfactory to the participants. All individuals want to be recognized as individuals at some level and want to assert themselves as such, but the pressure toward togetherness is very strong in our society. As a result, one spouse usually does more adapting in the relationship than the other. Of course, some degree of fusion exists in every intense emotional relationship. Whether or not it leads to dysfunction depends on the amount of perceived stress in the relationship and on how the fusion is handled. According to Bowen (1976) there are three common ways in which individuals in a marital relationship tend to handle the fusion between them: conflict, dysfunction in one spouse, and projection onto a child.

FUNCTIONAL FAMILY PATTERNS

Conflict

Marriage in our society is more than a legal sanction; it is an intense bonding between two individuals. The bonding is such that individuals expect, and are expected, to become a unit while maintaining their individuality. Some couples give up their sense of identity to "become one" only to find that neither they as persons nor the family unit mature. This situation is frequently described by newly married couples who appear for help anywhere from 6 months to 2 years after marriage and who report having lived together prior to marriage with no evidence of the conflict they now experience. The reports go something like this: "Before we were married, I did my thing and he did his. We took each other into consideration, but I didn't feel obligated to do what he wanted me to do. Now I feel like there isn't any *me* left." And the husband adds, "I have to tell her everything I do, every place I go; it's like living in a prison, not a home." Observation of these couples reveals that they fight over "every little thing." Another interesting phenomenon is that these husbands and wives are excellent observers of the behavior of the other but seem to have little appreciation of their own participation in and responsibility for the ongoing conflict. Statements such as "She *makes* me do it" or "I *have to* do this because of him" liberally sprinkle the conversation. One soon realizes that each is not necessarily attacking the other; the purpose is not to hurt or malign, but to save or maintain self. It is as though the only way to appreciate self is to minimize the importance of the other. This kind of conflict can go on for years without ever coming to the full consciousness of the individuals involved. Some people think that daily quarrels are what married life is all about. And as long as the tension and stress level stay within manageable system boundaries, the situation will continue without being labeled as a problem for the family. The following example illustrates such a marriage. Clinical assistance was sought only when there was a loss of a source of satisfaction.

Mr. and Mrs. M. were both professional people in their late thirties. They had been married about 12 years and had never had children. They were both musicians with a large orchestra and had spent a great deal of time moving from city to city when the orchestra was on tour. One day the local community mental health center received a frantic call from Mrs. M. requesting an immediate appointment. She stated, "You have to do something about my husband or I will kill myself." The intake worker gathered enough information on the phone to make the appointment with Mr. and Mrs. M., and both appeared the next afternoon for an evaluation. Mrs. M. had lost her job approximately 2 months previously. She had become increasingly unable to handle the instrument she was playing due to an arthritic condition in her hands and had been informed by the orchestra manager that she would no longer be able to play with the orchestra. She reported that, since then, life with Mr. M. had been "absolutely unbearable." He had screamed at her constantly that she should find another job and she had responded by throwing things at him. She was becoming concerned about the possibility of his abusing her physically.

As the couple talked, it became apparent that they did not agree on anything except the fact that she had lost her job. They bickered over every detail, each contradicting and interrupting the other. Since the intake worker realized that this was most probably a time of increased anxiety and stress in the relationship, she undertook to obtain a history of the relationship to assess the usual patterns of interaction. It was more of the same. Each reported that the other was argumentative, dissatisfied, and always looking for a fight. There was no indication that the relationship had ever been anything but conflictual, nor that the couple had been particularly distressed by this pattern in the past. It was only after the job crisis that either one had paid attention to the usual behavior. At this time, they wanted someone else to do something, and quickly.

Dysfunction in a Spouse

Another fairly common way for individuals to handle the fusion in the relationship between them is for one spouse to "give in" more than the other and become the overly adaptive one. Due to the status of women in our culture, it is (or has been until recently) expected that the woman give up whatever career plans she has for the sake of furthering her husband's career. Although our culture is beginning to change because of the impact of the women's movement, female adaptation, at least in the area of work, is still culturally sanctioned. In addition to societal pressures on one spouse or the other to adapt more to the relationship in terms of giving up aspirations or achievements, there is also emotional pressure for adaptation. The extreme of emotional adaptation is dysfunction, which may appear in the form of physical, mental, or emotional dysfunction. In many marital relationships one spouse is not as "strong" or as "capable" as the other and evidences the need to be taken care of and/or protected from life. That may not have been the way the relationship began, but the way it evolved. Chronic physical illness in one spouse may be evidence of system dysfunction. Usually the other spouse is competent, capable, and highly responsible. The same is true for families which contain an alcoholic spouse, a spouse who abuses drugs, or a spouse with "bad nerves." Since people tend to marry those at the same level of differentiation as themselves, one can assume that the highly responsible one is existing partly on "borrowed" self "lent" by the underfunctioning one. In families such as these, it is more productive to help the responsible spouse to do less of the caretaking than to help the less responsible one to become more responsible. The following case history is an example.

Mr. D. was admitted to the hospital for chronic low back pain. This was his fifth admission in 2 years, and the first following a repair of a ruptured disc 3 months previously. Mr. D., a minister by profession, was married and had three children. The nursing staff noted that Mr. D. appeared cooperative in following his treatment plan in that he verbally agreed to all suggestions offered by those responsible for his care. However, few suggestions were ever carried out. Mr. D. was in too much pain to do his prescribed exercises. He couldn't seem to get out of bed without coaxing and he always had something to do before he could take his medication or go to physical therapy. Mrs. D. appeared consistently annoyed or angry. She berated the nursing staff and told them they weren't paying enough attention to her husband. She hired and fired several physicians, who couldn't find anything specifically wrong with her husband's back, and managed to alienate nearly everyone who came in contact with her husband. She claimed she was the only one who could take care of him properly.

At the point at which she was about to sign him out (against medical advice) a nurse consultant was called in. The assessment was made that, while Mr. D. was a dedicated and respected minister, Mrs. D. took care of everything else. She had a part-time job, ran the house, chauffeured the children, did the yardwork, and was available to Mr. D. at all times for comfort and support. According to her, he could not even get out of bed in the morning to be at his office on time unless she spent about 15 to 30 minutes waking him up. Her anger was directed not only at the health care professionals, but also at Mr. D. for not being more responsible for his own care, even though she realized he would have to be "made" to participate. She said that she was also tired of having to take care of everything, including him, and felt virtually exhausted.

   The consultant suggested that it might be possible to find a way for Mrs. D. not to have to take care of everything and also pointed out that if Mrs. D. *was* doing everything, then it obviously wasn't necessary for Mr. D. to do *anything.* Mrs. D. was agreeable to a new approach and the plan decided upon was to be implemented immediately after discharge. It consisted of a small, beginning step, one which Mrs. D. chose herself. She decided she would no longer be willing to awaken her husband in the morning. If he overslept, he overslept, and would be late to whatever he had scheduled. Mrs. D. did implement the plan, and reported at a follow-up meeting with the consultant that it was one of the hardest things she had ever done, but she had managed to stick to it. Mr. D. had been extremely angry when she told him she was no longer going to wake him. He had arrived late at several meetings and had accused her of not caring about him or his work; as far as he was concerned, it was her fault. This was a predictable response and had been discussed with Mrs. D. prior to putting the plan into effect. Even though she had been prepared, she stated it was "really hard to take."

   After a few weeks, Mr. D. began paying attention to his alarm clock and managed to get himself up and dressed and out of the house on time. Mrs. D. decided to continue to work with the consultant on implementing other functional changes in her overresponsible pattern. Change of this particular type, that is, functional change, never initially "feels" right. In fact, family members report that it goes against what is supposed to happen, what usually happens, and what they expect to happen. This is one of the hallmarks of functional change. However, if the change can be maintained by one spouse in the face of system pressure to return to the usual way of functioning, the other spouse will eventually adapt.

Projection onto a Child

This phenomenon, according to Bowen (1976), happens to some degree in every family. Due to tension between the spouses, one spouse becomes more emotionally involved with one of the children than with any of the others. In most families, the spouse involved is the mother because mothers are socially designated to channel emotions. What occurs is that the mother invests more emotional time in one particular child. She thinks and worries about that child more, and she is in more frequent emotional contact with that child. Conversely, the child is more sensitive than the siblings to the moods of the mother and is more concerned about her than the rest of the siblings seem to be. The characteristics of this type of "worry system" are different from the realistic worry that each mother experiences periodically about each of her children. For example, if one child falls out of a tree, the mother is concerned and that worry is probably realistic. If, 6 months later, after the cast is removed and the arm is completely healed, the mother is still worried about the broken arm and is preventing the child from climbing

trees or engaging in similar activities because of the danger of getting
another broken arm, that worry may border on being unrealistic.

There is no way to predict which of the children the mother will be
most tied to, and vice versa. It may have to do with events surrounding
pregnancy, birth order, someone the child reminds her of at birth, whom
the child is named for, or the state of the marital relationship during the
child's infancy. A multitude of factors influence the selection of the child.
The outcome is that the child who is emotionally closest to the mother does
not have the opportunity to develop the independence enjoyed by the less
involved siblings. The child remains emotionally tied to the mother
throughout life and does not become as differentiated as the mother. This
closeness is not necessarily a positive experience. Many people have extremely negative feelings about one or both of their parents and at the same
time deny that their parents have or have had any influence on their lives.
Experience has shown that this is simply not so. A negative fusion with the
family of origin is just as intense and influential as a positive one, though a
positive one is certainly more tolerable for those involved.

As has been previously stated, all children learn to read the anxiety
level in the family, particularly in the mother, at an early age. The child who
is overly invested in the mother is even more sensitive to her anxieties and
tensions, and, as the following example shows, may undertake to protect
her by drawing attention to himself in times of increased stress.

Jimmy did not want to go to school. He screamed and cried every morning after breakfast and, when his father insisted he go, he actually became
physically ill with nausea and vomiting. Jimmy's mother saw her husband
off to work and assured him that she would get Jimmy to school. However,
she couldn't bear Jimmy's tears and obvious pain, so she kept him home.
Finally the teacher called to inquire after Jimmy's health. His mother
reported that he had been ill and then reluctantly added that he did not want
to go to school and that his illness seemed to be aggravated by the thought of
going. The boy's father was annoyed by the situation but did not consider
that he had any control over it since he had to leave for work before Jimmy
left for school. The teacher waited another few days and, when Jimmy did
not appear, again called the mother. This time the mother was more
distraught, and had absolutely no idea of what to do; she was worried about
Jimmy, but did want to force him to go to school when he was so upset. The
teacher suggested that the school nurse make a visit to see if she could be of
help. The mother agreed and an appointment was arranged.

The nurse assessed Jimmy's previous school and developmental history
and then investigated the present family situation. She discovered that the
mother was concerned about the upcoming surgery of her own mother, and
had found her husband unsympathetic and nonsupportive when she had attempted to discuss her fears. Jimmy, it seemed, was tuned in to his mother's

increased anxiety even though he had no idea what it was about and was exhibiting behavior which enabled him to be at home.

Based on the assessment, the nurse and mother worked out a plan whereby the mother would take Jimmy to school whether or not he wanted to go. She would also tell him what her recent worry was about. The mother was willing to follow the suggestion that she talk to her minister, whom she trusted and to whom she could reveal her fears about her own mother. Though this resolved the immediate situation, it was unlikely to have produced any functional change in the family. The mother continued to feel somewhat alienated from her husband, and nothing was done to change that relationship. Jimmy remained his mother's protector, and, if tension were to reappear in the system, he would probably develop another "problem." Over time, he could become a "problem child." To get Jimmy back to school was certainly an admirable goal, but it did nothing to change the functioning of the ongoing family system. In order to produce functional change, the important adult members of the family must be involved.

For descriptive purposes, the three functional family patterns have been discussed separately, but they can be found in any combination. It is more the exception than the rule to find only one functional pattern in a family. Commonly, one pattern predominates, and others become apparent under different conditions in the family system. Once the family assessment is made, the goals established, and the plans for change outlined, the next step is the implementation of functional change.

IMPLEMENTATION TECHNIQUES

The techniques chosen to implement functional adaptation depend on the selected theoretical framework, as well as on the components of the theoretical framework that are applicable to the family system under consideration. This statement may sound somewhat obvious, but it is necessary to reiterate it. Many well-written care plans, problem lists, and goals can be found, but investigation of how the plans were implemented reveals instances in which one would be hard-pressed to connect the action taken by the health care professional with the proposed plans. The point of implementation is the point at which many well-laid plans are set aside and professionals begin doing what seems best in the situation. Sometimes this works well and sometimes it does not. It is not until the evaluation is done (if it ever is) that one notices that the implementation did not coincide with the assessment and planning.

The most difficult thing to grasp about the implementation of change is that the health care professional does not really "do" anything; it is the family that "does the doing." And if one is used to "doing" things to clients (for example, in the form of physical procedures), it is often difficult to observe the frustration of families as they solve their problems. It is one thing to appreciate intellectually that one cannot change another person and something else to understand it emotionally and behaviorally. This difficulty is compounded by the fact that some well-meaning persons imply that one can change another individual if only one works hard enough or finds the right therapeutic "trick." Finding the right trick may rearrange some interactions for varying periods of time, but will not change the basic way individuals function. Only the individuals involved can do that. Therefore, the techniques that will be described have more to do with what the practitioner can help the family accomplish than with what the practitioner can do to a family.

In general, functional adaptation can be approached from two major paths in the systems framework. One can focus on the structural components of the system, for example, role function, output mechanisms, feedback loops, etc. Or, one can focus on the emotional forces that guide the structural forms. This implies paying attention to the process by which role function gets carried out, the process by which feedback loops are established and maintained, and the way in which (and by whom) decisions concerning output are made. Since function itself is a process and since a major goal is the maintenance of equilibrium, the focus here is on process techniques rather than on communicational or structural techniques.

Establish a Calm Environment

The first step in implementation is for the practitioner and the family to become calm enough to address the task. One immediate consideration involves how one introduces oneself. It can be assumed that the individual or family asking for help is anxious, or at least uncomfortable, and expects something positive from the professional.

One might start with an introduction and an explanation of one's professional orientation. This should not include detailed educational history, but merely some statement to the effect that "I am a nurse," "I am a physician," "I am a social worker," and so on.

The family may have already exhausted social and other support system resources before they approached the health care system. Therefore, at this time, a friendship or social relationship is not what is being sought. Use of first names presupposes a social relationship that does not really exist. Usually it is not appropriate to develop a social relationship in the course of a professional contact. If you have ever been hospitalized, recall your reaction when everyone from the physician to the person delivering your meals called you by your first name, giving no indication of who they were nor why they were entering your room. Unfortunately, being a patient often means accepting a childlike position which is not designed to communicate dignity or respect. The use of last names, at least initially, communicates recognition of the professional nature of a relationship and acknowledges that clients are adults with mature behaviors and responsibilities.

The family, or one of its members, presents a problem which has not been resolved by the usual functional mechanisms in the system. This failure evokes an increase in the anxiety level of the family, and produces what looks like random or ineffectual behavior. This may not necessarily be the case, but an effective evaluation must wait until the anxiety level is low enough to observe the usual ways in which the family functions. There are a variety of ways in which one can help a family lower the level of anxiety in its system. One way is to ask what has already been done, or what coping measures were used in the past when tension was extremely high. Another method is to focus on seemingly less anxious members and investigate their knowledge of anxiety-relieving behaviors.

It is relatively nonproductive to spend time exploring feelings such as anger, depression, hurt, and love; this only leads into a philosophical discussion of the nature of the feeling or to a justification of the feeling. It is far more productive to focus on the context which evoked the feeling. This provides an opportunity for speaker and listeners to understand which situations evoke which specific responses.

Because the experience of anxiety tends to preclude rational thinking, one of the most helpful techniques is to focus on the thinking processes in order to assist the family to reach a rational level of problem solving. This entails being clear about the questions asked, and careful of the language used in asking them. It is imperative to ask factual questions instead of judgmental ones. In general, questions requiring a "yes" or "no" answer reflect far more work on the part of the questioner than on the part of the respondent, and should be avoided. Questions such as "What was going on?" "Who was there?" "What did you say?" "What did he say?" "What did you make of that?" all invoke rational processes and ask the respondent to think about what happened or is happening. He or she is asked to step outside the framework of immediate reactions, and to look at the total picture. One should also focus on the individual respondent and refrain from asking that person to make judgments about the behavior of others. If it is necessary to collect data about the behavior of others, it should be kept in mind that the information is filtered through the perceptions and subjective responses of the informant and may not be congruent with observations that the questioner would make if the others were present.

Any technique for helping the family system lower its anxiety level is equivalent to providing an opportunity for it to do so. Family members may not, however, seize the opportunity and there is no way they can be made to do so. Any technique that is chosen should also be used by the professional. One must recognize and identify one's own anxiety, and understand what factors evoke anxiety and what factors alleviate it before attempting to help others do the same. There is no way to understand the anxiety of others unless one can appreciate the nature of one's own.

Allow Families to Help Themselves

Once their level of anxiety has been lowered, many families will thank you for your time and effort and go away. Others will continue to work even after anxiety diminishes. Unfortunately, the lowering of anxiety (often equated with symptom relief) is sometimes considered sufficient change by both the family and the health care professional. This is not necessarily so. Family members may have learned some useful things during the course of relieving distress, but they have not learned to change functional patterns. Changing a functional pattern occurs only with concerted effort and over time. The following family histories and discussion of outcomes illustrate the differences between relief of anxiety and functional adaptation.

Mr. and Mrs. M., the conflictual couple described earlier in this chapter, agreed to attend four more sessions at the clinic with the stated goal of helping Mrs. M. become calm enough to find some kind of work that she could do, given her physical impairment. Although hesitant, Mr. M. agreed to attend. During the next four sessions the examination focused on the conditions under which arguments began, the reaction of each spouse, and ways in which each could refrain from hurling insults and accusations at the other. At the end of four sessions, Mr. M. appeared visibly calmer, stated that he thought things were going better at home, and announced that his practice schedule for the orchestra was such that he could no longer find time to come. Mrs. M. agreed that things were better and although she had not met her goal of finding a job, she thought that she, too, would stop. Three weeks later, she again called the clinic and requested another appointment. At that time, she confessed that, although things had been better at home, she had a nagging sense of some unfinished business. She was interested in spending more time in trying to understand her contribution to the ongoing conflict in the relationship. She agreed to an open contract with the health care professional so as to define and modify her role in the marital relationship. This was easier said than done. While Mrs. M. had years of experience in observing and commenting on the behavior of her husband, she had spent little or no time observing herself. She presented herself in such a way that it was easy to understand how others might consider her helpless. Due to the arthritis in her hands, she could not obtain a job, nor could she sew, an activity that she really enjoyed. Since her husband used the car, she could not go anywhere during the day unless her husband took her, and she had few social contacts.

One thing the professional might have done was to make suggestions and busily give advice to Mrs. M. about what she could do to solve any one of the problems she had identified. That, however, would have been participating in the ongoing functional pattern which Mrs. M. had already said she wanted to identify and modify. Therefore, the professional did not offer suggestions or advice. Instead, questions were asked which elicited Mrs. M.'s ideas of her alternatives. What had she thought of? What had she tried? What had other people that she knew done? What sounded reasonable to her? There were times when the professional was accused of being not at all helpful, but, within a few months, Mrs. M. had figured out how to get the car by herself. That was her initial step in recognizing that her usual pattern was to get other people, especially her husband, to help her, and that there were many things that she could do by herself for herself without the aid of others. This then led to a consideration of what she might do on her own, and where she realistically needed help. Once she had made those decisions, she began to put some plans into effect. One was to teach music to children. Although she could not play well enough to participate in the orchestra, she could do well enough to give lessons.

In the course of the sessions, the professional did some teaching about systems and the way in which they operate. This helped to prepare Mrs. M. for some of her own reactions—and her husband's—to her new behaviors. Her husband was furious when she first suggested he find a carpool for work so that she could have the car 3 days a week, but she did not retreat and, finally, he agreed. After about 6 months she reported that the orchestra was going on tour and she would be leaving the city with her husband, but intended to continue to work both while she was gone and when she returned. She said that her husband's anger still evoked a great deal of fear in her, but that, instead of fighting back, she could sometimes manage to stay calm and not participate in an argument.

Initially, it looked as if this couple would get some relief from the immediate situational crisis and then go on their way. They did get some relief, and Mr. M., who was not experiencing the same amount of pressure as his wife, did leave. Mrs. M. appeared to go with him, which turned out to be part of her usual pattern: she did what she thought he wanted her to do and then gave him a hard time about it. However, something must have impressed her during those four sessions, because she rethought the situation and decided to do some work on her own. This is evidence of a well-motivated family member, confirmed in this instance by the decision not to continue the pattern of just going along with the husband. Mrs. M. then began planning and implementing some early functional change. It is of importance to note that the work was done on problems identified by the client and not on what the professional thought should be changed. Often health care professionals make the assumption that they know the direction a family or a family member should take in setting and/or reaching goals. They may be right, but if the family is not willing to go in that direction, the family is then labeled as "resistant." It would be far more useful if the professional became aware of how the family was being coerced instead of thinking about how recalcitrant it was.

The Use of Suggestions and Advice

In the above example, based on assessment of the functional pattern of the client, suggestions and advice were not given. There are times when the decision is made to give suggestions to families. When there is a real block in the thinking process or when a series of attempted alternatives has produced no useful results, it is realistic to share with a family what other families have tried and found useful. Professionals should present such suggestions not as ways in which they think the family ought to go, but rather as ways that other people have tried and found useful. This ameliorates the tendency of the family to see professionals as the ones with all the answers and also keeps professionals themselves from thinking that they *have* all the answers (and some do think so). It also prevents the family from saying "I tried what you told me to do and it didn't work."

Of course, one cannot give suggestions unless one has alternatives in mind. A professional who is in the position of not being able to think of suggestions or alternatives, whether the family asks for them or not, is in trouble. This is because the professional is seeing the situation in exactly the same way the family does and, like the family, is anxious, frustrated, and upset. In such a situation, the professional should get some consultation or supervision, whatever it takes to open up some options. The value of being a professional is not in having answers, but in being able to view the situation from a different perspective from that of the family. And that enables one to ask all kinds of illuminating questions that the family itself never would have thought of asking.

Opening a Closed System

When perceived stress occurs in the form of the loss of a family member or the addition of a new member, dysfunction may become apparent. The dysfunction may be temporary or it may become chronic. Intervention can be useful in opening the family system and assisting in the establishment of a new level of functional equilibrium.

Mr. P. was diagnosed as having hypertension when he dropped in at a public health sponsored clinic held in his neighborhood school. The public health nurse who spoke with him about the findings from his tests suggested that he see his local family physician for follow-up. Mr. P. was visibly shaken and promised to make an appointment with his doctor. A few days later, the nurse received a call from Mrs. P. asking what had happened at the clinic. She stated that her husband had come home and told her he was ill, taken to his bed, and would not get up to dress, eat, or go to work. Mrs. P. had attempted to contact their physician, but he had so far been unavailable. She was worried and wanted to obtain some information about the nature of her husband's illness. The public health nurse agreed to make a home visit to talk with the couple.

When she arrived, she found that there were three preschoolers in the home as well as Mrs. P.'s father, who had been living with the family since the death of his wife 3 months previously. Mrs. P.'s father was in excellent health and very handy around the house; he had taken over many of the household chores since his arrival, much to Mrs. P.'s relief. The nurse also learned that he was dependent on Mr. and Mrs. P. for financial support.

Mrs. P. appeared worried about her husband. He had always been well, she reported, with no illnesses, not even a cold, in the last several years, and she couldn't understand what was going on. She went on to say that they all had been under something of a strain since her father had moved in with them. He was lively and energetic, and had very definite ideas of how the children should be raised and how things should be done around the house. He hardly ever mentioned his wife, while Mrs. P. was still in the process of grieving for her mother. In addition, Mrs. P. reported that her husband had had to take on another job , part-time, to meet the expense of having his father-in-law live with them and of getting the oldest child ready for school. What would the family do, she wondered, if he were ill and could not continue to work?

When the nurse arrived at Mr. P.'s bedside, he looked and sounded depressed. He didn't feel like getting up; in fact, he didn't feel like doing anything, and was convinced he was going to die. The nurse acknowledged the possibility and stated that everyone had to die sometime. She went on to ask why he thought he was going to die just then. He responded that he had been told the other night that he had an incurable disease. Although nobody had told him that, he had read that hypertension was incurable and therefore believed he was going to die. The nurse first responded with information about the nature of hypertension and the need for further medical investigation of his kind of hypertension. She then went on to relate to him some of the things Mrs. P. had told her about their current situation and asked for his thoughts about what was going on in the family. He said he thought that, except for money, his father-in-law had pretty much taken over the house, the children, his wife, and his responsibilities. And his wife wasn't much help either; she was crying all the time about her mother. Nobody seemed to be paying the slightest attention to him. The nurse asked if he had told his wife the things he had just told her and he said that he had not. Mrs. P. was then called into the room and the suggestion was made that perhaps there were some things that the two of them needed to discuss. The nurse then said she would be available if they needed her in the future, concluded her visit, and left.

This family was in the throes of a forced homeostatic shift, resulting from the introduction of a new member. From the information available it is not possible to say whether the family would make the necessary adjustments without one or more members becoming chronically dysfunctional, but the likelihood of them doing so with help from the health care system was good. The nurse made some useful interventions that would lay the groundwork for functional adaptation if the family chose to pay attention to them. She did not get caught up in trying to get Mr. P. out of the bed and to the doctor, though she did present information which would guide him in that direction. She also did not challenge his conviction that he was going to die. She indeed affirmed that he *would* die some time and went on to investigate just why that was an issue at this point. By doing so she avoided an argument and/or power struggle with Mr. P. about the state of his health. It would have been useless in this situation (as it is in most situations) to contradict his statement, which was based on his emotional response to his current life situation and not on any objective data. There is a distinct difference between giving information and proving oneself right; a considerable number of health care workers fail to appreciate the difference. It is practically impossible for people to learn when they are in a state of high anxiety, so that if one assesses a high state of anxiety one should delay teaching until the anxiety level goes down. It is a reasonable understanding, but the constraints of time, the need to get the job done and, occasionally, the need to demonstrate how competent one is get in the way of completing the assessment phase before beginning implementation. Then, when feedback should alert the professional that the learner is not paying attention, the teacher ignores the signals and soon gets caught up in an argument. When one is involved in an argument or power struggle, the appropriate thing to do is stop it regardless of how wrong or misinformed one's protagonist may be. This is not the time for arguments. A good rule of thumb is that information imparted in times of calm leads to discussion; information imparted in times of emotional reactiveness leads to arguments. The nurse in the above example imparted information without asking Mr. P. to do anything with it and without trying to convince him he *should* do something with it. At the time, taking action was not the priority.

Based on the data collected from Mrs. P., the nurse suspected that there was more going on in the family system than was apparent. When she elicited from Mr. P. that he perceived himself to be neglected and unnecessary, her suspicion was confirmed. The next order of business was to get the two important people in the system, the husband and wife, talking openly to each other about the current issues and their reactions. She provided that opportunity and they appeared to take it. She did not choose to investigate whether or not it would be helpful for her to be present during the exchange and perhaps she might have done that. She did, however, make herself available for consultation at a future time.

The addition of any new member to the family system entails a functional adaptation. It may be a more productive adaptation or it may produce dysfunction in the system. In one sense, Mrs. P.'s father was not a "new" family member, since he had been around for years, but he had just moved into the home. The more planning and negotiating done before a move like this, the better things are apt to function in the system. From the information given, it seemed that there had not been much negotiation about who was going to be responsible for what and who was responsible to whom. For the family to proceed on a positive adaptive course, those negotiations would have to be initiated.

Symptom Relief

Work systems are as emotionally laden as family systems. The following example illustrates a common pattern: symptom relief without any functional change.

Ms. B. was admitted to the hospital for plastic surgery on her nose. The night before the scheduled operation, the anesthetist paid a visit to her room to discuss anesthesia and recovery. During the conversation Ms. B. became hysterical, demanded to see her physician, and stated that she would not be put to sleep by "that man." She was given tranquilizing medication for sleep. The next morning she was still upset and kept repeating she did not want to be put to sleep. She accepted preoperative medication and was taken to the surgical suite. After talking with her briefly, her physician decided to cancel the surgery and requested she be returned to her room. She told the staff upon her return that the physician had told her she was "spoiled and silly" and that he would not do surgery that day because she was so upset. She became tearful and began screaming at the staff. The nursing supervisor was called because the staff could not "handle" Ms. B.

The supervisor spent about an hour with Ms. B., then sought out the physician and anesthetist and talked with them. Surgery was rescheduled for the following morning.

Professionals are a part of work systems, which have the same characteristics and same emotional components, though not the same degree of emotional intensity, that exist in families. When Ms. B. became upset, she was passed around from person to person until someone who was willing to take responsibility, and had the authority to do so, stepped in to get the problem straightened out. The person with the authority who can stay calm is the one who gets the work done in a system and has the leverage to institute change in the system. It should be noted that the person who appears to have the power and the person who does have the power may be two different people. Therefore, change should be planned and implemented with the help of those who have the power to institute change and to resist the forces that react against it.

In the example given, no functional change occurred. The supervisor had the authority, and she used it to resolve the immediate crisis, to provide symptom relief as it were, and not to take any different sort of stand. Had she worked with the nursing staff to "handle" the patient, that might have been the beginning of a functional change. Had she met with the nursing staff for inservice education following the incident and perhaps instituted workshops on dealing with behaviors that the staff found problematic, that might have been a step toward functional change. As it was, there was no discernible difference in the process, even though the anxiety in the system was relieved.

Shifting Focus from Child to Family

As previously stated, children may signal distress in the family system. Mrs. N. took her daughter Priscilla to her pediatrician for help with a behavior problem. Priscilla, who was 8 years old, would not eat, though she appeared healthy and alert with no signs of malnutrition. The pediatrician was sure that Priscilla was getting plenty to eat, but she obviously wasn't eating what and when her mother wanted her to.

History taking revealed that Mrs. N. was presently 3 months pregnant with an unplanned child. The family consisted of Mr. N., a lawyer, Mrs. N., a schoolteacher, Priscilla, and her 6-year-old brother, Tim. Mrs. N. had recently started graduate school against the wishes of her husband. Mr. N. had never approved of his wife working, but had tolerated it because it supplemented the family income. The family was currently comfortable financially and Mrs. N. had decided to resume her education. Mr. N. could see no need for her to do so and was strongly opposed to her returning to school. The children were excited about their mother's going to school and often asked to study with her at night. Mrs. N. had discovered that she was pregnant when she had gone for her yearly examination and was trying to decide whether or not to have a therapeutic abortion. She had discussed the matter with her husband and he was against the abortion. In fact, he was overjoyed at the thought of another child and added that now Mrs. N. could stay home and take care of the children like a real mother. In addition to all this, Priscilla had refused to eat. The mother reported that she and Priscilla had always gotten along well. Priscilla was a compliant child who gave her mother no trouble and did as she was told. Mrs. N. asked her repeatedly what the matter was, but the child simply stated that she was not hungry.

Physical examination of Priscilla proved negative. The pediatrician said that she would call Mrs. N. when the results of the serological tests returned, but she doubted that she would find anything amiss. She then sent Priscilla into the playroom and talked with Mrs. N. Mrs. N. became increasingly tense when talking about her own condition and the difficulty she was having making a decision about what to do. She thought she might need some kind of professional help, but did not know where to go or whom to ask. The pediatrician stated that she would be willing to work with Mrs. N. on the problem of Priscilla's eating, but that she would refer her to a colleague for help with the other family problems. She also suggested that it might be a good idea for Mr. N. to be involved, and Mrs. N. said she would consider it. The two of them then worked out a plan whereby Mrs. N. decided not to pay attention to Priscilla's eating. Mrs. N. would serve the food as usual, but would not make any kind of issue if Priscilla ate or not. The ease with which Mrs. N. formulated such a plan indicated that Priscilla's problem was only a signal that there was something else going on in the family system that needed attention.

Once attention had been directed to the family, Priscilla resumed eating. Mrs. N. did talk with her husband, and together they sought the services of a family counselor. The most pressing problem as they defined it was whether to proceed with the pregnancy or to terminate it. With the aid of the counselor, the family reviewed the conditions under which the previous pregnancies had occurred, what disruptions in the marital relationship they had entailed, and how this pregnancy would predictably alter the family system. The counselor consistently encouraged the couple to think about how they had made decisions in the past and what kinds of considerations should go into making the present decision. Although anxiety and distress were evident and pervasive, the counselor did not focus on them directly, but rather attempted to engage the thinking processes. The couple did agree to continue the pregnancy and to have the child. Mrs. N. decided she could delay graduate school until the child was about six months old, but that she would continue to take courses in spite of Mr. N.'s disapproval until she was ready to deliver. She was clear about her career goals and also was sure she could combine being a wife and mother with having a career. Mr. N. grudgingly agreed.

In this family, functional adaptation had begun. The family appeared to function at a fairly high level of differentiation and the situational stresses produced a temporary dysfunction. It is interesting to note how many times children are the ones who call attention to increased stress in the family system. Though there is nothing they can do about it per se, they *can* manage to direct the family's attention to the fact that something is going on. If the health care professional is sensitive to thinking in terms of families, problems with children can no longer be seen as concerning only the children. One begins to appreciate that children live in families, that families are systems, and that symptoms are signals of system distress. The child may need attention, but the emphasis should not be on the child, but on the family as a functional unit.

For families willing to work on improving the level of their functional adaptation, this is an arduous, sometimes painful, but eventually rewarding process. Once patterns of adaptation are identified and some modifications started, the exploration of the origin of the patterns begins. Since every individual is raised in a family system, patterns originate in the family of origin. If Mr. and Mrs. N. wished to do so, they could be encouraged to investigate the relationships between them and their families of origin so as to gain understanding of their current functional patterns. Not only can one only change oneself, but one can only change things that one understands in a conscious, rational way; otherwise change is not lasting.

SUMMARY

Implementation through functional adaptation is based on a specific theoretical framework. The framework guides the assessment and planning of changes in adaptive patterns. The changes should be ones that the family identifies as necessary and helpful to the family system, and not necessarily those that the professional thinks would be good for the family. Change is a relatively long-term process and is different from symptom relief. The homeostatic forces in the family operate to maintain the status quo and to resist changes in the functioning of the system or in members within the system. Systems concepts apply not only to families, but also to work relationships and social relationships.

Anxiety and stress play a major part in the work of functional adaptation. Anxiety, when it reaches a certain level, precludes thinking and learning and, therefore, must be kept within manageable limits in order to institute change. Any time change is introduced, the system will automatically react with increased anxiety and resistance to the change. Techniques for lowering the anxiety of the system are available, but there is no guarantee that they will work unless the professional who is using them is calm.

If the professional is calm, whatever techniques are used will become more effective. Once the system anxiety is within manageable limits, the family may equate that situation with effective change and consider the problem solved. This may be true for a while, but chances are that, as the perceived stress escalates, the problem will reappear.

People who are least likely to bring problems in living to the attention of health care agencies are those who are more emotionally differentiated. They are people with a more reasonable balance between their rational and emotional processes. However, every family has the potential for dysfunction given enough stress in the system.

Once the system is calm, the work of functional adaptation involves identifying the usual functional patterns and observing the role the self plays in perpetuating those patterns. It is always easier to observe the behavior of others than it is to observe one's own. The next step is to choose to take a different position or a different stand than usual. This different behavior never seems natural or right at first, because it is awkward and difficult to try something new. However, if one is convinced that the changed behavior will eventually lead to improved functioning, one perseveres until the behavior gets new results. The system will then reorganize around the new behavior. It is helpful if the person doing the changing is an important member of the system in terms of having the responsibility and the power to change it. Children in family systems do not have that power and a focus on them does not produce functional change in the family.

Throughout implementation, the professional has a responsibility to teach the family about how systems operate and what can be expected to happen at each step along the way. This not only gives family members useful information for assessing and planning, and for evaluating their own behavior, it also prepares them for system responses and pressures. Information should be given when the system is tranquil enough to allow thought and discussion. Information given when anxiety is high leads to inattention, discounting of information, arguments, and power struggles. Professionals who assist families in the task of improving functional adaptation should be in touch with their own anxiety, what evokes it, and how they handle it. They should confine themselves to working on goals that the family identifies and should direct inquiry into alternatives and options to expand the family perspective if it seems restricted.

REFERENCES

Bowen, M. Theory in the practice of psychotherapy. In P. J. Guerin (Ed.), *Family therapy.* New York: Gardner Press, 1976.

Duvall, E. M. *Family development* (5th ed.). Philadelphia: Lippincott, 1977.

Jackson, D. D. The question of family homeostasis. In D. D. Jackson (Ed.), *Communication, family, and marriage.* Palo Alto, Calif.: Science & Behavior Books, 1970.

Peplau, H. E. A working definition of anxiety. In S. F. Burd & M. A. Marshall (Eds.), *Some clinical approaches to psychiatric nursing.* New York: Macmillan, 1963.

Chapter 19

Behavioral Intervention of Family Feedback Process

Sally M. O'Neill

Every social system has its own contingencies, its instigating conditions, and its particular method of reinforcement (Atthowe, 1966). The family system is no exception. The instigating conditions and contingencies in this case are generated by family members and are the principal determinants of feedback, of how energies are expended, and of whether or not the goals of the family system are achieved.

The purpose of this chapter is to discuss a behavioral approach that can be used in the analysis and modification of interaction and feedback between parents and children, and to suggest a methodology for remediating clinical concerns associated with feedback within the family system.

BEHAVIORAL CONCEPTS

The central focus of any behavioral approach is *operant behavior,* that is, voluntary behavior which operates on the environment, causing consequences. These consequences, in turn, affect the recurrence of the specific operant which caused them. The sequence is:

operant behavior ⟶ consequences ⟶ recurrence or nonrecurrence of operant behavior

Operant behavior is distinguished from respondent, or reflex, behavior as shown in the list that follows.

Operant behavior	Respondent behavior
Voluntary	Reflex activity, i.e., knee jerk, eye blink
Controlled by stimulus that follows it, technically termed stimulus consequences, commonly called consequences or contingencies	Controlled by stimulus that precedes it

The process by which individuals learn the extent to which they can control and be controlled by their environment is termed *operant conditioning.* This chapter will focus on interaction behaviors in which family members are operants, which instigate consequences (feedback) and are, in turn, controlled by that feedback.

Consequences are defined by the concepts reinforcement and punishment. *Reinforcement* is the process in which consequences (reinforcers) occur which *increase* the behaviors they follow. *Punishment* is the process in which consequences (punishers) occur which *decrease* the behaviors they follow. Reinforcers and punishers are always operationally defined by their effect on an individual's behavior. If reinforcers do not increase an individual's behavior, they are not reinforcing for that individual. Similarly, if punishers do not decrease the behaviors they follow, they are not punishing for that individual.

There are two types of reinforcers:

1 *Positive reinforcers,* which are desirable consequences that are added to the environment as a result of a specific operant behavior. Positive reinforcers include
   a primary reinforcers—those which answer biological needs, such as food, water, warmth, sex, etc.
   b secondary reinforcers—those which become reinforcing because they were paired with a primary reinforcer during an individual's reinforcement history. These include toys, tokens, money, praise, attention, etc.
2 *Negative reinforcers,* which can be defined as the removal or absence of something aversive to an individual. Negative reinforcers increase behaviors which avoid or terminate something aversive. An example is the absence of noise after a mother stops her baby from crying by put-

ting a pacifier in its mouth; the absence of noise will reinforce the individual in doing whatever he or she did to terminate the noise.

It is important to view reinforcers in a mathematical way, i.e., as the addition (+) or absence (-) of consequences, rather than to place a "good" or "bad" value judgment on positive or negative reinforcers. Think of positive reinforcers as R+: the addition of a consequence that is viewed as desirable by the individual who receives it. Think of negative reinforcers as R-: the absence of something aversive, something that the individual has been able to remove or subtract from the environment.

There are also two types of punishers:

1 *The addition of an aversive consequence* as the result of a behavior. Such punishers include spankings, yelling, nagging, angry looks, etc.

2 *The extinction,* i.e., *removal or subtraction of a positive reinforcer,* for example, ignoring a behavior which has previously received attention.

	Addition	Subtraction
desirable consequence	positive reinforcement	extinction
aversive event	punishment	negative reinforcement

CONSEQUENCES VIEWED AS INTERACTIVE PROCESSES

Reinforcers and/or punishers can be identified in any interaction between family members. Although the examples in this chapter are typical of parent-child interactions, the same kind of consequences occur in interactions between adults. The important consideration is that each family member provides consequences for every other family member.

Parent-child interaction is a reciprocal process. It includes parents' expressions of attitudes, values, interests, and beliefs, and their care-taking behaviors, as well as children's individual growth patterns, learning potential, and ability to incorporate increasingly complex experiences into their current stage of thinking and functioning.

Events occur in sequence on an interaction continuum between parents and children in which each response to an action can become the cause of future behaviors. It is by this interactive process that both parents and children learn new behaviors (O'Neil, 1977). Behaviors are both the cause and effect of other behaviors.

Consider the following examples:

Situation 1. A mother takes her child into a grocery store. The child starts crying for some candy. The mother is embarrassed by the crying, but says "no." The child screams and the mother immediately gives her a candy bar. The child stops crying.

In this situation, the child was positively reinforced for crying by receiving candy. The mother was negatively reinforced for giving the candy because the crying stopped.

Situation 2. On another occasion, this mother took her child into the store, and the child cried for candy. Her mother went about her shopping and ignored the crying. After a short while the crying stopped.

Situation 3. On a third occasion, the mother took her child into the grocery store and the child cried. The mother became angry and spanked her. The child screamed for a few seconds, then stopped crying.

In each situation the mother was negatively reinforced for stopping the crying, regardless of the method she used. However, the child suffered a variety of consequences for her crying behavior, among them an occasional positive reinforcement (candy bar) for crying. This occasional or intermittent positive reinforcement could exert very powerful control over the maintenance of her crying behavior. In addition, because each method the mother used seemed to work some of the time, she was negatively reinforced to be inconsistent in her approach. To analyze further why this pattern of mother-child interaction was maintained over such a long period of time it is important to consider how reinforcers may be scheduled, and the effect of these schedules on behavior.

Continuous reinforcement is used when teaching a new behavior or when increasing the rate, duration, or intensity of an existing behavior. Reinforcement follows every occurrence of the desired behavior. Following this period of continuous reinforcement, a schedule of intermittent reinforcement is used to maintain the desired behavior. An *intermittent reinforcement schedule* involves the gradual increase in the number of behaviors required in order for reinforcement to occur. Thus, the number of reinforcers are gradually decreased. Intermittent scheduling is important because it strengthens behaviors and ensures their resistance to extinction. The greater the interval between reinforcers, the less likely it is that a behavior will decrease if the reinforcers are discontinued.

It is important to note that intermittent reinforcement is equally effective for desirable and undesirable behaviors. In the previous example, the intermittent reinforcement (candy) that the child received for crying in the grocery maintained her crying behavior.

RECIPROCATION—FEEDBACK AMONG FAMILY MEMBERS

In Kozloff's (1973) attempt to describe interactions in families with autistic children, the family was studied as a system of structured exchanges. Kozloff's use of the term "structured" meant that patterns of interaction were relatively stable and recurrent. He used "system" to indicate that "the exchanges do not exist in isolation, but influence one another."

The exchange was used as the basic unit of analysis, and consisted of two main classes of responses: initiations and reciprocations. Kozloff viewed parent-initiated exchanges as having three steps: (1) the parent initiates with an exchange signal (i.e., directive, question, contract); (2) the child engages in some response (appropriate or inappropriate behavior); and (3) the parent completes the exchange with a reciprocation (reward, ignore, punish). On the other hand, Kozloff viewed child-initiated exchanges as having only two steps: (1) the child initiates by engaging in some response (appropriate or inappropriate behavior); (2) the parent then completes the exchange with a reciprocation (reward, ignore, punish).

It is interesting to note that Kozloff did not add a third step to child-initiated exchanges—reciprocation by child to parent. Nevertheless, Kozloff's work is an important contribution to the development of a standard set of variables to describe family interaction patterns. Such a set of variables is essential if one is to modify therapeutically either child or parent behavior, and thereby restructure family interaction patterns.

Kozloff's approach further suggests that *reciprocation* is a useful term for feedback between family members as distinguished from feedback that the family system receives from the suprasystem (neighbors, school, etc.). Feedback among family members is clinically assessed by analyzing specific reciprocations within the family.

A number of investigators have documented the effects of child behavior on parents, treating the child's behavior as the independent variable and parental behaviors as the dependent variables (Bell, 1968). However, while a variety of child characteristics and behaviors have been identified and studied, none have been viewed as reinforcers, or punishers, to parents.

In order to understand why family interaction patterns have long-term stability it now seems important to take into account that in all exchanges parents receive reciprocation (reinforcers, ignoring, punishers) from their children. The intermittent scheduling of reinforcers to parents may well account for much of the long-term maintenance of disruptive and/or ineffective parent-initiated exchange patterns. Consider the following parent-child exchange:

1 Mother pours milk into a glass saying, "Here's your milk."

2 Child starts crying "I want soda."

3 Mother says, "You can't have soda; now drink your milk."

4 Child cries louder, pushes glass of milk away.

5 Mother pushes milk toward child. "Drink your milk; it's good for you."

6 Child screams, throws milk to floor.

7 Mother says, "OK, you can have soda now, but you must drink your milk later." Gives child soda, then cleans up mess.

8 Child stops crying, drinks soda.

In this situation the child responds to the parent initiation by crying for soda and not drinking milk; the mother reciprocates (*punishes*) by insisting that the child drink milk; the child reciprocates (*punishes*) by crying louder and pushing the glass away; the mother reciprocates (*punishes*) by pushing the glass toward the child and coaxing the child to drink; the child reciprocates (*punishes*) by screaming, and throwing the glass; the mother reciprocates (*positively reinforces*) by giving the child soda; the child reciprocates (*negatively reinforces* the mother) by stopping crying. (Remember, negative reinforcement is the absence or removal of a punisher.)

Obviously the child was reinforced for crying by getting the soda, and the mother was reinforced for giving the soda because the crying stopped. But, not only were they both reinforced for the final behaviors which immediately preceded the reinforcers, they were also reinforced for enduring the sequence of punishing interactions which occurred prior to the reinforcement. In other words, they were reinforced for engaging in and maintaining the whole exchange. In addition, as a result of the reinforcement, they are both likely to engage in similar exchanges in the future. Repeated interactions of this sort generally result in a stable exchange pattern. When reciprocations of long duration occur, such as in this situation, they become accelerated. In the clinical situation, both parent and child seem compelled to respond to each other's punishing responses; neither one is able to change the pattern to one of positive cooperation until, finally, the parent usually gives in one more time. Since punishment occurs repeatedly within the exchange, and since punishment always evokes emotional responses such as anger, parents generally give in because they are afraid of their anger toward the child. They report feeling out of control of most situations involving their child, and may often resort to spanking, followed by giving the child what he or she wanted in the first place.

All behavior is rational when viewed and understood in the content of its occurrence. As a result of an individual's direct or vicarious experiences, behavior comes to be regulated by antecedent stimulus events that convey information about probable consequences of certain actions in given situations (O'Neil, McLaughlin, & Knapp, 1977). These cues, which provide information about reinforcing consequences, are termed *discriminative stimuli.* Initiations which are part of stable exchange patterns become such discriminative stimuli. Initiations become signals which tell family members which exchange pattern is now in effect and which behaviors will be reinforced. For instance, if the previous exchange with the milk and the soda are repeated, the cues are the mother pouring the milk and saying, "Here's your milk." The child will quickly learn that when the cues occur, if she cries enough, she will probably receive the soda. Furthermore, in an effort to control the situation, the parent may suggest as she is pouring the milk, "You have to drink your milk; you will not get soda this time." The child cries anyway, louder and longer than before. To terminate the crying, the parent again gives in and replaces the milk with soda. Instead of discouraging the child, the parent has "set the child up" with the stronger cue (*discriminative stimulus*) by verbally including more reminders of the exchange.

Acceleration of reciprocation is most often seen in clinical situations that center around disruptive child behaviors which the child initiates and the parent finds difficult to control. An example of this is found in the following exchange.

1   Three-year-old Judy gets on the hearth to play.

2   Mother says, "No, Judy, you can't play there."

3   Judy keeps on playing.

4   Mother removes Judy from the hearth. "No, Judy, I don't want you to play there."

5   Judy cries, looks at her mother, gets back on hearth.

6   Mother says, "No, Judy, you know you can't play there; if the fire were going, you would get hurt. Now, I want you to play somewhere else."

7   Judy cries louder, goes back on the hearth with her toy.

8   Mother removes Judy, spanks her.

9   Screaming, Judy goes back on the hearth.

10   Mother says, "Oh, damn! I don't know what to do with you; I guess you can play there for now."

11   Judy slowly stops crying and continues to play.

In this situation, once again, both mother and child were reinforced not only for the behaviors that finally ended the exchange, but for enduring the entire exchange. The child was positively reinforced for crying and going back to the hearth. The mother was negatively reinforced for stopping the crying.

In order to remediate this kind of feedback clinically, the mother must understand how her reinforcers occur in this situation. A strategy is then developed whereby she can be reinforced for controlling the situation. The following strategy was used successfully in this example:

1   Judy started playing on the hearth.

2   Mother removed Judy and said, "No."

3   Judy returned to hearth, whining.

4   Mother removed Judy to her room for a 5-minute time-out period.

5   Judy screamed for 2 minutes, then quieted.

6   Mother opened Judy's door. "You can come out now, if you feel better."

7   Judy came out, began playing.

8   Mother hugged her.

9   Judy hugged her back and continued to play, smiling.

The most useful strategy in breaking up accelerated reciprocation is that of *time-out* (*extinction*) since it removes all reciprocation. In this case, the child received no positive reinforcement for disruptive behavior. The mother was still negatively reinforced because she terminated the disruptive behavior (playing on the hearth) and avoided the entire crying exchange. She had, in effect, been reinforced for being in control of the situation.

Just as accelerated reciprocation can be a manifestation of feedback, so, too, can *decelerated reciprocation.* This occurs when either parent or child receives little or no feedback, and behaviors which support interaction are extinguished (decreased). This frequently occurs when a child is handicapped, for example, with deafness, blindness, or some other condition which inhibits the child from learning appropriate responses to the parents' overtures and initiations. In addition to the child's lack of responsiveness, the parents feelings about the handicapping condition itself, may impair the quantity and quality of their interactions with the child.

Deceleration of reciprocation can also occur when parents and child engage in such punishing interactions that one or the other simply no longer responds, or avoids interaction altogether. This occurs most often when either the child (usually an adolescent) or the parent can leave home.

The impairment in feedback that is most commonly observed clinically is probably a combination of accelerated and decelerated reciprocation.

When a child exhibits many aversive behaviors such as unprovoked whining, throwing food, or biting and pinching, the parents may be so involved with coping with these disruptions that they pay little attention to the child's "good," or appropriate, behaviors. Therefore, reciprocations around disruptive behaviors become accelerated while reciprocations that focus on appropriate behavior or acquisition of developmental tasks become decelerated and sometimes nonexistent. The example that follows was observed during a clinical evaluation.

Peter, a 3-year-old, exhibited disruptive behaviors, such as whining, pinching, biting, throwing food during meals. He also had many developmentally appropriate skills common to 3-year-olds. While it was difficult to know just how his disruptive behaviors began, it was clear at the time of observation that he received a great deal of parental attention because of them.

1 Father announces dinner and attempts to steer Peter toward the table.

2 Peter starts whining but accompanies father and climbs into his chair. Once seated there, he reaches out and pinches father.

3 Father says, "Why did you do that? Here are some peas." He looks at Peter.

4 Peter eats some peas, then tips plate over and bangs spoon on table.

5 "Peter, stop that. Here's your plate; want a sandwich?" Looks at Peter.

6 Peter whines, tries to get down from chair.

7 "No, Peter, it's time to eat. Here's a peanut-butter sandwich."

8 Peter sits quietly, munching on sandwich.

9 No comment or eye contact from father.

10 Peter throws the remains of sandwich at father, then hits father.

11 "Peter, why are you doing that? Tell me what you want. Do you want to get down?"

12 Peter gets down, gets a puzzle, and proceeds to assemble it correctly.

13 No comment from father for approximately 10 minutes.

14 Peter approaches father and bites him on the arm.

15 "Peter, why did you do that? Was that a love bite? Well, I love you too." (Hugs Peter.)

16 Peter then proceeds to sit on father's lap and eat what is left on father's plate.

17 Father holds Peter and helps him to eat.

In this exchange, it is apparent that reciprocation for disruptive behaviors was recurrent and that there were no parental responses for appropriate eating or for assembling the puzzle. Further observations revealed that this was a stable exchange pattern between Peter and his parents.

Assessment of feedback must necessarily:

1   Define the family's goals including both long- and short-term goals which are specific to a given family's life-styles and which consider the needs of each member
2   Identify and specify problems that inhibit the achievement of family goals
3   Identify and specify exchange patterns (behaviors and consequences) which support impaired feedback
4   Determine and specify treatment goals

Intervention then becomes a matter of helping family members to become aware of their interactions and to actively modify the reinforcement contingencies that are perpetuating their present exchange patterns. Intervention requires developing and implementing simple and easy strategies that parents can employ to produce immediate results, as well as longer-term plans to achieve lasting parental competence.

When optimal feedback exists, family members frequently reinforce each other for behaviors that are supportive of a happy, healthy, family constellation. However, the pattern of reciprocal feedback that a particular family develops may support maladaptive and ineffective behavior. When much of the energy within a family is directed toward supporting maladaptive behaviors little is left to achieve family goals.

In discussing their situation, Peter's parents reported that:

1   They felt unable to control Peter's disruptive behavior
2   They felt that Peter's developmental progress was not increasing
3   They often resorted to spanking Peter when Peter bit or pinched them
4   Generally felt that they were incompetent parents

They indicated that Peter responded appropriately to other people, but when his parents were present his behavior seemed to disintegrate.

For this family, parental goals related to Peter included:

1   Promoting his development; since he could talk, but usually did not with them, they wanted to assist him with talking
2   Eliminating his inappropriate behaviors
3   Promoting "good times" together; not expending their energy in fighting with him

It is obvious even from the sample exchange between Peter and his father that their exchange pattern was incompatible with the attainment of these goals. Clinical intervention consisted of sharing recorded observations with Peter's parents, paying special attention to:

1   The length of time they endured Peter's disruptions
2   The reinforcers Peter received for those behaviors

3 The reinforcers the parents got when his disruptions stopped, even if only momentarily

4 The age-appropriate behaviors Peter displayed

5 The utilization of a simple time-out procedure for disruptions

A discussion followed of how opportunities could be arranged to promote these skills and of what would be the appropriate reinforcement. Another major area of discussion centered around how Peter's parents could take advantage of and encourage mutually positively reinforcing interchanges with Peter. These could occur at special play times as well as whenever he was engaging in behaviors which supported positive interaction.

Peter's parents learned to set limits on his disruptions either by "timing Peter out" in his room for a few minutes, or by simply leaving the room themselves. Another observation made one month later looked like this:

1 Father announces dinner.

2 Peter climbs into his chair.

3 Mother says "Good for you, Peter. Have some chicken."

4 Peter serves himself chicken and vegetables.

5 Father talks with Peter about playing ball after dinner.

6 Peter eats—talks with father.

7 Mother joins conversation, and tells Peter, "Such a big boy, eating so well."

8 Peter continues eating throughout meal, talking with parents.

9 Father, looking at Peter's empty dish, says, "Are you all finished, Peter?"

10 "All finished," says Peter.

11 "OK, let's go play ball for a while, Peter."

12 "Yep, let's play ball, Daddy." Goes with father outside.

This work with Peter's family exemplifies one approach to the assessment of feedback within a family system, and demonstrates effective strategies of intervention. It is important to consider specific assessment and intervention procedures within the total context of family life-style values and functioning strategies. Intervention undertaken without an adequate assessment, which should include the articulation of the family's goals, will usually be ineffective for all concerned. On the other hand, it also seems inadequate to base intervention on assessment data that does not identify the interaction patterns that support the behaviors of family members.

SUMMARY

The main concepts of operant behavior were discussed, and were integrated into a systems approach to families. An in-depth analysis of feedback within the family was offered. Assessment of feedback includes the definition of short- and long-term goals and the identification of problems which inhibit achievement of family goals, identification of exchange patterns which support impaired feedback, and the determination of treatment goals. Intervention is accomplished through assisting family members to identify and actively modify the reinforcement contingencies that perpetuate existing exchange patterns.

REFERENCES

Atthowe, J. M. Behavioral innovation: An all-encompassing system of intervention. In D. Harshberger & R. Maley (Eds.), *Behavior analysis and system analysis: An integrative approach to mental health program.* New York: Academic Press, 1966.

Bell R. Q. A reinterpretation of direction of effects in studies of socialization. *Psychology Review,* 1968, **75,** 81–95.

Kozloff, M. A. *Reaching the autistic child: A parent training program.* Champaign, Ill.: Research Press, 1973.

O'Neil, S. Behavior management of feeding. In P. Pipes (Ed.), *Nutrition in infancy and childhood.* St. Louis: Mosby, 1977.

O' Neil, S., McLaughlin, B., & Knapp, M. E. *Behavioral approaches to children with developmental delay.* St. Louis: Mosby, 1977.

Part Five

Family
Directions

Chapter 20

Community Needs
Assessment

Marilyn Peddicord Whitley
Jean R. Miller

The purpose of family-centered health care delivery is not merely to help families cope with existing conditions, but to detect the precursors of dysfunction and to intervene, whenever possible, before maladaptive patterns appear. The prevention of family difficulties in a primary sense may be defined as intervention aimed at avoiding the development of dysfunction. Unfortunately, interventions may not always be introduced until after maladaptive patterns have already emerged. Therefore, a health care professional must adopt measures designed to interrupt or stop the progress of the developing dysfunction. In other words, the interventions made at this point are at the level of secondary prevention. When maladaptive patterns are deeply entrenched in the family system, the health professional endeavors to reduce the dysfunctional effects of irreversible events.

Primary, secondary, and tertiary prevention can be clearly differentiated in work with families. Primary prevention involves altering susceptibility to dysfunction or reducing exposure to risk for susceptible families. Secondary prevention involves the early detection of dysfunction and its reversal. Tertiary prevention is concerned with the alleviation of disability resulting from earlier patterns of dysfunction and focuses on the restoration, to the greatest possible extent, of adaptive family functioning.

Although prevention at all levels may be implemented with individual families, many families do not have sustained contact with health professionals or with the health care delivery system. Some of these families may be at risk, but the risk factor is unknown to the families or to the community of which they are part. If large numbers of families are to derive benefit from prevention programs, whether primary, secondary, or tertiary, the health needs of communities must be systematically assessed.

In such an assessment, a circumscribed community replaces the individual family as the object of professional concern. Approaching the community as client is a means of serving individual as well as collective families, since there is always feedback between the community social system and the smaller family systems of which the community is comprised.

In this chapter some family needs will be identified so as to demonstrate the feasibility of constructing prevention programs based on systematically collected and objectively analyzed data. It is important to identify needs when selecting and studying target populations, formulating responsive objectives, and devising community program activities based on the assessment of needs. A further step, which is of equal importance, is the evaluation of program activities which are or have been offered (Reinhardt & Chatlin, 1977). For example, one segment of a community may need help with parenting issues, while another may need assistance in dealing with problems related to loss, loneliness, and aging. The complex process of need identification, and the methods used for analyzing the collected data are among the components of community assessment dealt with in this chapter.

In order to prevent a problem, one must first discover its presence and dimensions. Moreover, prevention of a problem is rarely effective unless the precipitants, nature, and consequences of the problem are well understood. The etiology and classification of individual family dysfunctions cannot be reduced to simplistic terms. It is the complexity of family life that makes the prevention of either small- or large-scale family problems extremely difficult. However, certain conditions seem to predispose families to difficulties. The public health model categorizes predisposing conditions as environmental, host-related, or agent-related, and provides a foundation on which the community assessment of family issues may be constructed.

ENVIRONMENTAL, HOST, AND AGENT-RELATED CONDITIONS

Environmental aspects of family life include conditions created by variables such as income, education, socioeconomic class, race, and living space. Families living in disadvantaged areas tend to be more restricted socially and to engage in fewer extrafamilial community activities. Although environmental stressors make some families more vulnerable than others to health problems, individual family strengths may counteract negative environmental conditions (Zautra & Simons, 1978). Even though the relationship between environmental stressors and family problems is not always direct, evidence suggests that an amelioration of adverse environmental conditions may prevent dysfunction in many families.

Host-related factors refer to conditions within the family, which are sometimes related to structure and sometimes to function. The number of single-parent families in a community is an example of a host-related factor that results from family structure. Single-parent families often require specific services such as counseling or child care facilities. It is somewhat more difficult to obtain reliable information on family function in the collective sense. The extent of functional problems may be deduced from the number of families represented in juvenile court, but specific problems in the realm of family function are less easy to measure. In some cases, family members clearly recognize their need for help, and are able to articulate this need and approach community agencies. More often, however, problems of family functioning cannot be accurately defined by the families involved. This means that community assessment is frequently of a quantitative and general nature, and does not encompass the specific needs of individual families. This is not to detract from the importance of community assessment; indeed, it is an essential prerequisite for family program planning.

In community assessment a decision must be made: (1) to collect information about conditions affecting family functioning, (2) to collect information about actual family functioning, or (3) to collect both types of information so that relationships between antecedent conditions and family functioning may be documented. For example, it might be assumed, based on data from previous studies, that crowded living conditions are related to family enmeshment or to protective disengagement among family members. A choice might then be made to gather data only about the number of families presently living under conditions described for the purpose of the investigation as "crowded." Alternatively, investigators might decide to obtain the data described above, but also to note the number of families living under defined crowded conditions who exhibit characteristics of enmeshment or disengagement in their operations. If there is a question of the relationship between spatial crowding and family enmeshment or disengagement, it becomes useful to collect information on all three variables. It may be practical to identify only those households which exist under crowded conditions for the purpose of assisting those families over time. Usually the scope of community assessment is restricted by limited resources of time, money, and personnel rather than by limited interest on the part of the investigators.

Agent-related conditions are attacks from outside forces against which the family lacks adequate protection. Disasters such as war, flood, fire, and accident disrupt family organization and destroy family and community resources. Employers or occupations that demand a disproportionate amount of an employed parent's life are other examples of agent-related conditions that affect family life. Although agent-related conditions cannot always be controlled or prevented, their effects may be diminished through early identification of associated risks, and through subsequent intervention.

A preliminary step, then, in assessing community needs is to decide what conditions should be investigated. This decision usually is based on community history, a review of literature related to the suspected problems, and relevant data already available in the community being studied. As was indicated earlier, the public health approach undergirded by basic epidemiological techniques may be used to discern patterns and describe conditions in a population of any size. Assessing needs and planning appropriate prevention programs usually are done in the following sequence:

1   Define the community
2   Measure the rate or amount (morbidity) of dysfunction in the community
3   Apply information about the natural history of the dysfunction in question by identifying and classifying the community according to susceptible, presymptomatic, and dysfunctional families
4   Use information about the stages of disability due to dysfunction to note actual functional deficit and duration of disability
5   Apply the concepts of primary, secondary, and tertiary prevention in planning and executing a prevention program (Mausner & Bahn, 1974)

The defined population is the community of interest, delineated by discrete boundaries such as a mental health catchment area, a school district, or an area served by a particular public or private agency. If the defined population consists of a large number of families, it may be necessary to obtain a sample of families that is representative of the total population under consideration. There are a number of ways to sample a population and anyone implementing a large-scale needs assessment program should be aware of the different sampling methods. The simple random sample is the basis of most sampling plans and is most commonly used. In this type of sample, every family has an equal chance, or probability, of being selected. However, random sampling can only be used when all the families in the population of interest can be identified. Since the procedure is costly and time-consuming, other types of approaches for obtaining information about families in a defined community may be employed.

NEEDS ASSESSMENT APPROACHES

Seigel, Attkisson, and Cohn (1974) divided needs assessment approaches into the community nonsurvey, the social and health indicators, and the community survey approaches. Warheit, Bell, and Schwab (1974) subdivided these categories into five specific approaches as follows:

1 The *key informant* approach
2 The *community forum* approach
3 The *rates-under-treatment* approach
4 The *social indicators* approach
5 The *field survey* approach

These approaches may be used independently or in various combinations.

The key informant approach is based on the opinions of those who already know the needs and health services utilization patterns of the community. Such individuals include administrative and clinical staff of health centers, public officials, and clergypersons. Information is relatively easy and inexpensive to obtain in this manner, but the possible bias of individual views should be kept in mind.

The community forum approach is similar to the key informant approach except that opinions are solicited from all segments of the population. Members of the community are invited to attend a meeting, or series of meetings, in which the needs of the community are discussed. Again this is a relatively easy and inexpensive approach which may contribute greatly to future program involvement. Its potential drawbacks stem from impressionistic information, unrepresentative attendance, the possibility of negative outcomes, and unrealistic expectations of participants.

The rates-under-treatment approach is based on the number of persons who utilize health care services in the community. Community needs are estimated by ascertaining the number of people who have received care. Agency records often include data about the presenting problem(s), the frequency and duration of treatment, and sociodemographic characteristics. The availability of data at a relatively low cost is an advantage of this approach, but great care must be taken to guarantee the anonymity and confidentiality of the persons who received the care from the designated agencies. A disadvantage of this approach is that the assessment is based on data regarding persons who obtained care in the identified community. Other persons may have gone elsewhere for help or may not have sought help despite unmet needs. Unmet needs for which services are not available would not be detected by the rates-under-treatment approach.

The social indicators approach is based on selected factors, or indicators, which have been found to correlate with persons and families in need. Inferences of need are drawn from descriptive statistics found in public reports and records. Common indicators are the spatial distribution of people and institutions, sociodemographic characteristics, social behavior and well-being of people, and general social conditions. Specific indicators of disorganized families include divorce, single-parent families, child abuse, spouse abuse, and overcrowding. The availability of data from existing records in the public domain makes this approach feasible in most communities. A disadvantage is that often there is no direct relationship between the indicator and the associated need. For example, single-parent families may be an indicator of family instability in some groups, but not in others. It is dangerous to infer that a factor such as low socioeconomic status is an overall indicator of family instability, since some lower-class families function as well or better than some upper-class families. The choice of indicators and the corresponding interpretation must therefore be made with great care.

The survey approach is based on data obtained from a sample or an entire population living in a defined community. Data usually is collected through telephone or personal interviews or through mailed questionnaires. When it is not possible to contact each family in the population, a method must be devised to obtain a representative sample of the population. Any good sample must meet four broad criteria (Kish, 1965).

1 The sample should be selected based on the goals of the survey. If the goal is to assess the needs of all families in the community, the sample should be taken from the entire population of families. If, however, the needs of disorganized families only are to be assessed, the sample should be obtained from all disorganized families rather than all families in the community.

2 The sampling design should be such that an estimate can be made of sampling variability as expressed by the standard error.

3 The plan for obtaining the sample should be clearly described and practical to implement.

4 The costs should be economical in relation to the results.

The questions asked in a survey should be designed so that they have a direct relationship to the goals of the survey. The questions should be stated in a way that is clear to all segments of the sample. The format of the questions can be either structured or unstructured; however, the analysis of the answers that is to follow should be kept in mind when designing the questions. Consideration should be given to the respondents' reactions to the questions, the ease of coding the data after it is obtained, and the desired statistical method for analyzing the data.

The survey approach is best used to obtain specific information from families. It can be helpful in determining the needs of marginal families who are in equilibrium but who might benefit from outside assistance. The effectiveness of this approach depends, however, on the willingness of the respondents to answer the questions. If the return rate is poor, this can affect the validity and reliability of the results even though the original sampling design was representative of the population. Also, the high cost of this approach should be weighed in relation to the outcomes. In many instances the expense is acceptable, since this may be the only way to obtain the desired information.

PREVALENCE RATES

There are many ways to analyze data collected through the various needs assessment approaches. The discussion in the remainder of this chapter will be limited to calculating the rate of morbidity or family dysfunction in a defined population by using prevalence rates. In order to establish prevalence rates the professional needs to know the number of families in the community defined as dysfunctional by a preexisting set of criteria at some point in time. The rate is then established by dividing the number of dysfunctional families by the sum total of families in the community. The equation looks like this:

$$\text{Prevalence rate} = \frac{\text{number of existing cases of dysfunction}}{\text{total number of families in community}}$$
at a point in time

For example, the defined population might be the local school district, which serves 20,000 families. The defined dysfunction could be expressed as "inability to prepare children for school." This could be determined by the inability of any one child in a family to make a satisfactory adjustment to kindergarten in the combined areas of social, academic, and emotional skills.

Prevalence information is computed by establishing diagnostic criteria and applying them to all families in the district in a particular time frame. For example, suppose that of the 20,000 families served by the district on December 1, 500 had at least one child who had not made satisfactory adjustment in kindergarten. The rate would be: $\frac{500}{20,000} = .025$; that is, 25 families per 1000 in the district were unable to present a kindergartner with adequate skills for adjustment to school as defined by the criteria.

If one wished to change the focus of interest to only those families at actual risk, that is, families with kindergartners in the present year, such a calculation could be done by use of the same formula for prevalence rates. One need only "shrink" the denominator to the population at risk and the numerator to cases from that denominator. The formula would look like this:

$$\text{Prevalence rate} = \frac{\text{number of cases of dysfunction found in kindergartners}}{\text{number of families with kindergartners}}$$
$$\text{at a defined point in time}$$

Suppose that there are 400 families in the district who have kindergarten children in a particular school year. Using present diagnostic criteria, 50 out of 400 families have a child who is unable to make a satisfactory adjustment. That is, $\frac{50}{400} = .125$, or 125 out of 1000 families, have the dysfunction called "inability to prepare children for school" this school year.

Calculating prevalence rates over a period of several school years allows the health professional to observe fluctuations from year to year and helps establish priorities when designing a prevention program aimed at families with preschoolers. Prevalence rates are not based only on new cases (incidence)—they also show the amount of residual dysfunction in the community (duration). If a program is implemented that helps to reduce either the occurrence of cases or the length of time a case lasts, this will be reflected in prevalence rates. Therefore, it is advisable to gather new data from the entire district every few years to see whether the prevalence of the dysfunction has been lowered. The entire process is completed by comparing the rates in one community with those of a similar community or of all similar communities in the state or the nation. In many areas of family dysfunction, however, rates for comparison are not available.

When the amount of dysfunction in a community has been assessed, the next step is to discover what is known about the natural history of that particular dysfunction. In some areas of family dysfunction, e.g., situational and developmental crises, historical data are readily available. In other areas of family dysfunction, such as child abuse, abandonment, or drug abuse, data are inadequate or unreliable.

In the example of the kindergarten children, it is useful to remember that some of the families identified as dysfunctional may have been dysfunctional over several generations, while others may have had a single causative factor with which they were unable to cope or find adequate help for. It is the job of the person interested in prevention to discern the stage of disability, since stages dictate the intensity of prevention needed.

CLINICAL EXAMPLE: PLANNING THE PREVENTION PROGRAM

The kindergarten example lends itself to considering prevention. After the assessment, the health professional knows that, in a particular school year, 50 families out of every 400 who have kindergarten children were unable to present a child capable of adjusting to the district's standards in kindergarten. Given that the criteria are sound and the data collection methods accurate, a closer look at those 50 families seems warranted. Just who are they, where do they live, what is their economic level, of what race are they, how many adults are in the home, what kind of a history does each family have in regard to past generation's ability to perform in school, etc.?

Let us suppose that consideration of those criteria led to the discovery that 30 of the 50 families were members of ethnic groups of color, were headed by a single parent with less than a high school education, had no income other than public assistance, and lived in a housing project. For those 30 families it would seem reasonable to plan a primary prevention program aimed at trying to reduce their susceptibility to dysfunction. Some of the options are: increasing the family head's educational and job training levels, helping the family find a less crowded neighborhood in which to raise their children, or providing an educational program for the children and their parents before entry into school. The health care provider in this example might choose the last option and try to get a Head Start program begun in the area. This would be a primary prevention program.

For 10 of the 50 families, the health provider found no commonalities regarding residence or the economic or educational level of the parents. Most were two-parent families. Since no common risk factors were identified, it might be decided that these 10 families would benefit most from a secondary prevention program in which reversal of the newly detected dysfunction was attempted. The health provider might organize an educational program that involved acquisition of social skills through structured group play for the children while upgrading the parents' level of knowledge about growth and development. Extra emphasis on increased academic opportunity at school would also be encouraged at home through choice of family time together (e.g., increase reading, educational outings, and educational television).

The remaining 10 families seemed to have serious difficulties in many areas not amenable to educational approaches. Some of the parents were abusers of alcohol, some were child abusers, some were away from home for long periods of time due to work-related causes, some were mentally ill, some physically ill, and some had a combination of several of these factors. In short, these families would need a very different program from that of the others surveyed. For this group the health provider might consider a family therapy program to provide tertiary prevention aimed at restoring family functioning sufficiently to allow the children to adjust to school. This program would last longer and would have to be supportive in many more areas than the first two programs.

SUMMARY

Prevention programs begin with a clear understanding of the needs of the community. Needs were broadly classified as environmental, host, and agent-related conditions. The assessment of these conditions can be made through one or more of the following needs assessment approaches: key information, community forum, rates-under-treatment, social indicators, and field survey. Data obtained from these approaches can be used to determine prevalence and incidence of dysfunctional family conditions.

These steps, of course, are reductionistic. Public health planners cannot plan and execute a prevention program of any kind without considering many extraneous factors such as administrative support, economic backing, community acceptance, and available resources. However, to avoid prevention programs solely because of obstacles constitutes a grave disservice to the families served by a professionally staffed agency.

REFERENCES

Fox, J. P., Hall, C. E., & Elveback, L. R. *Epidemiology, man and disease.* New York; Macmillan, 1970.

Kish, L. *Survey sampling.* New York: Wiley, 1965.

Mausner, J. S., & Bahn, A. K. *Epidemiology: An introductory text.* Philadelphia: Saunders, 1974.

Reinhardt, A. M., & Chatlin, E. D. Assessment of health needs in a community: The basis for program planning. In A. M. Reinhardt & M. D. Quinn (Eds.), *Current practice in family centered community nusing* (Vol. 1). St. Louis: Mosby, 1977.

Siegel, L. M., Attkisson, C. C., & Cohn, A. H. *Mental health needs assessment: Strategies and techniques.* Washington, D. C.: National Institute of Mental Health, 1974.

Warheit, G. J., Bell, R. A., & Schwab, J. J. *Planning for changes: Needs assessment approaches.* Washington, D. C.: National Institute of Mental Health, 1974.

Zautra, A., & Simmons, L. S. An assessment of a community's mental health needs. *American Journal of Community Psychology,* 1978, **6**, 351–362.

Chapter 21

Anticipatory Family Guidance

Jean R. Miller

The overall goal of preventive health education for families is to provide
family members with skills that will maximize their potential for healthy living. *Anticipatory guidance,* a form of preventive health education, helps individuals anticipate difficult situations which might arise and teaches them
how to prevent problems, or cope with them if they do arise. During each
stage of the family life cycle, families are faced with certain predictable problems which affect interpersonal relationships. Many families are capable of
coping with critical tasks without external aid, but others are able to adjust
more quickly and easily if they have received anticipatory guidance. The
predictability of certain critical tasks during the family life cycle permits the
broad use of anticipatory guidance as a preventive technique. An approach
for anticipating potential family problems will be suggested in this chapter.
Problem solving is presented as a procedure which health professionals can
share with families in need of anticipatory guidance, and methods for
teaching problem solving to families are included.

Opportunities for anticipatory guidance in family relationships can be found in the broad areas of couple communication, parent-child interaction, and family responses to stresses such as chronic illness. Many programs already exist which endeavor to provide preventive health education for healthy families. Such programs include marriage encounter sessions for couples, support groups for single parents, and parent-training courses such as Gordon's (1977) Parent Effectiveness Training. Special purpose programs are also available for families with ill members, but these usually focus on adaptation to existing problems.

Except in the case of well-child visits, health professionals are likely to have most of their contacts with families which have ill members. This does not necessarily mean that such families are having relationship problems; it implies only that they may be more susceptible to the disequilibrium that can result from long periods of illness in a family member. Families facing chronic or terminal illness have the greatest need for the health professional's understanding of the relationship between physical and psychosocial consequences. Current knowledge of the dangers of over- or under-involvement (*enmeshment* versus *disengagement*) associated with chronic illness, and of the stages of grief, provides direction for anticipatory guidance. However, much additional research is needed to define the risks to family functioning and to identify the family configurations most susceptible to problems associated with chronic illness and death.

THE PROBLEM-SOLVING APPROACH

Teaching families merely to comprehend the risks associated with chronic illness or death is insufficient, since this information may increase rather than decrease anxiety. Families need to be warned of specific problems to be faced and told how these problems may be handled. Families also need assistance in evaluating information so that effective decisions can be made as problem situations arise. Pridham, Hansen, and Conrad (1977) formulated a problem-solving approach as a method for teaching persons how to face and adapt to stressors. The value of the problem-solving approach is that families can be taught to handle expected as well as unexpected problems. The seven phases of problem solving suggested by Pridham et al. are (1) scanning, (2) formulating, (3) appraising, (4) developing willingness or readiness to solve problems, (5) planning, (6) implementing, and (7) evaluating. These phases can be adapted for use with families as well as with individual patients.

Families can be alerted to potential problems by discussing with them some of the problems they conceivably will face. It is helpful for families to know what behaviors and attitudes frequently precede or follow various problems. For example, signs of overinvolvement or enmeshment between family members might include rising tension in the system because a parent is spending most of his or her time with an ill child while neglecting the spouse and the other children. Another sign of enmeshment which the family should learn to recognize is the overdependence of an ill member on another member. In this situation, the growth of the dependent member and of the supportive member may be equally impaired.

During the formulating phase, families need to explore factors or events which are distressful to one or more members. Reactive feelings may be expressed in this phase, but members also need to remind one another to be specific in locating the sources of stress. When possible, various aspects of the problematic issue should be explored.

Family members next need to appraise the issue and determine if it is important enough to warrant intensive exploration. When one member of the family is unwilling or unready to solve problems, attention needs to be given to that member. This is essential because the family system is profoundly influenced by each member, and resistance on the part of one member can be detrimental to an adaptive solution. The readiness to solve problems is linked to the values placed on a desired outcome, since values affect how information is processed and how decisions to act are made. Resistant family members may need the time and the opportunity to explore a variety of behaviors before they are ready to engage in problem-solving activities. The interrelationship of knowledge, values, and behavior makes it necessary to shift emphasis according to the needs and goals of all family members. Changes in behavior are the most desired outcome, but behavior is dependent upon what families want or value, and how they perceive the desired outcome (Laufman & Weinstein, 1978).

The next stage of the problem-solving approach is planning how the problem(s) will be solved. This means determining what changes will be made by whom, when, and in what order. For example, if several family members believe they are not getting enough recreational time because of the responsibility of caring for an ill member, the comprehensive plan should indicate how much recreational time is desired, how this time could be arranged, whom the plan would affect, and when the plan would be enacted.

The implementing phase, according to Pridham, et al., may include as many as four subphases: orienting, guiding, developing decision rules and problem-solving strategies, and practicing. During the first, or orienting, subphase, family members discuss their understanding of or feelings about the issue and what they hope to achieve from resolving the issue. During the second, or guiding subphase, the family may want assistance regarding alternative approaches, although the solutions suggested by family members often provide an adequate range of choices. In the third subphase, the plan of action is selected and clarified. Specific strategies are chosen for obtaining the expected goals. In some cases, families may next want to practice the plan of action before putting it into action. This is the fourth subphase. In this situation family members may engage in role playing to see how they would interact with one another under various circumstances.

The final phase in the program-solving sequence is the evaluating phase, in which the family discusses the selected strategies to determine if they are clear and appropriate. Subsequently, family members compare the goals they have attained with the goals they had expected to attain. It is important that expected outcomes be clearly defined so that the family has an accurate assessment of progress. "Feeling better" is a pleasing evaluation, but the progress of the family is more likely to be reinforced if specific changes can be identified. Such adjustments as the mother being freed of responsibility for two afternoons each week instead of none, or the number of family quarrels decreasing from ten to three each week can be rewarding to the family if the progress is clearly noted.

TEACHING STRATEGIES

Learning how to solve anticipated problems of family functioning can be accomplished through several methods. The selection of teaching methods should be based on criteria which take into consideration the abilities of the health professional and family, the type of family problem(s), environmental conditions for learning, the number of family members and their background, and the relationship between the health professional and the family members (Hyman, 1974). The teaching method should be such that the health professional is comfortable with it and the learners are capable of benefiting from it. It would be unwise for a health professional to read a cognitive lecture on solving family problems to a family that has had little formal education and little experience with formal statements. The subject matter also dictates the teaching method, since different methods may be adopted depending on whether knowledge, values, or behaviors are being taught. The number of learners and the time and place where the learning occurs will determine whether small group discussion or a combination of lecturing with discussion is chosen. If the learners have little background in the subject matter to be presented, they need to be familiarized with basic terms before they are encouraged to solve problems through discussion. Finally, the teaching method chosen should take account of the relationship between the health professional and learner. Open discussion of family situations requires mutual trust between health professionals and families.

Four commonly used teaching methods are independent reading, lecture-discussion, group discussion, and role playing.

Independent Reading

Recently there has been a proliferation of self-help and health promotion books which have had a wide appeal. In a study of consumer preferences for learning methods, subjects from all socioeconomic classes indicated that they preferred reading about approaches to parent-child interaction to discussing such matters with health professionals, or watching movies or slide-tape shows on the subject (Miller, Roghmann, & Saunders, 1979). Although the reasons for this response are unclear, they may be related to economic factors or to consumers' perception of the roles of health professionals. Pamphlets and reading material of one kind or another have been displayed in clinics, doctors' offices, and hospitals for many years, but the effectiveness of pamphlets in promoting health behaviors is questionable (Miller & Pless, 1977). Although reading materials are the least expensive form of preventive health education, the limited number of reliable books on family functioning and anticipatory guidance designed for consumer reading restricts their usefulness.

Lecture-discussion

The lecture presentation is an efficient and interesting way to convey knowledge, but it is difficult to assess the level of learning which occurs. Through information received from the lecture method, patients and their families are likely to comprehend the risks to family functioning associated with illness and death, and learn of some appropriate approaches for handling related problems; they are, however, unlikely to apply this knowledge to their own situation unless applications are suggested in the lecture. Health professionals using the lecture approach need to present information and then provide a situational model for applying, analyzing, and synthesizing it. This can be done by using examples in which the lecturer demonstrates problem solving on issues which are relevant to the learners. When using the lecture method, it is important to convey the purpose of instruction clearly through a careful review of the key points covered. The content must be presented in a stimulating manner, and a summary should be made at the end of the presentation. Active learner participation should be encouraged throughout the lecture by the use of questions and demonstrations.

Group Discussion

The discussion method is most effective when used with small groups consisting of a single family or of members from several families. Discussion groups are best designed to teach alternative ways of handling possible problems rather than to explore deeply those problems which already exist. Therefore, participants should be encouraged to discuss issues rather than their personal opinions and responses. In the area of family relationships, it is helpful if, before coming to the group, members read material related to the issues to be discussed. If adequate materials are available and if all members have prepared for the discussion through prior study, the group can proceed easily through the sequential steps developed by Hill (1977, p. 23). These are:*

1 Define terms and concepts used in the study materials.
2 State the overall purpose of the assigned readings.
3 Identify major themes and/or subtopics.
4 Allocate time for discussion of each theme
5 Discuss the major themes and subtopics
6 Integrate the material with other knowledge.
7 Apply the material to relevant family problems.
8 Evaluate the way the study material was presented.
9 Evaluate group and individual performance

Past experience with small groups has shown that, all too often, the group leader was expected to perform tasks and roles for which group members should have been responsible (Hill, 1977). More recently group members are being encouraged to perform all the tasks and roles which facilitate a discussion in which all participate. Hill (1977) has defined the sequence of task roles which must be performed in any group discussion by any member. According to this sequence, someone in the group must initiate the discussion; give and ask for information; give and ask for reactions; restate and give examples; confront and test reality; and clarify, synthesize, and summarize. In the beginning sessions it is the leader's responsibility to teach the group how to perform these roles so that individual members become capable of exchanging and distributing responsibilities. Group members also need to accept the overall task roles of directing the discussion through the nine major steps listed above, keeping watch on the time, evaluating group and individual performance, and setting standards for the level of discussion. Finally, members need, when necessary, to encourage free expression in order to regulate tension (Hill, 1977). In this group context, health professionals relinguish leadership tasks or roles in order to become active group members. This fosters group interaction that clarifies thinking through the assumption of tasks which promote effective group process.

*This data is from "Group Cognitive Map" in *Learning thru Discussion: Guide for Leaders and Members of Discussion Groups* by Wm. Fawcett Hill, © 1977, 1969, 1962 by the Author, p. 23. By permission of the Publisher, Sage Publications, Inc. (Beverly Hills/ London).

Role Playing

Role playing is an effective teaching method which can be used to supplement lectures and discussions. Role playing may be done through simulations, sociodramas, and dramatizations, and it has the advantage of engaging families in experiential learning. *Simulations* are replications of family behavioral processes such as the reenactment of past behaviors. *Sociodramas* encourage group problem solving through the spontaneous enactment of real-life situations. This differs somewhat from *dramatization,* which follows a script of role enactment decided on in advance by family members in collaboration with the health professional.

Role playing is an effective technique for clarifying the steps of problem solving and encouraging their application. In addition to gaining insight about family behavior and processes, family members learn to cooperate with one another by understanding the reciprocal nature of role enactment. Role playing also reveals family behavioral patterns to the health professional. These patterns can then be evaluated and the progress of the family determined.

The health professional is responsible for introducing certain measures to enhance productive role playing (Hyman, 1974). First, the health professional must prepare the group by briefly describing the situation to be enacted. Second, he or she should delineate the problem situation by explaining the scenario or presenting the roles. It is essential to make sure that participants understand the situation which is to be enacted. Third, players are selected to act out the agreed-upon situation. If possible, volunteers should be sought, since volunteers tend to be more spontaneous than appointed players. Fourth, the players begin to enact the situation. Fifth, the health professional may interrupt the role playing either at his or her discretion, or when the players request it, or when the acting appears significant or insignificant, or when some discussion of the action is needed. Sixth, the health professional should debrief, or review, the enactment by asking how family members responded to the role playing and whether problem solving went well or poorly. Finally, the health professional should summarize, generalize, and conclude, with the help of the participants.

Family Sculpting Another type of role playing is family sculpting. This differs from simulations, sociodramas, and dramatizations in that it is a nonverbal exercise in which family members physically arrange themselves in positions which symbolize their emotional relationships with one another. Family members' posture and their spatial relationships express behavior and feelings as these exist within the family. The goals of sculpting are to teach families how to (1) observe their own interaction, (2) notice problems in relationships rather than in individuals, and (3) develop an awareness of family behavioral patterns which have continued from one generation to the next. The main advantages of family sculpting are that it forces families to communicate with one another without intellectualizing, becoming defensive, or projecting blame; it also compels families to view themselves as a system in which each person affects every other person. Family sculpting can be used as an educational method to detect problems before they escalate into crisis proportions (Papp, Silverstein, & Carter, 1973).

HEALTH BELIEF MODEL

No discussion of preventive health education would be complete without some mention of the Health Belief Model (Becker, Drachman, & Kirscht, 1974). This model explicates the factors which affect the likelihood that individuals will follow recommendations for preventive health action. The model has generally been used in the prevention of physical problems, but the major variables are applicable to psychosocial problems as well. The principal variables covered by the theory are perceptions of cues to action, perceived susceptibility, perceived severity, perceived benefits, and perceived barriers to action. Perceptions of cues to action include the influence of advice and teaching programs, newspaper or magazine articles, and mass media campaigns. According to the theory, a family must feel susceptible to a relationship problem in the system and must view this as serious before the recommended preventive action will be followed. The family must also perceive the benefits to be derived from taking action as greater than the barriers to taking action. For instance, families must view the goal of healthy communication as being worth the effort involved in obtaining anticipatory guidance. Additional variables which are deemed important by the Health Belief Model in assessing family receptivity to preventive recommendations are: (1) general health motivation, (2) resusceptibility to the problem, (3) general faith in health care providers and the health care system, and (4) practitioner-patient relationships (Becker, 1977). Each of these variables requires research in order to determine to what extent it predicts preventive health behaviors. Further research also is needed to adapt this model for individuals to use with families.

SUMMARY

Anticipatory guidance was defined as a viable form of preventive health education for families. The need for offering specific guidance whenever possible was stressed. It is, however, difficult to predict fully the problems which families might conceivably experience throughout the family life cycle. A problem-solving approach was suggested as an effective means of coping with unexpected problems. The problem-solving phases of scanning, formulating, appraising, developing willingness or readiness to solve problems, planning, implementing, and evaluating were enumerated and described.

Four teaching strategies—independent reading, lecture-discussion, group discussion, and role playing—were discussed and their advantages were compared. The need to consider factors related to family values and preferences when selecting a teaching method was emphasized.

Finally, the elements of the Health Belief Model were enumerated. This theory has applicability for predicting family health behaviors associated with family functioning; however, much research must be undertaken in order to establish clearly the risks families may face in various circumstances and the degree to which the Health Belief Model can predict necessary family preventive action.

REFERENCES

Becker, M. H. Recent studies of the Health Belief Model. Presentation at the workshop/symposium on compliance. Hamilton, Ontario, Canada, May 25, 1977.

Becker, M. H., Drachman, R. H., and Kirscht, J. P. A new approach to explaining sick-role behavior in low-income populations. *American Journal of Public Health,* 1974, **64**, 205–216.

Gordon, T. Parent effectiveness training: A preventive program and its delivery system. In G. W. Albee and J. M. Joffe (Eds.), Primary prevention of psychopathology. (Vol. I: The issues). Hanover, N.H.: University Press of New England, 1977.

Hill, W. F. Learning thru discussion. Beverly Hills, Calif.: Sage Publications, 1977.

Hyman, R. T. Ways of teaching (2nd ed.). Philadelphia: Lippincott, 1974.

Laufman, L., & Weinstein, J. Values and prevention. *Health values: Achieving High Level Wellness,* 1978 **2**(5), 270–273.

Miller, J. R., & Pless, I. B. Child automobile restraints: Evaluation of health education. *Pediatrics,* 1977, **59**(6) 907–911.

Miller, J. R., Roghmann, K., & Saunders, S. Consumer preferences for health teaching methods. Unpublished manuscript, University of Rochester, 1979.

Papp, P., Silverstein, O., & Carter, E. Family sculpting in preventive work with "well families." *Family Process,* 1973, **12**(1), 197–212.

Pridham, K. F., Hansen, M. F., & Conrad, H. H. Anticipatory care as problem-solving in family medicine and nursing. *The Journal of Family Practice,* 1977, **4**(6), 1077–1081.

Chapter 22

Maintenance of Family Equilibrium

Marilyn L. deGive

FACTORS WHICH AFFECT FAMILY ADAPTABILITY

How effectively a family unit can maintain equilibrium when faced with stress-inducing events depends upon a number of complex factors. The socioeconomic position of the family, its kinship network, its history as a functioning unit, or its stage in the family life cycle all have an effect on recovery and reorganization. If the professional is to help families adapt to stressful life events, salient variables must be studied in a framework which takes account of changes over time in all facets of family life.

Continual changes within families are a constant threat to family health maintenance. Changes in number of members, roles, or settings require flexibility and adjustment in order for the family to survive. Over the course of the family's life cycle, internal resources will vary according to the economic, social, and emotional status of the family unit. How appropriately the family modifies its boundaries, protects its structure, and propagates its values will ultimately determine the extent of the stress produced by change.

The vulnerability of the modern nuclear family to inner turmoil and external societal pressure is one of the major reasons for the decreased adaptability to stress exhibited by most familial units. "Problems and exigencies beset American families from wedding day to dissolution day," Hill (1958, p. 140) wrote in his classic article, "Social Stresses on the Family." However, the role of family values, cohesion, and other resources in deterring a family from dissolution and failure during stressful periods still remains to be empirically evaluated.

The concept of the family as an arena of interacting personalities organized into positions and roles assumes a prominent place in the evaluation of intrafamilial response to stress and crisis (Hill, 1958). The conflict between role expectations and role performance, patterns of internal decision making, and the familial system of values and of norms provide the necessary material for the assessment of a family's coping patterns during health and illness. Because today's family is more dependent upon external resources for the socialization of its members and the protection of its boundaries, and for assistance with its tasks, a degree of flexibility in environmental transaction is essential for the maintenance of the family's structural integrity.

The family can be viewed as a complex social system consisting of intricately related positions with multiple sets of roles and norms (Hill, 1958) and having a variety of objectives. These objectives can be considered as a series of developmental tasks which must be successfully fulfilled if health maintenance and progress through the family life cycle is to be achieved (Rowe, 1971). Different developmental tasks face individual family members and the unit as a whole at set transition points in the development of a family. The completion of these tasks leads to satisfaction and to success with later tasks; failure to complete the tasks causes unhappiness in the family, difficulty with future tasks, and disapproval by society. Thus, the point at which a stressor bisects the life cycle of a family can lead to an increase in familial vulnerability if a transitional crisis is already occurring within the family organizational structure (Hymovich, 1973).

The adaptability potential of a family varies with its ability to retain and to utilize its experiences, its inherent strengths, and its patterns of bonding. During a stressful event, the health maintenance of the family unit is threatened; the security derived from accustomed means of dealing with conflict may disappear; and the expected responses in family interactions may not be forthcoming. The family unit thus flounders under the tension of a situation that can rapidly reach crisis proportions. To assist a family in mobilizing its intrinsic resources to combat the threat of a stressor event, four principal factors in a number of variations must be considered. These

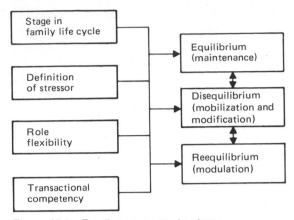

Figure 22-1 Family responses to stress.

are the stressor, the family's definition of the event, the family's resources, and the stage of the developmental life cycle that the family is experiencing (Hill, 1958; Hymovich, 1973).

In any period of stress, for example, stress caused by the illness of a family member, the force of the event is seen in the resulting disequilibrium in familiar structure and in the often inevitable failure to carry out role responsibilities (Hill, 1958). The changes induced by stress *must* be coped with by the family unit. If the family cannot assimilate such changes by mobilizing its resources, dysfunctional patterns of behavior will result (Satir, 1971). Symptoms of disequilibrium in family functioning occur when *dysfunction* leads to *nonfunction* in necessary areas of role allocation, task completion, and decision making. The primary goal must then be the reorganization of the familial unit to regain equilibrium in order to survive. The course of a nuclear family through the changes induced by its readaptation to stress is diagrammed in Figure 22-1.

The initial stage, that of equilibrium, can best be understood by viewing the family unit as a system *in process,* rather than one *in pure equilibrium* (Schvaneveldt, 1973). Since the family's equilibrium is dependent upon the complementarity of roles, i.e., "a role does not exist in isolation, but is patterned to gear in with that of a role partner" (Robischon & Scott, 1973), any small change in normal family life necessitates changes in interior role sets, individual behavior patterns, and general communication pathways. Thus, a family unit must have a certain flexibility or the seemingly ordinary events of the day would throw it into chaos. In most instances, the family is able to balance forces within itself to attain both unity and working order. Family equilibrium is accomplished through setting and fulfilling task objectives, exchanging information within the established pathways of intrafamilial communication and controlling permeability to outside influence from the community and society at large.

The result of the stressor event, and the way the family defines it, may or may not lead to the second system state, *disequilibrium*. At this point, mobilization of resources and modification of structural role definitions are important. The permeability of the family's boundary to the outside environment, the family's potential for absorbing assistance from beyond the intrafamilial organization, and its success at assimilating additional crisis-meeting resources offered by the external world, i.e., the family's transactional competency, become critical factors. Social agencies, kinship patterns, friendship ties, and health and social services personnel can be evaluated in this situation by the extent to which they succeed in alleviating the stress imposed by the event on the family unit. The family's previous experience with outside resources in similar crises, its religious affiliation with church or synagogue, and its economic and social status in the larger community all affect the extent of the crisis and, thus, the family's ability to move into the third stage, that of recovery or reequilibrium.

Another variable which is intimately involved with progress toward family reequilibrium is role flexibility. Roles refer to the pattern of wants and goals, feelings, beliefs, attitudes, values, and actions which members of a family expect to characterize the typical occupant of a position (Robischon & Scott, 1973). Roles are linked to various positions in the family, for example, the "father" position. With the disablement of a family member, the group must either move to restructure its system of positions and roles to adapt to the change in behavioral expectations and performances, or collapse under the strain imposed by a rigid familial structure and an inoperative set of norms. Unless the family group is able to exercise role flexibility, it will be unable to adjust to the crisis-provoking event, to define the illness in realistic terms, or to mobilize its energies and resources to combat the stress imposed. Thus, the problem is not so much how the family defines the crisis, but whether it is able to deal with it in the concrete terms of continued role performance for maintenance of the familial unit.

It is important to remember that the stressor event may be any situation ranging from the death of a family member to the marriage of the last child. A family disturbance in equilibrium may thus be stimulated by change in the family constellation, which then leads to changes in both family organization and interactive patterns (Beatman, 1957). The demand is placed on the family to reorganize its relationships, adapt its functions, and alter its lines of communication, i.e., to modulate its previous patterns of functioning, so that the health of the family group will be maintained. Such adaptive measures may be long-term or short-lived; they may lead to such gross alterations in familial internal structure that a relapse into disequilibrium will occur; they may also establish the primary group at a lower or higher level of task achievement, decision making, or role allocation than the one that prevailed before the stress occurred. In any event, because most families continue to strive toward resolution of conflict, diminution of

Role flexibility (internal resource)	Transactional competency (external resource)	Predicted prognosis
↑	↑	+
↑	↓	±
↓	↑	∓
↓	↓	−

Key

↑ High score

↓ Low score

Figure 22-2   Predicted prognosis for family modulation of stress.

stress, and reorganization of internal structure, each family is likely to move gradually toward the final stage of reequilibrium or recovery, in which the energy of the family unit is once more directed toward the maintenance of group cohesion and integrity. For family units unable to deal effectively with stress, a continuation of the stage of disequilibrium becomes inevitable.

How successful families will be in modulating a family crisis depends upon previous role assignments. Families in which roles have been apportioned equitably and appropriately in the past are most likely to make smooth adaptations in times of stress. Proper role assignment and a good communication system both contribute to the establishment of reequilibrium (Goldberg, 1973).

The resources of role flexibility and transactional competency can be assessed together to aid in the prediction of familial success at reequilibrium stages. A variety of results are possible, as shown in Figure 22-2.

High scores on both variables indicate a compensated family whose needs for professional intervention are likely to be short-term. Such a family should be helped to express feelings about the stressor event and about changes in power relationships and role responsibilities. It also should be encouraged to utilize familial resources in order to increase flexibility for coping with stress. The next category is a high score on role flexibility, but a low score on transactional competency. In such a case, professional intervention might not be accepted by the familial unit. Thus, the family would have to resolve its feelings of rejection before supportive intervention could be implemented. Because of the high transactional competency in the third category, an aggressive family intervention might be instituted. The poorly operating family units in the last category (low score on both variables) require limited objectives and a specifically goal-directed approach toward solving only one part of a larger family problem.

As Figure 22-1 shows, the movement of families through the three stages of stress-induced change toward a recovery of equilibrium can be predicted in terms of two sets of variables.

    1 Factors *internal* to the family, i.e., role flexibility, other familial resources, stage of the developmental life cycle, and the family's definition of the event itself
    2 Factors *external* to the family, i.e., the unit's transactional competency with their kinship network, their community, and society at large

COPING PATTERNS IN FAMILIES

Family coping mechanisms consist of any response to external life strains that serves to prevent, avoid, or control emotional and physical distress (Pearlen & Schooler, 1978). If the family unit is confronted with a stressor event, and if the variables discussed above are considered, the maintenance of family equilibrium may still be in question. Unless the family unit is able to mobilize and identify its resources, to assess and effect structural change, and to modulate and adapt its functioning, it will become enmeshed in conflict and will never attain the reorganization necessary for its survival. Under stressful conditions, families seek answers to the following questions:

    1 How can the distress be relieved?
    2 How can a sense of worth be maintained?
    3 How can a rewarding continuation of interpersonal relationships be maintained?
    4 How can the requirements of the stressful task be met or utilized?
(Hamburg & Adams, 1967, p. 277)

Each nuclear unit must devise its own adaptive process, i.e., its own repertoire of coping mechanisms to avert, diminish, or attack the sources(s) of stress. Coping mechanisms may be both externally and internally directed, i.e., offensive and defensive in nature. Internally, roles must be reallocated, decisions must be made, tasks must be reapportioned, and communication pathways must be altered. Externally, familial boundaries—whether with schools, church or synagogue, business, government, hospitals, or friends and relatives—must be adjusted and reassessed. There are set stages in familial coping progress; differences arise primarily in each unit's ability to mobilize resources for the assimilation of change and the attainment of reequilibrium (Figure 22-3).

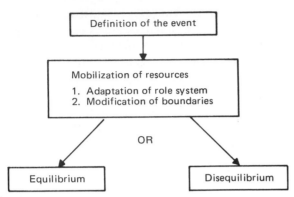

Figure 22-3   Family coping process.

Because individual families vary primarily in the extent of their resources and their ability to mobilize them, their external and internal coping mechanisms should be carefully examined. The *external* variable, i.e., the modification of family boundaries which affect relationships with others outside the family, parallels the transactional competency discussed earlier in this chapter. In this case, however, family supportive resources can be more clearly identified. By exchanging information with the outside environment, adjusting internal response to stress as a result of the feedback received, and allowing and inviting supportive services, the nuclear family increases its available resources and, consequently, its base of power to deal with a stressful event (Hill, 1958). The importance of friends and relatives outside the immediate family in helping the group adapt and adjust to a crisis was determined by Croog, Lipson, and Levine (1972) in a study of 345 men who suffered a myocardial infarction. Although its conclusions were drawn in terms of individuals, the study's emphasis on the need for social interaction to promote external resource utilization and accessibility parallels the family's requirement for boundary openness during stress. It was found that individuals whose social relationships were characterized by mutual visiting and emotional and material support were likely to receive aid from a variety of sources during times of severe illness.

Other external resources to be considered are the family's economic ties to the larger society, their transexperiential contacts with available community services, and their social and kinship relationships. As Speck and Rueveni (1969) noted, the extended family still plays a significant role in nuclear families in the American culture.

The *internal* variable, i.e., the adaptation of internal role systems, assumes even greater importance than the external one as a predictor of families' ability to cope with stress. Without predetermined pathways for conflict resolution or accepted means of decision making, and without bonding for mutual support and empathy, the family unit is vulnerable to the disorganization and disequilibrium that accompany a stressor event. Stress requires a reallocation of roles within the family and a standardization of these roles on a more or less permanent basis (Hill, 1958). The adequacy of role performances on the part of family participants, the precrisis determination of role behaviors and positions (Bahr & Rollins, 1971), and the ongoing structure of power and authority in the primary group all affect and are affected by the stress of crisis. Fink (1968), in studying a sample of disabled women, found changes in the way the disabled women related to others and in how others related to them.

When a disturbance in the equilibrium of role structure occurs, the family has to adapt to the forces of change, attempt variations in previous patterns, and move toward a new balance in interpersonal relationships. How effective the family's attempts to reestablish its structural integration will be dependent primarily on how flexible and interchangeable its role and positional systems are. Adaptation is facilitated when flexibility in roles and function apportionment is characteristic of the family.

The end result of appropriate utilization of resources by the family unit, as illustrated in Figure 22-3, is a decrease in stress and a return to health maintenance. Families who are unable or unwilling to mobilize their strengths to achieve greater flexibility and increased boundary permeability will experience disorganization and defeat.

This pattern of defeat and inadequacy is found in many families who are unable to cope with any stress at all. When the capacity to meet obstacles and to shift course has been exhausted, the family unit has usually had a history of failure to adapt its functioning to the changes wrought by internal and external forces. Each new stress conjures up past experiences of failure to reorganize and to reattain a sense of cohesion and integrity. As Hill (1958) has stated, successful coping strengthens a family, while failure weakens family morale and structure.

Each family thus must learn to surmount innumerable crises during its life cycle, and to reorganize, and reestablish equilibrium in its internal structure; it must also strive to prevent the stress inherent in continued failure and defeat.

The challenge to the health practitioner lies in examining the stages the family system goes through, from homeostasis through change and reorganization, and in translating these concepts into practice. The coping abilities of individual families, i.e., their success or failure in maintaining the health of the family unit, are a function of the recognition and the utilization of resources both internal and external to the family. It is by identifying familial resources and helping to mobilize them that practitioners of every discipline can best achieve positive results in family intervention.

CLINICAL EXAMPLE: MOBILIZATION OF RESOURCES
IN A FAMILY WITH STRUCTURAL-FUNCTIONAL PROBLEMS

The Adams family was referred to the community health nursing agency for: (1) home evaluation of safety features, (2) planning for the necessary physical therapy equipment for activities of daily living, (3) physical-behavioral assessment of Mrs. Adams; and (4) general medical supervision of the family group as a whole.

On the initial visit, the nurse became acquainted with the entire family constellation. Mr. Adams, a 46-year-old white male, had been unemployed for several months due to exacerbation of a chronic back ailment. The family had consequently been living on disability checks for several weeks, since their savings account and financial resources had been depleted. Mrs. Adams, a 42-year-old white female, was returning home from a small community hospital with some residual disability (a left-sided hemiparesis) after having suffered a cardiovascular accident (CVA) 6 weeks previously. In addition, she had a history of poorly controlled hypertension, gastric ulcer, adult onset diabetes mellitus, and obesity. Since Mrs. Adams's hospitalization, Mr. Adams's mother had come to live with the family. Age 68, the grandmother had a long history of depression, and was receiving ongoing treatment at the local mental health center. The two children, a boy, aged 11, and a girl, aged 6, appeared to be in good physical health, but had been without medical supervision for several years because of the family's precarious financial situation.

The Adams home was quite small and cluttered, with the children having to share a room since the arrival of their grandmother. The kitchen was well equipped, but no alterations in layout had been effected there or in the bathroom, despite the predischarge visit to the Adams home made by the hospital's physical therapist and her subsequent suggestions to Mr. Adams. The family was having great difficulty financially; they had not yet received their Medicaid coverage, and were being held responsible for large medical bills that they were obviously unable to pay. Meal preparation and food shopping were sporadic and poorly planned. In addition, Mr. Adams had been informed by the school principal that the oldest child had not been to school for 2 weeks. Mr. Adams expressed much dissatisfaction with the family's present situation and was overwhelmed by the prospect of his wife's return, particularly since she would now be requiring additional care. Mrs. Adams spoke of being "frightened" of coming home; she was especially fearful of no longer being "part of the family."

Assessment

In assessing the family's health status, the nurse evaluated intrafamilial communication patterns, decision-making processes, interchangeability of roles, stage of the family's life cycle, participation in community and kinship network activities, and past history of dealing with stress. This was accomplished through a series of group interviews and ongoing process recordings of family visits. In addition, the nurse administered a tool known as the Family Coping Index (1964) to the entire family group.

Mrs. Adams was also fully evaluated by the nurse, the agency physical therapist, and the occupational therapist. The goals were stabilization of her physical condition, institution of a rehabilitation program, and adaptation of the home setting for Mrs. Adams's independence, despite her residual left-side hemiparesis.

At the point at which the nurse met the Adams family, the group appeared to be engulfed in the stage of disequilibrium. Mrs. Adams's illness, the grandmother's consequent relocation to the family residence, Mr. Adams's inability to return to work, and the oldest child's truancy all were events that had forced this family into immobility. Failure to combat the original stressor event (the CVA), and to readapt its role structure to the consequent changes this incident required, not only increased the family's vulnerability to future problems, but also made such problems inevitable.

The Adams family seemed to be incapable of sorting out its objectives as a unit, of reassigning tasks once performed by Mrs. Adams to other role sets, or of adapting a familial structure to the return of Mrs. Adams and the arrival of the grandmother. Its role flexibility thus was severely limited.

On the other hand, further talks with the family identified some strong resources in transactional competence. The Adams's had long-standing religious ties to their parish church and had formerly been active participants in church and parochial school functions. Both Mr. and Mrs. Adams had several siblings living in the community who were frequent, concerned visitors to the home. In addition, Mrs. Adams's physician was deeply involved in attempting to secure Medicaid coverage for the family; he had also referred the family to the community health nursing agency and to the local poststroke rehabilitation group.

Thus, although the Adams's were structurally lacking in cohesion and in stability at the time of assessment, their functioning as a family unit was still important to them and to many individuals and groups outside of the family itself. The Adams's would belong most appropriately in the third category (see Figure 22-2) of families under stress, i.e., those exhibiting low role flexibility (decreased internal resources), but high transactional competency (increased external resources). The Adams family continued to demonstrate great eagerness to work with various community agencies in the hope of achieving some familial equilibrium.

Intervention

Often, "network therapy" is a most effective therapeutic intervention (Speck & Rueveni, 1969). Network therapy involves calling upon the entire spectrum of the involved family's outside contacts to assist the family in working out its problems. A meeting of concerned relatives and friends provided many benefits to the Adams family. Besides allowing the family to see that there were many caring people outside of its primary group, two of these meetings, held at the Adams home, brought forth concrete options. Mr. Adams was offered a temporary job in a cousin's hardware store until his back problem could be more fully evaluated and more permanent employment plans could be made. In addition, Mr. Adams's mother was relocated to his brother's home, which offered more room and more resources for her care.

Once these two problems had been resolved, the nurse proceeded to deal with the department of social services. Despite Mr. Adams's part-time position, the family's medical coverage, as well as continued disability benefits, were assured. The institution of medical benefits made ongoing medical supervision for the children and Mr. and Mrs. Adams an immediate reality. With greater financial stability, and the convenient adaptations made in the kitchen and bathroom, the Adams family was able to begin group meetings with the nurse to work through much of the unresolved conflict in role changes and communication pathways engendered by Mrs. Adams's CVA.

The oldest child's truancy remained an ongoing problem. However, after several months of group meetings, the family as a whole gained more insight into the causes of familial disorganization and greater confidence in handling future stresses. Mr. Adams assumed many more of the homemaking tasks initially, but was increasingly sensitive to Mrs. Adams's needs to participate in these functions as well. Having Mrs. Adams at home allowed the children to return to a seminormal family situation, despite their mother's continuing impairment (Mrs. Adams ultimately was able to ambulate independently with the use of a quad cane). The children themselves were expected to perform more daily tasks for maintenance of the family unit, and they gradually began to accept these increased responsibilities.

A posttest with the Family Coping Index 3 months after the initial visit showed a marked improvement in conflict resolution and role flexibility within the primary group. Although follow-up visits continue, the family, through the mobilization of both internal and external resources, is considered to have partially recovered from the stressor events and to be in a state of reequilibrium for the present time.

SUMMARY

Two major variables, role flexibility and transactional competency, were defined as predictors of a family's ability to maintain equilibrium through changing life events. The process of family coping was described as a series of stages in which the family defines the meaning of the change and mobilizes its resources by adapting its internal role system and modifying its boundaries. Depending on how successful the process is, the family subsequently either maintains a state of well-being, with alleviation of stress, or becomes disorganized and defeated with minimal or no alleviation of stress.

REFERENCES

Bahr, S., & Rollins, B. Crisis and conjugal power. *Journal of Marriage and the Family,* 1971, **33,** 360–370.

Beatman, F. L. Family interaction: Its significance for diagnosis and treatment. *Social Casework,* 1957, **38,** 111–118.

Croog, S. H. The family as a source of stress. In S. Levine & N. A. Scotch (Eds.), *Social stress.* Chicago: Aldine, 1970.

Croog, S. H., Lipson, A. A., & Levine, S. Help patterns in severe illness: The role of kin network, non-family resources and institutions. *Journal of Marriage and the Family,* 1972, **34,** 32–41.

Family Coping Index. Unpublished tool, Richmond Visiting Nurse Association, John Hopkins School of Hygiene and Public Health and the City Health Dement, Richmond, Virginia, 1964.

Fink, S. Physical disability and problems in marriage. *Journal of Marriage and the Family,* 1968, **30,** 64–73.

Goldberg, S. Family tasks and reactions in the crisis of death. *Social Casework,* 1973, **34,** 398–403.

Hamburg, D., & Adams, J. A perspective on coping behavior. *Archives of General Psychiatry,* 1967, **17,** 277.

Hill, R. Social stresses on the family. *Social Casework,* 1958, **39,** 139–150.

Hymovich, D. The family with a young child. In D. Hymovich & M. Barnard (Eds.), *Family health care.* New York: McGraw-Hill, 1973.

Pearlen, L. J., & Schooler, C. The structure of coping. *Journal of Health and Social Behavior,* 1978, **19,** 2–21.

Robischon, P., & Scott, D. Role theory and its application in family nursing. In A. Reinhardt & M. Quinn (Eds.), *Family-centered community nursing.* St. Louis: Mosby, 1973.

Rowe, G. The developmental conceptual framework to the study of the family. In F. M. Nye & F. I. Berardo (Eds.), *Emerging conceptual frameworks in family analysis.* New York: Macmillan, 1971.

Satir, V. M. The family as a treatment unit. In J. Haley (Ed.), *Changing families.* New York: Grune & Stratton, 1971.

Schvaneveldt, J. D. The interactional framework in the study of the family. In A. Reinhardt & M. Quinn (Eds.), *Family-centered community nursing.* St. Louis: Mosby, 1973.

Speck, R., & Rueveni, U. Network therapy—a developing concept. *Family Process,* 1969, **8,** 182–191.

Chapter 23

Development of Family Conceptual Frameworks

Mary-'Vesta Marston
Bianca M. Chambers

Health professionals frequently use several conceptual frameworks to assist them in working with families. At this time no single conceptual framework is sufficient to guide family assessment and intervention. The purpose of this chapter is to delineate elements necessary for a conceptual framework that is both theoretically valid and clinically reliable. Concepts from developmental, interactionist, and systems theory will be used to illustrate the important elements of any conceptual framework. Finally, key concepts from these three theoretical frameworks will be combined with additional constructs to formulate an alternative, eclectic approach to family-focused care.

Some confusion exists about the definition and use of theoretical and conceptual frameworks in family practice; often the two terms are used interchangeably. For the purposes of this chapter, a conceptual framework is not necessarily synonymous with a theoretical framework. A *family conceptual framework* is defined here as a set of loosely related concepts and assumptions not yet scientifically validated through nursing research (Hill & Hansen, 1960). According to Reilly (1975), a conceptual framework is

416

primarily derived from both empirical data and intuition. A family conceptual framework should serve as a guide to clinical practice until sufficient data are obtained to validate it as theory. Thus, a family conceptual framework may be regarded as a rudimentary stage in theory development.

Well-developed and tested family theories which can be used as bases for practice are not yet available. However, to recommend the exclusive use of current family conceptual frameworks invites premature closure for alternative viewpoints in this area. At present it is desirable for professionals to build their own frameworks for family practice using hypotheses currently presented in the literature. The approach suggested is similar to that of Glaser and Strauss's Grounded theory (1967). According to this formulation, clinical practice can provide the data for building theory, which in turn can be tested in practice.

To be useful to a professional engaged in clinical practice, any family conceptual framework should include the following components:

1 Concepts believed essential to practice, suggested by the literature or by clinical experiences, should be listed. The selected concepts require operational definitions so that careful guidelines can be established for making family assessments.

2 The selected concepts should be interrelated, although in the early stages of developing a conceptual framework they may stand in unstructured and tentative relationships to each other.

3 The set of assumptions on which the framework is based must be explicit. The list of chosen concepts, the interrelationships between concepts, and the assumptions underlying these interrelationships provide a basic framework which the health care provider, in collaboration with the family, can use to determine goals related to outcomes of the intervention.

4 Interventions should be based on available theories and models from relevant disciplines. Examples include Roy's Adaptation theory (1974), behavior modification, and the Health Belief model (Becker, Drachman, & Kirscht, 1974). It is important that the professional be familiar with a wide range of theories and models. Planned interventions should be compatible with the underlying concepts and assumptions of the theoretical model.

5 Criteria for success must be established in order to evaluate the effectiveness of the interventions. Examples of successful outcomes might include: greater knowledge of desirable behaviors or of treatment for an acute disability; actual adherence to a therapeutic regimen; improved control of a chronic condition, e.g., family adjustments when a member has hypertension, diabetes, or glaucoma; family involvement in mental health therapy; or family capacity to accommodate the addition of a new member. The extent to which outcome criteria are met and evaluated provides clues as to whether additional concepts may be required in order to provide further theoretical bases for the evaluation of intervention.

THEORETICAL ELEMENTS FROM THREE
CONCEPTUAL FRAMEWORKS

While developmental, interactionist, and systems theory frameworks have aided countless theorists and clinicians, this does not obviate the need to integrate key concepts from various other frameworks in order to build theory.

Developmental Framework

Erickson's (1959) theory delineates eight stages in the development of the individual. Maturation is essential for the individual to pass from one developmental stage to the next, and is predicated on successful mastery of the critical tasks of the preceding stage. As a unity of interacting individuals, the family also passes through developmental stages with critical tasks specific to each stage. Successful passage from one family developmental stage to the next encourages growth of individual family members and cyclic family progression.

Duvall (1977) regarded family developmental tasks as growth responsibilities accomplished in order to satisfy biological requirements, cultural imperatives, and aspirations. The criteria Duvall used to divide the family life cycle into stages were "(1) plurality patterns; (2) age of the oldest child; (3) school placement of the oldest child; and (4) functions and status of families before children come, and after they leave" (p. 145). Duvall's eight stages of the family life cycle follow.

> **I** Married couples (without children)
> **II** Childbearing families (oldest child birth–30 months)
> **III** Families with preschool children (oldest child 2½–6 years)
> **IV** Families with school children (oldest child 6–13 years)
> **V** Families with teenagers (oldest child 13–20 years)
> **VI** Families launching young adults (first child gone to last child's leaving home)
> **VII** Middle-aged parents (empty nest to retirement)
> **VIII** Aging family members (retirement to death of both spouses) (p. 144).

Duvall wrote that "a family developmental task arises at any point in a family's life when the needs of one or more family members converge with the expectations of society in terms of family performance" (p. 177). At different stages in the life cycle some specific family developmental tasks may take priority over others. Duvall listed the following family developmental tasks as basic to all families:

1 Providing shelter, food, clothing, health care, etc., for its members.

2 Meeting family costs and allocating such resources as time, space, facilities, etc., according to each member's needs.

3 Determining who does what in the support, management, and care of the home and its members.

4 Assuring each member's socialization through the internalization of increasingly mature roles in the family and beyond.

5 Establishing ways of interacting, communicating, expressing affection, aggression, sexuality, etc., within limits acceptable to society.

6 Bearing (or adopting) and rearing children; incorporating and releasing family members appropriately.

7 Relating to school, church, work, community life; establishing policies for including in-laws, relatives, guests, friends, mass media, etc.

8 Maintaining morale and motivation, rewarding achievement, meeting personal and family crises, setting attainable goals, and developing family loyalties and values (pp. 176–177).

Hill and Rodgers (1964) stated that the most frequently used concepts in family development theory deal with definitions of the family, family structure, family functioning, and family patterns or "sequential regularities." Position refers to the location of the family member in the family structure such as the positions of wife-mother or son-brother. Role refers to the actual and expected behaviors associated with a position and defined by the norms of the culture. Examples include parenting, homemaking, and providing financial support. A norm refers to rules or standards shared by family members and by society at large. Rhodes (1977) superimposed a systems theory approach on the developmental framework, describing the family as a social system with the following characteristics:

1 Family members occupy family positions which are interdependent so that a change in one results in a change in the others.

2 The family is a "boundary-maintaining unit with varying degrees of rigidity and permeability in defining the family and nonfamily world" (p. 302).

3 The family adapts, seeks equilibrium, and has repetitive patterns of interaction over time.

4 The family meets the external needs of society as well as the internal needs of its members.

Rhodes (1977) proposed a six-stage developmental life cycle which is somewhat simpler than Duvall's. Rhodes's stages are as follows:

I *Intimacy versus idealization or disillusionment* (Relationship development period prior to advent of children)

II *Replenishment versus turning inward* (Childbearing period from birth of first child to time last child enters school)

III *Companionship versus isolation* (Families with teenage children)

IV *Regrouping versus binding or expulsion* (Families with children in the process of leaving home to establish themselves independently)

V *Rediscovery versus despair* (First postparental period after departure of last child)

IV *Mutual aid versus uselessness* (Second postparental period—retirement to death)

Recently, increased attention has been given to the importance of healthful life-styles. Bruhn, Cordova, Williams, and Fuentes (1977) distinguished between good health and wellness. They view wellness as a "continually evolving and changing process related to the developmental stages of man and the individual's completion of certain developmental tasks" (p. 209). It has been suggested (Bruhn et al., 1977; Bruhn & Cordova, 1977) that certain "wellness tasks" are specific to each stage of the Eriksonian life cycle. Wellness is a condition which continues over time, requiring the individual's initiative, decision making and activity; wellness is dependent upon ability to accomplish the critical tasks of each stage. The presence of some clinical symptoms does not negate wellness in other areas. For example, the wellness tasks for early adulthood include commitment to the marriage partner and the assumption of long-term responsibilities for the family; selecting a career and making a commitment to membership in social groups and organizations; incorporating health habits and practices into one's life-style; and learning the importance and place of noncommitment (Bruhn et al., 1977, p. 216).

Wellness tasks have been assigned to the individual life stages of Erikson. However, one of the characteristics of a developmental task is that it can rarely be accomplished in isolation; successful resolution is dependent on interpersonal contact. Wellness tasks may easily be identified in families at various stages of the family life cycle. For example, the development of personal autonomy in a family with growing children has been reported by Pratt (1976) to be associated with good health practices plus the ability on the part of members to negotiate the health care system.

The developmental conceptual framework is appropriate for the majority of families in America. However, because of its emphasis on alterations in family size and on the socialization of the young, this framework may be less useful in assessing alternate or atypical family constellations. Some professionals prefer to emphasize interactions within the family; others choose an explicit systems approach. The developmental framework does not minimize the importance of interactionist or systems concepts. It merely places emphasis on developmental stages and tasks. By itself, the developmental framework provides the professional with a set of guidelines for family assessment. Further elaboration of wellness tasks for developmental stages of individuals and families may enhance the value of the framework. An important limitation of the developmental framework is its lack of theoretical foundation on which to base interventions once the assessment has been accomplished.

Interactionist Framework

Increased attention is being devoted to defining aspects of interaction, verbal and nonverbal, which are associated with desirable outcomes. The quality of interpersonal relationships within the family, and between the professional and the family, is also of significance in potentiating desirable outcomes relative to health and illness issues.

The interactionist framework has its roots in symbolic interactionism, and focuses on the internal functioning of the family (Schvaneveldt, 1966). According to Stryker (1964), this framework is useful for addressing problems related to socialization and personality organization. The interactionist framework is concerned with communication processes and role performance of family members, and with interactions between members of a family. Family members stimulate each other, and the behavior of one family member is both cause and effect of the behaviors of other family members. Members act according to the way they define the situation. During the process of family socialization, situations are structured for each individual, and common meanings eventually emerge.

Hill and Hansen (1960) listed three major assumptions of the interactionist framework, which are as follows:

1 Social conduct is most immediately a function of the social milieu.
2 A human is an independent actor as well as a reactor to his or her situation.
3 The basic autonomous unit is the acting individual in a social setting.

The applicability of the interactionist framework to families is readily apparent. However, this framework is not without limitations as a foundation for family assessment and intervention.

Central to the concept of interpersonal interaction is the idea that interactions involve more than one person. Thus, the family is a system in which each member influences the actions of all the other members. Also, families interact with social suprasystems. The family of today is dependent upon society's technology to meet its needs. Therefore, it is necessary to consider external forces that influence family socialization.

Schvaneveldt (1966) noted that interaction is a process rather than a state. The value of family assessment is increased by utilizing knowledge of the context in which interaction occurs. This means that being aware of the family developmental stage is basic to assessing interaction processes. In this framework each person is viewed as a developing member in a changing group. Using this framework, members of helping professions can isolate specific problems as family members interact with each other and with the larger society. Thus, the usefulness and applicability of the interactionist framework is expanded by the addition of concepts from developmental and systems theory.

Systems Theory Framework

The family was described in Chapter 1 as a social system possessing characteristics of wholeness, nonsummativity, and equifinality. Major concepts such as family goals, family structure, boundaries, function, feedback, energy, and suprasystem were presented. In formulating an eclectic model, some amplification of systems theory concepts is in order.

According to Chin (1974), "The analytic model of system demands that we treat the phenomena and the concepts for organizing the phenomena as if there existed organization, interaction, interdependency, integration of parts and elements" (p. 49). The boundary determines what belongs inside and what belongs outside a particular system. Varying degrees of permeability exist in different kinds of systems; as a result, the degree to which matter, energy, or information are exchanged will also vary. Systems may experience stress or tension caused by internal interactions of members or external factors in the environment. In interacting with the environment, the family system receives information, or feedback, which is used in its operations. Systems theory assumes that a system tends toward a state of equilibrium, or balance, between forces within the system and those impinging on it from the outside. Systems resist disturbances and attempt to restore balance with the end result of a new equilibrium based on status quo or on change.

The developmental framework provides the means to assess the developmental stage of a family and the corresponding tasks it faces. Developmental tasks influence the total functioning of the family system, and must be carefully taken into account. An interactionist framework describes the communication processes and role performances within the family system and with the environmental suprasystem. Without utilizing concepts provided by the systems framework, there is no way to assess how the parts interact.

AN INTEGRATED FRAMEWORK

Because of limitations inherent in the developmental, interactionist, and systems frameworks, an eclectic framework is suggested which combines selected concepts from each of the frameworks with some new concepts. This new conceptual framework provides an example which might be emulated by practitioners seeking guidelines for clinical practice. To be useful, a conceptual framework must be understandable, pragmatic, and generalizable. Its scope must be broad enough to encompass many needs and situations; moreover, it should possess a sound theoretical foundation.

For the purposes of an integrated framework, *family* is defined as an organization of human beings united through kinship, sharing a common biological-psychological, sociocultural, and environmental milieu. A *family member* is one of a group of unique individuals with commonalities and differences in needs and goals. *Organization* refers to two or more individuals united in the purposeful activities or socialization; it is a dynamic, interacting system (Kantor & Lehr, 1975). *Kinship* refers to bonds established between family members through marriage, birth and/or adoption.

Health care providers interact therapeutically with clients. Family work requires the ability to recognize the myriad features of a family organization, its strengths and weaknesses, and its readiness to accept or reject a helping relationship. The health professional's purpose is to promote a family's positive adaptation to *time, territory,* and *technology* so that it can meet its own core needs of *existence, relatedness,* and *growth.*

Assessment

The proposed framework contains three core needs concepts—existence, relatedness, and growth—as well as three resource dimensions—time, territory, and technology. How a family meets its basic core needs through its resource dimensions provides the clinician with data for assessment and intervention.

Basic core needs are behavioral motivators, and they are defined as needs for existence, relatedness, and growth. The basic core needs for *existence* refer to the maintenance of material and physiological needs. They include not only the basic drives for food, water, rest, and activity, but also the safety needs of security, stability, dependency, protection, freedom from fear, anxiety, and chaos, and formal structure providing order, law, and limits (Maslow, 1970). *Relatedness* needs involve relationships with significant other people. Relatedness incorporates both social and esteem needs, and is largely influenced by the degree of sharing or mutuality present in personal interactions. The exchange of acceptance, confirmation, understanding, and influence are elements. The essential conditions for relatedness involve willingness to share thoughts and feelings (in the positive affective state and in the negative states of anger and hostility) as fully as possible (Alderfer, 1969). *Growth* needs are synonymous with the need for self-actualization. Growth needs involve individual family members in achieving creative, productive goals for themselves and for their environment. The interactions within families provide the opportunities necessary for members to fully realize their potentialities (Alderfer, 1969).

Resource dimensions are the domains within which the core needs are met. *Time* is defined as a quantifiable dimension which is sequential and developmental to the family life cycle (Kantor & Lehr, 1975). *Territory* refers to the dimension of bounded and unbounded distance-regulating space in which family interactions take place (Kantor & Lehr, 1975). Both personal and family space are needed for regulating physical and interpersonal interactions. *Technology* refers to the family's ability to use individual and collective energy to allocate resources to meet its core needs. The family's capacity to act and to maintain itself is dependent on successful use of energy and resources.

This integrated framework requires a number of supporting concepts. *Socialization* refers to the process by which a family, through its interaction in time and territory, and with technology (Tosi & Hammer, 1977), teaches its members the behavior necessary to survive and be effective in the society of which they are a part. The process is accomplished by meeting the core needs of each member for existence, relatedness, and growth (Huse & Bowditch, 1977). *Teaching/learning* is a socialization process in families that involves verbal and nonverbal, and direct and indirect activities, which transmit family and social norms values. Learning is accomplished when norms and values are incorporated into the behavior of family members both collectively and individually. *Society/culture* refers to the social system in which the family lives and interacts. *Norms/values* are beliefs related to meeting the core needs of human beings. Norms and values determine the family's expectations, priorities, and goals.

Families are subjected to pressures from within and without; as dynamic systems families are always in the process of becoming. The primary function and responsibility of the family is the socialization of its members. Recognizing and meeting the core needs of existence, relatedness, and growth are basic to the well-being of the family. To assess how these needs are met, the professional must consider the dimensional influences of time, territory, and technology. Figure 23-1 portrays a systems model of the family, which incorporates the concepts that have just been defined.

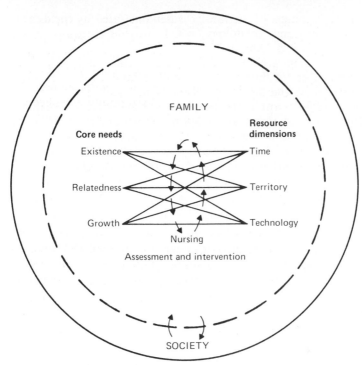

Figure 23-1 Family conceptual framework.

The values and assumptions underlying the proposed integrated framework are as follows:

1 Humans are biopsychosocial beings who operate within environmental constraints (Roy, 1974).

2 Human beings have needs in each of three spheres—biological, psychological, and social—and these needs serve as stimuli for behavior.

3 The behavior of humans is purposeful and goal-achieving; it seeks to satisfy the core needs of existence, relatedness, and growth.

4 The family unit serves as the first and primary mode for satisfying core needs through the socialization process.

5 Needs satisfaction serves as a further stimulus for goal achievement. One is never completely satisfied.

6 The family, as a collective unit, fosters personality development in each of its members by reducing need tension and generating the tension necessary for positive adaptation (Kluckhohn & Murray, 1967).

7 Socialization takes place within a cultural context and is essential to the life of a community (Anderson & Carter, 1974). The family is a subsystem of the community.

8 The cultural context of the family is demonstrated by the dimensions of time, territory, and technology, which provide access to family norms and values (Kantor & Lehr, 1975).

9 Norms and values are influenced by society and the family.

10 The family's use of time, territory, and technology defines roles, communication patterns, and the power of the family and its members.

11 Individual status within the family hierarchy, decision making, concepts of property, and rights and responsibilities are expressions of roles, communications, and power.

12 The family's capacity to act and its power to maintain itself lies in its ability to use energy and resources to meet its core needs. Also, the family is subject to societal influences.

Intervention

The proposed framework provides adequate guidelines for assessing family functioning. However, a conceptual framework does not of itself provide the theoretical foundations for intervention (Sedgwick, 1974). Other theories (Roy, 1974; White, 1974; Dagar, 1964) may be used as bases for intervention. None of these theories by itself provides a firm basis for nursing intervention, but together they are adequate. Roy's Adaptation theory (1974) was based upon manipulating the four human subsystems: physiologic, self-concept, role function, and interdependence. Stimuli which bear on the individual or family may be focal, contextual, or background. *Focal* stimuli are those which act immediately on the individual or family, e.g., pain or pregnancy. *Contextual* stimuli are the locations or situations in which the focal stimuli are operative, e.g., the hospital room of an individual patient or the immediate extended family of a pregnant woman. *Background* stimuli are attitudes, beliefs, and values from the individual's past experience and from the larger society. The aim of intervention is to influence focal, contextual, and/or background stimuli so that the individual or family can make adaptive responses in physiologic, self-concept, role function or interdependence subsystems. Although Roy's theory is concerned with individuals, it can also be useful when the family is the client. In most respects this theory is also congruent with a systems approach.

White asserted that adaptation is part of "the whole tapestry of living . . . it is a striving toward acceptable compromise" (1974, p. 52). This postulate forms the basis of the relationships of human beings with their environment. It is a function of all living systems, and allows for growth and autonomy. To accomplish adaptation several conditions are necessary:

1 The individual and/or family must secure adequate information about the environment to serve as a guide to action.

2   The individual or family system's internal organization must be balanced. Information must be available at a rate which can be assimilated.

3   The individual or family must have freedom of action or autonomy. A range of choices must be available in order to permit adaptive responses.

White emphasized the importance of self-esteem and stated, "No adaptive strategy that is careless of the level of self-esteem is likely to be any good" (p. 61). White further proposed that intervention based on the above strategies required the helper to be cognizant of the client's potential for action. Although White's theory was directed toward individuals, it is also useful with families.

Dager (1964) regarded socialization as an adaptive process, which might be explained through the analysis of human interactions. Assumptions basic to Dager's theory include the following:

1   Individuals are born with "tabula rasa," or the empty slate.

2   The basic unit of study is interaction because both the individual and society stem from interactional processes.

3   Humans attempt to put order into their world and thus are dependent upon their ability to organize the physical and social environment.

The source of all socialization is human interaction; conceptualization of self is dependent on one's interactions with others. The family serves as the individual's first socialization modality. Dager proposed that "family organization has always been related to fulfillment of the needs of the individual and to fulfillment of the needs of the larger society" (p. 776). With the decline of the extended family in modern society, intervention in the socialization process falls within the province of alternative institutions.

Family interventions founded on systems and interactional frameworks provide the bases for operationalizing many of the concepts presented. The core needs of existence, relatedness, and growth are similar to Roy's subsystems of man (physiologic, self-concept, role function, and interdependence). The concepts of time, territory, and technology serve as additional tools for assessing and planning strategies for adaptation. How a family uses its time, space, and resources provides clues for intervention. Finally, Dager proposed that intervention is required in today's society in order to ease the socialization process. Professionals must appraise their own problem-solving abilities and those of clients in trying to meet the overriding goal espoused by all three theories. This goal is the successful adaptation of family members to each other and to the larger environment with which the family interacts.

CLINICAL EXAMPLE: THE EXPECTANT FAMILY

Assessment of the Norton family focused on the core needs of the family within the resource dimensions of time, territory, and technology available to the family. Kay was a married, healthy 23-year-old woman who had had two uncomplicated, full-term deliveries of healthy girls, now 3 years and 18 months old. Kay's family of origin included four younger siblings. Prior to her marriage, Kay had completed one year of college. She had always enjoyed and found satisfaction in her role of full-time wife and mother. Kay and her husband had recently learned that she was expecting twins in July. This disclosure explained her sudden weight gain of 10 pounds in 1 month, and the information alleviated her initial fears that something was wrong with her pregnancy. It also meant that the family was faced with an unexpected situation (*focal stimulus*) of greater proportion than was originally known.

Ted, the father, aged 35, was in excellent health and was a self-employed farmer. At age 20, after his father's sudden death from a coronary, he had assumed responsibility for his family of origin, leaving agricultural college to take over the family farming business. Ted, who was the oldest of five siblings, operated a successful farm and produce stand with his two brothers. Economically, the farm stand supported three families. Ted's two sisters were deaf-mutes who had made successful adaptations to their disability. Their disability was suspected to be of genetic origin (*residual stimulus*). This had been of concern to Kay and Ted during the previous pregnancies; however, their two children had been given audio testing and no hearing deficits had been detected.

Kay and Ted had been married for 4 years and were accepting of the addition of another child, even though they had originally planned to limit their family to two offspring. They had recently moved to a new home and were in the process of planning extensive renovations. Financial resources had been allocated for the renovations without regard for another pregnancy. (These variables comprise the *contextual stimuli*.)

Kay's first concern centered on her ability to carry twins to term without having to spend the last 6 weeks in bed. She was dismayed to learn that this might be a possibility. Secondly, she was concerned about her ability to continue to give her two daughters the attention she thought necessary. Thirdly, she was concerned about the impact this pregnancy might have on her relationship with her husband. She wondered whether her limited energy would permit her to meet all the demands placed on her (*feelings of internal disorganization*). She worried about how she would cope after the twins arrived and what changes in living arrangements and housekeeping responsibilities would be needed (*need for freedom of action and need to maintain autonomy*).

The rural visiting nurse discussed how the family might adapt to the arrival of the twins in terms of meeting the family's needs for existence, relatedness, and growth, and how family space and resources could be allocated to satisfy these needs. Much of the discussion was exploratory. For example, what was the possibility of obtaining a live-in mother's helper prior to the delivery? Could the house renovations be revised to accommodate the expected additional family members? Would it be feasible to enroll one child in nursery school 2 or 3 days a week in the fall? How could Kay and Ted reserve some time for themselves (*socializaton of all family members*)? The nurse emphasized Kay's immediate need for sustained prenatal care and for more frequent contact with her physician than in the past in order to obtain information that would enable her to plan realistically.

With help, Kay began pacing her activity levels, primarily focusing on the needs of her two young daughters. A part-time housekeeper was found to take over the heavy cleaning and some of the light housekeeping activities as well. House renovation plans were altered so that the basement would provide a large play area for the children, as well as a new laundry. The room previously planned as a playroom was redesigned as a bedroom/den. A young woman from Canada was engaged for a year to live in as a mother's helper. Plans were made to register the older daughter in nursery school 2 days a week in the fall. This would give Kay more time with her younger children and expand social opportunities for the oldest child. Ted voiced concern about depleting the family's savings, but was optimistic about having a good growing season despite the late spring. "We've changed our spending priorities—no trip south next winter, but we'll manage a short vacation to Maine after harvest time to view the foliage." Ted's cooperation in setting new family priorities was crucial to family equilibrium and to Kay's peace of mind. The joint planning undertaken by Ted and Kay added a rich new dimension to their relationship.

SUMMARY

It is important to base family assessments on conceptual frameworks, and to base interventions on sound theoretical frameworks. In the framework which has been proposed in this chapter, both assessment and intervention occur at the point of interaction of the six concepts of existence, relatedness, growth, time, territory, and technology. In the case illustration, interventions were directed toward influencing the focal, contextual, and residual stimuli to permit adaptation in the appropriate subsystems. The clinical example also demonstrated the need to process information in order to mobilize the resources of a well-functioning family organization, to uncover the availability of various options, and to encourage the family to make decisions autonomously so that successful adaptation might occur.

Health care professionals helped this family meet its socialization responsibilities by recognizing its strengths and limitations; family members did their part by showing willingness to draw the necessary resources from the environment and from each other in order to fulfill members' needs.

Considerable work remains to be done in formulating conceptual frameworks which can be tested in a variety of family settings. More attention must be paid to the use of other theoretical bases for family intervention in addition to those alluded to in the clinical example. Health care professionals should be encouraged to develop integrated conceptual frameworks that utilize the criteria outlined at the beginning of this chapter, and to select concepts which are compatible and coherent by using an eclectic approach to family intervention based upon verifiable frameworks.

REFERENCES

Alderfer, C. An empirical test of a new theory of human needs. *Organizational Behavior and Human Performance,* 1969, **4,** 142–175.

Anderson, R. E., & Carter, I. E. *Human behavior in the social environment: A social systems approach.* Chicago: Aldine, 1974.

Becker, M. H., Drachman, R. H., and Kirscht, J. P. A new approach to explaining sick-role behavior in low-income populations. *American Journal of Public Health,* 1974, **64,** 205–216.

Bruhn, J. G., & Cordova, F. D. A developmental approach to learning wellness behavior. Part I: Infancy to early adolescence. *Health Values,* 1977, **1**(6), 246–254.

Bruhn, J. G., Cordova, F. D., Williams, J. A., & Fuentes, R. G. The wellness process. *Journal of Community Health,* 1977, **2**(3), 209–221.

Chin, R. The utility of systems models and developmental models for practitioners. In J. P. Riehl & Sr. C. Roy (Eds.), *Conceptual models for nursing practice.* New York: Appleton-Century-Crofts, 1974.

Dager, E. Z. Socialization and personality development in the child. In H. T. Christensen (Ed.), *Handbook of marriage and the family.* Chicago: Rand McNally, 1964.

Duvall, E. M. *Marriage and family development* (5th ed.). Philadelphia: Lippincott, 1977.

Erikson, E. H. Identity and the life cycle. *Psychological Issues,* **1**(1), Monograph 1, New York: International Universities Press, 1959.

Glaser, B. G., & Strauss, A. L. *The discovery of grounded theory: Strategies for quantitative research.* Chicago: Aldine, 1967.

Hill, R., & Hansen, D. A. The identification of conceptual frameworks utilized in family study. *Marriage and Family Living,* 1960, **22,** 299–311.

Hill, R., & Rodgers, R. H. The developmental approach. In H. T. Christensen (Ed.), *Handbook of marriage and the family.* Chicago: Rand McNally, 1964.

Huse, E., & Bowditch, J. *Behavior in organizations.* Reading, Mass.: Addison-Wesley, 1977.

Kantor, D., & Lehr, W. *Inside the family.* New York: Harper & Row, 1975.

Kluckhohn, C., & Murray, H.A. Personality formation: The determinants. In E. Kluckhohn, H. A. Murray, & D. Schneider (Eds.), *Personality in nature, society and culture* (2nd ed.). New York: Knopf, 1967.

Maslow, A. *Motivation and personality.* New York: Harper & Row, 1970.

Pratt, L. *Family structure and effective health behavior: The energized family.* Boston: Houghton Mifflin, 1976.

Reilly, D. E. Why a conceptual framework? *Nursing Outlook,* 1975, **23**(8), 566–569.

Rhodes, S. L. A developmental approach to the life cycle of the family. *Social Casework,* 1977, **58**(2), 301–311.

Rowe, G. P. The developmental conceptual framework to the study of the family. In F. I. Nye & F. M. Berardo (Eds.), *Emerging conceptual frameworks in family analysis.* New York: Macmillan, 1966.

Roy, Sr. C. The Roy adaptation model. In J. P. Riehl & Sr. C. Roy (Eds.), *Conceptual models for nursing practice.* New York: Appleton-Century-Crofts, 1974.

Schvaneveldt, J. D. The interactional framework in the study of the family. In F. I. Nye & F. M. Berardo (Eds.), *Emerging conceptual frameworks in family analysis.* New York: Macmillan, 1966.

Sedgwick, R. The family as a system: Network of relationships. *Psychiatric Nursing and Mental Health Services,* March–April 1974, 17–20.

Stryker, S. The interactional and situational approaches. In H. T. Christensen (Ed.), *Handbook of marriage and the family.* Chicago: Rand McNally, 1964.

Tosi, H., & Hammer, W. C. *Organizational behavior and management: A contingency approach.* Chicago: St. Clair Press, 1977.

Travelbee, J. *Interpersonal aspects of nursing.* Philadelphia: Davis, 1975.

White, R. Strategies of adaptation: An attempt at systematic description. In G. B. Coelho, J. E. Adams, & D. A. Hamburg (Eds.), *Coping and adaptation.* New York: Basic Books, 1974.

Chapter 24

Evaluation of Family Progress

Jean R. Miller
Ellen H. Janosik

Family-focused care may be an idea whose time has come, but the problem of evaluating the process and outcomes of family intervention remains difficult. Intervention is often based on principles from several theoretical frameworks, which makes it difficult to document the effectiveness of a particular approach. While many outcomes of physical care can be systematically monitored, the outcomes of family system care may be harder to determine. Some progress has been made in evaluating outcomes of family care, but documentation of the effects of family intervention is at present incomplete. In the absence of definitive measures, one may begin the evaluation process by examining practitioner performance according to certain predetermined standards.

EVALUATION OF PRACTITIONER PERFORMANCE

Evaluative efforts may begin with the performance of the practitioner, based on the assumption that family intervention by skilled practitioners facilitates therapeutic change. Cleghorn and Levin (1973) wrote that an effective practitioner is one who can develop a collaborative relationship with the family in the initial interview. Through guidance from the practitioner the expectations of the family are clarified in the early stages of work, so that a therapeutic alliance is established which successfully allays family dissension and fear. According to Cleghorn and Levine, the skilled practitioner demonstrates perceptual, conceptual, and executive skills when working with families. In this context, *perceptual skills* are defined as the ability to perceive the effect of family interactions on individual members and on the system. A practitioner possessing *conceptual skills* will be aware of the implicit rules of behavior which make family interactions predictable. It is the application of conceptual skills which enables the practitioner to convey to the family that relationships and interactions are patterned and reciprocal. The *executive skills* of a family practitioner include the ability to demonstrate to families just how their system works so as to persuade them to alter their dysfunctional transactional patterns.

The practitioner who has mastered these levels of skills may be considered capable of mobilizing the reparative capacities of the family. When standards are adopted to evaluate practitioner skills, the progress of the family is not attributed to specific changes in the system, but rather to improved communication and collaborative problem solving largely generated by the skilled practitioner.

More recently, Garrigan and Bambrick (1977) identified competencies, objectives, and criteria for evaluating novice therapists. The four competencies, which are outlined below, are broad enough to be applied in many situations in which families require assistance.

1   Competence in assessing family interaction by incorporating family systems theory and relationship patterns
2   Competence in formulating a treatment contract based on issues which each family member is willing to negotiate
3   Competence in engaging the family on an issue
4   Competence in redefining or terminating the contract, when indicated

Certain perceptual/conceptual and therapeutic skill objectives were presented by Garrigan and Bambrick under each competency. One example of a perceptual/conceptual objective was that the practitioner should be able to identify patterned sequences of pathological relating between family members. Therapeutic skill objectives included the ability to obtain data about the presenting problem, to refocus the family's attention on specific issues which had potential for resolution, to encourage family members to amend areas of conflict in a controlled fashion, and to seal the family's ability to negotiate present issues.

The evaluation of practitioner performances based on the above objectives (among others suggested by Garrigan and Bambrick) constitutes a beginning step. However, the evaluation of more specific behaviors suggested by various theoretical frameworks is also important. For instance, there are several ways of obtaining data about a presenting problem. A practitioner who is using a structural approach might obtain data through assessing *patterns* of communication between members, while a practitioner using an interactionist approach might make the assessment based on the *content* of the communication. In both instances the practitioner may be credited with making an assessment; nevertheless, there remains the question of the genuine accuracy and reliability of the two approaches. As the practice of family-focused care evolves, the evaluation of specific therapeutic behaviors associated with each theoretical framework will command further attention.

FAMILY OUTCOMES

Defining the outcomes of family intervention is an activity in which both practitioner and family should participate; however, this becomes difficult when there is discrepancy between the dysfunction identified by the family and that determined by the practitioner. In such instances, it may be advisable for the practitioner to address the dysfunction presented by the family, even though the parameters of the problem are perceived differently by the practitioner, whose aim is to locate the causes of dysfunction in the system rather than in any individual. It is essential to reconcile the practitioner's assessment of the problem with the family's assessment during the planning phases of treatment.

The idiosyncratic nature of the family complaint may puzzle the practitioner. Often behaviors which appear relatively inoffensive are labeled as intolerable by the family, while bizarre behaviors are considered ordinary. Family history, family norms, and family values determine which behaviors are allowed and which disallowed. Families usually ask for help only when they believe the integrity of the system is threatened by the behaviors of one or more members. A beginning practitioner may erroneously impose certain ideas of appropriate behavior on the family, whereas a more experienced practitioner tends to accept the wisdom of facilitating change which is acceptable to the family.

Families who come to the attention of a practitioner usually are operating in ways which the family has labeled problematic. Some of the family-applied labels may seem accurate to the practitioner, but others may not. In the latter case, a practitioner may try to help the family redefine system operations according to a new set of values which the practitioner believes will prove more functional. In rare cases, the family is in complete agreement with the redefinition, but more often a compromise must be reached between the family's perception of the problem and that of the practitioner. Goal setting is usually a complex issue which requires both family and practitioner to make concessions in order to preserve the therapy system. The family must be willing to accept some guidance from the practitioner, while the latter must balance idealistic goals against the realistic capacity of the system to adapt to change.

Although the practitioner assumes the responsibility for introducing change, it is the family that has the power to accept or reject it. The practitioner is only responsible for the therapy system; the family remains accountable for its own destiny. Therefore, accommodation must be made between what the family wants to change and what the practitioner wants to see changed. During the planning phase of family treatment specific goals must be formulated so that the family has a sense of direction and accomplishment as these goals are approached. Without specific, agreed-upon goals neither the family nor the practitioner possesses measurement standards against which progress may be evaluated.

In negotiating goals with the family, the practitioner may categorize tasks as finite or continuous (Ferber & Ranz, 1972). *Finite tasks* are those in which success or failure is easily ascertained; a finite task might be a clear-cut goal such as leaving home or finding a new job. *Continuous* or *ongoing tasks* are comprised of processes which must be undertaken over long periods. Here task accomplishment often fluctuates over a period of time so that success or failure in continuous tasks may be difficult to determine. Progression followed by regression may become a recurring sequence which makes goal attainment obscure. Guiding a family toward a finite goal usually means that there is considerable agreement between participants and practitioner on what the goal is, and what behaviors are needed to accomplish it. Working on a continuing goal may involve protracted negotiations, as the practitioner repeatedly intervenes to reinforce new, adaptive operations and to eliminate old patterns which emerge again. The ongoing nature of a continuing goal rules out the possibility of decisive goal attainment. Instead of expecting unequivocal achievement, the practitioner and the family must learn to evaluate incremental gains or losses in working toward a continuous goal.

Family intervention has been described as an attempt to alter pathogenic relationships in the system, with change occurring as a result of "bargaining." Through the technique of bargaining, practitioner and family reach agreement on: (1) the type of change which will occur, (2) the rate at which change will occur, and (3) the extent of change which will occur (Zuk, 1968). In addition, Zuk warned that some families in treatment modify their operations somewhat in order to forestall the practitioner's zeal for greater change. This constitutes a subtle form of resistance which is not readily apparent in evaluating treatment, but which works to the detriment of family progress. In some respects the tendency of families to modify minor operations so as to preserve major ones is a replication of the pseudomutuality which characterizes apparently harmonious families whose members collude to avoid genuine transformation of maladaptive family dynamics.

Once the goals of treatment are determined, methods for evaluating progress must be decided on. There are a number of ways to obtain the information needed for evaluation; they include subjective reports by the family and/or outside observers and objective behavioral methods measured by the family and/or outside observers. Data obtained by different methods may not always agree, since each method generates different types of information. Data from each source should be used selectively during the treatment process. Selective use of data does not necessarily mean that extraneous information obtained through various methods is discredited; however, judgment is needed to select the evaluative data that is appropriate to the problems presented, and to weigh the credibility of the family and outside observers.

Self-report methods such as interviews, questionnaires, and standardized tests are more commonly employed than objective methods. Self-reports allow families to relate their subjective experiences and express their emotions. Practitioners may also contribute their perceptions of the family situation through self-report methods. Cromwell, Olson, and Fournier (1976a, 1976b) classified available self-report measures as nonprojective personality tests, projective personality tests, perceived interaction measures, and inferred interaction measures. The unit of assessment (individual, marital dyad, partial family, whole family) must be taken into consideration when selecting evaluative measures, since specific instruments have been developed for use with individuals and with various combinations of family members. Further information about available measures may be found in reviews by Straus (1969), Riskin and Faunce (1972), and Cromwell, Olson, and Fournier (1976a, 1976b).

Objective methods refer to the evaluation of measurable behaviors. The family and/or practitioner record(s) progress by counting specific predetermined behaviors which the family wants to modify. Monitoring by the family in the home setting is feasible, but practitioners generally do their monitoring in less than natural settings. Families may be asked to perform problem-solving, decision-making, or conflict resolution tasks, as non-biased observers monitor the interactions. In such situations the number of times each family member speaks to another might be recorded along with the number of times the interaction is construed by observers as supportive or destructive. Objective evaluation of interaction is a complex process which researchers are still trying to refine for clinical use.

Another method for quantifying family outcomes is goal attainment scaling, which was developed by Kiresuk and Sherman (1968) and tested with families by Woodward, Santa-Barbara, Levin, and Epstein (1978). Problem areas are listed across the top of the scale, as shown in Table 24-1, and possible outcomes are given vertically below each problem. Outcomes can be designated as: (1) most unfavorable, (2) expected, and (3) best anticipated. Corresponding values of -2, 0, and $+2$ are assigned within each category of outcomes. More levels can be included if desired. The behavioral or measurable descriptions of outcomes related to each problem are based on what a given family can be expected to attain in light of its capabilities and limitations. A check mark is placed on the attained level at predetermined intervals. Ease of scoring and accuracy of assessment depend on how measurable the different levels are. In addition to the objectivity of the scale, other advantages of goal attainment scaling include the wide range of problems which can be assessed, the variety of levels which can be included, and the potential for positive reinforcement of desirable behaviors. When a family measures its performance against known objectives, the discrepancies between performance and goals serve as a self-

Table 24-1 Goal Attainment Scaling

Outcome	PROBLEMS							
	Arguments over finances				Indecision regarding use of leisure time			
		3/1	3/7			3/1	3/7	
Most unfavorable outcome	3 or more arguments each week	X			Makes no plans each week	X		
Expected level of treatment success	2 arguments each week		X		Makes 1 plan each week but does not follow through			
Best anticipated outcome	0 or 1 argument each week				Makes 2 or more plans and follows through		X	

correcting stimulus. In systems theory terms, goal attainment scaling provides a feedback mechanism for self-correcting family systems.

The evaluation of outcomes through valid and reliable methods should include the extent to which goals were reached, as well as the degree of consumer satisfaction, compliance, and symptom relief (Linn & Linn, 1975). Families' perception of care is important since continuance in treatment is dependent in most instances on satisfaction. Clear information, personal interest, accessibility of care, and convenience are factors that affect the degree of consumer satisfaction; however, the measurement of satisfaction continues to be difficult.

Family compliance refers in part to the degree to which families actually behave in the way they say they will behave. For instance, a father may say he is going to spend more time at home to attain specific communication goals, but if he does not keep his word, improvement is not likely to occur. Mutually developed treatment programs are based on the assumption that families endeavor to reach the planned objectives. When there is noncompliance with the plan, goal attainment falls short. In such cases, it is not totally accurate to say the therapeutic approach was inadequate since the agreed-upon plan was not implemented by the family.

Finally, evaluations should indicate the extent to which families have experienced relief from symptoms such as anger, jealousy, and selfishness. Satisfaction with family relationships may result from behavioral changes or subjective experiences, but objective evaluation is needed to ascertain whether the disruptive effects of the presenting problem have been decreased or eliminated.

FUTURE ISSUES

Applying general systems theory to families has eliminated some ambiguity by locating pathogenic factors, not in an identified patient, but in the field created by familial and ecological forces. However, the application of general systems concepts to family work has not greatly simplified treatment evaluation. One drawback to the use of general systems theory in family work may be its universal applicability, which is also one of its strengths. Although Ackerman (1972) described systems theory as encompassing the "totality of relationships," he wrote that clinical realities demanded that systems theory be reduced to less than universal generalizations. Therefore, he dichotomized systems theory into a mechanistic model and an organismic model. The mechanistic model limits itself to the properties of systems, while the organismic model views the individual as a subsystem within a system, and thus attends to human values as well. Ackerman recommended that practitioners choose the organismic model so as to avoid the reductionism which causes practitioners to see only the properties of systems, while individual members fade into obscurity. In his argument, Ackerman did not accept statistical evaluation as totally adequate, since statistics provide only facts rather than incontrovertible truths. The effectiveness of treatment methods is dependent on refining and testing the theoretical constructs on which the treatment is based.

In questioning the claims of improvement made by practitioners and families, Ackerman decried the lack of a unified body of family theory and what he described as excessive experimentation in the techniques of family work. He believed that the development of uniform procedures which would permit adequate testing of theoretical concepts and therapeutic effectiveness was more important than preoccupation with techniques.

Concepts serve to organize outcome behaviors under a comprehensive heading, but behaviors associated with concepts must be stated in specific rather than general terms. For example, most clinicians agree that the concept of double bind can be defined as a communicational problem in which a message, A, is sent, to which an appropriate response is B or C. Simultaneously, message A′ is transmitted to which neither response B nor response C is appropriate. Behaviors associated with this definition of double bind include statements by family members which confuse the recipients, because conflicting messages are sent and there is no congruence between what is said and the context in which it is being said. Many families have a repertoire of double-bind messages such as: "Nothing is bothering me, but it wouldn't do any good to tell you, anyway." After the clinician and family agree on an operational definition of a double-bind message, certain outcomes of treatment may be evaluated by counting the number of times double-bind messages are transmitted in the family over a given period of time. The effect of a double-bind message on the recipients can also be evaluated by counting the number of times the victim either confronts the sender regarding the lack of clarity in the message, tries to respond to the inconsistent message, or withdraws from further involvement so that incoming messages can be ignored. The procedures described can be used to evaluate definable changes in family communication.

The difficulty of operationalizing concepts in behavioral terms is implicit in the example of the double bind. There are so many ways to communicate double-bind messages that it is virtually impossible to include all messages which can be said to place recipients in a double bind. While clinicians and families often sense that progress has been made, more sophisticated quantitative measures are needed in order to validate advances in the theory and technique of family counseling.

The need for adequate family assessment instruments may be questioned in view of the many family instruments that have been developed over the last 50 years. When one inspects existing instruments, however, one finds few that have been adequately designed and tested for use by health professionals dealing with families who seek primary care. Most instruments have been designed either for use with families having psychiatrically ill members, or for pure research purposes.

These are a number of reasons why these instruments have not been used extensively by nonpsychiatric practitioners. Many of the instruments are time-consuming and expensive to administer. Others have not been tested for validity and reliability; when instruments have been tested, the results often have been questionable. Moreover, the sensitivity of many of the instruments has been insufficient to guide ongoing assessment and intervention. Furthermore, many of the instruments have been developed for individual family members and marital dyads rather than for the family as a unit. Valid, reliable, and practical measurement instruments are urgently needed for the future.

SUMMARY

Typologies relating to structure and function have already been developed to classify pathogenic families, and some concepts such as scapegoating or the double bind are widely applied in family work. The organization and functioning of families must be conceptualized, not to serve a medical diagnostic model, but to reach agreement on assessment criteria, mutual objectives, and therapeutic interventions. Conceptual frameworks applicable to both healthy and pathogenic families must be subjected to rigorous research methodology, so that tested relationships between concepts can be used with assurance to guide family assessment and intervention.

Subjective and objective methods for evaluating family progress provide complementary information. As family theories are developed and tested, measures of supporting concepts can become the means for evaluating outcomes of intervention. Valid and reliable instruments that are easily implemented in clinical settings need further development. In the meantime, many structural and functional relationships can be identified by practitioners and families through the use of family maps, genograms, sociograms, and other selected existing instruments. The challenges presented by family-focused care are numerous and are not to be taken lightly. Present evaluation guidelines are not adequate for the task, but some interim procedures and methods have been suggested that may be of help to the family practitioner.

REFERENCES

Ackerman, N. W. The growing edge of family therapy. In C. J. Sager & H. S. Kaplan (Eds.), *Progress in group and family therapy.* New York: Brunner/Mazel, 1972.

Cleghorn, J. M., & Levin, S. Training family therapists by setting learning objectives. *American Journal of Orthopsychiatry,* April 1973, **43**(3), 439–446.

Cromwell, R. E., Olson, D. H. L., & Fournier, D. G. Diagnosis and evaluation in marital and family counseling. In D. H. L. Olson (Ed.), *Treating relationships.* Lake Mills, Iowa: Graphic Publishing, 1976.

Cromwell, R. E., Olson, D. H. L., & Fournier, D. G. Tools and techniques for diagnosis and evaluation in marital and family therapy. *Family Process,* March 1976, **15**(1), 1–49.

Ferber, A., & Ranz, J. How to succeed in family therapy. In A. Ferber (Ed.), *The book of family therapy.* New York: Science House, 1972.

Garrigan, J. J., & Bambrick, A. F. Introducing novice therapists to "go-between" techniques of family therapy. *Family Process,* 1977, **16**(2), 237–246.

Kiresuk, T. J., & Sherman, R. E. Goal attainment scaling: A general method for evaluating comprehensive community mental health programs. *Community Mental Health Journal,* 1968, **4**, 443.

Linn, M. W., & Linn, B. S. Narrowing the gap between medical and mental health evaluation. *Medical Care,* July 1975, **13**(7), 607–614.

Riskin, J., & Faunce, E. E. An evaluative review of family interaction research. *Family Process,* 1972, **11**(4), 365–455.

Straus, M. A. Family measurement techniques: Abstracts of published instruments, 1935–1965. Minneapolis: University of Minnesota Press, 1969.

Woodward, C. A., Santa-Barbara, J., Levin, S., & Epstein, N. B. The role of goal attainment scaling in evaluating family therapy outcome. *American Journal of Orthopsychiatry,* July 1978, **48**(3), 464–476.

Zuk, G. The side taking function in family therapy. *American Journal of Orthopsychiatry,* April 1968, **38**(3), 553–559.

Name Index

Subject Index